# PALEO
## COMFORT FOODS

Homestyle Cooking for a Gluten-Free Kitchen

Julie & Charles Mayfield

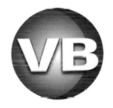

VICTORY BELT PUBLISHING INC.

Las Vegas

First Published in 2011 by Victory Belt Publishing.

ISBN 13: 978-1-936608-93-5

This book is for educational purposes. The publisher and authors of this instructional book are not responsible in any manner whatsoever for any adverse effects arising directly or indirectly as a result of the information provided in this book.

Victory Belt ® is a registered trademark of Victory Belt Publishing Inc.

Cover Layout by Mark Adams

Cover Design by Brian Rule

Printed in USA

RRD 07-13

# contents

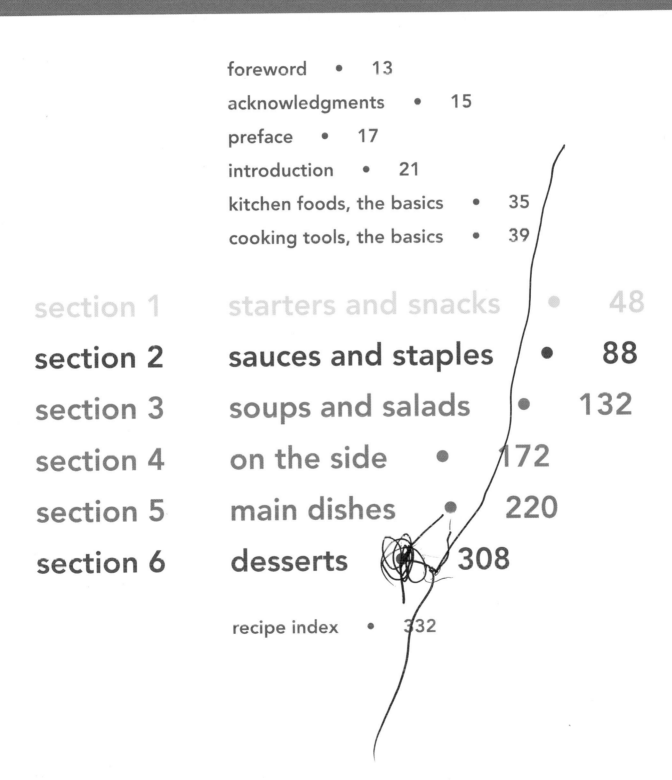

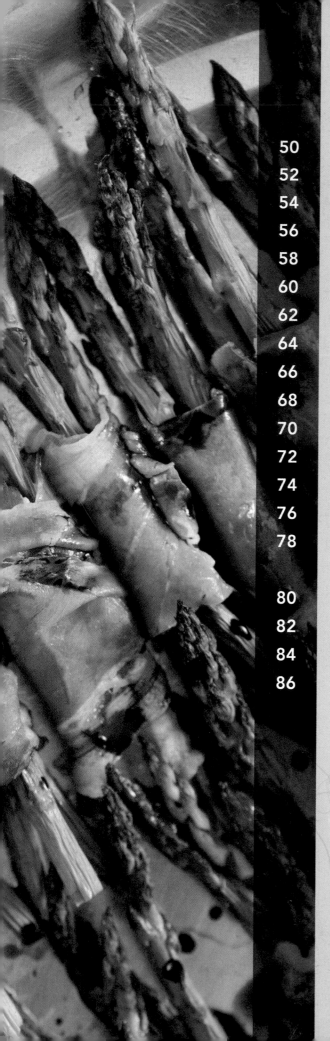

# starters and snacks

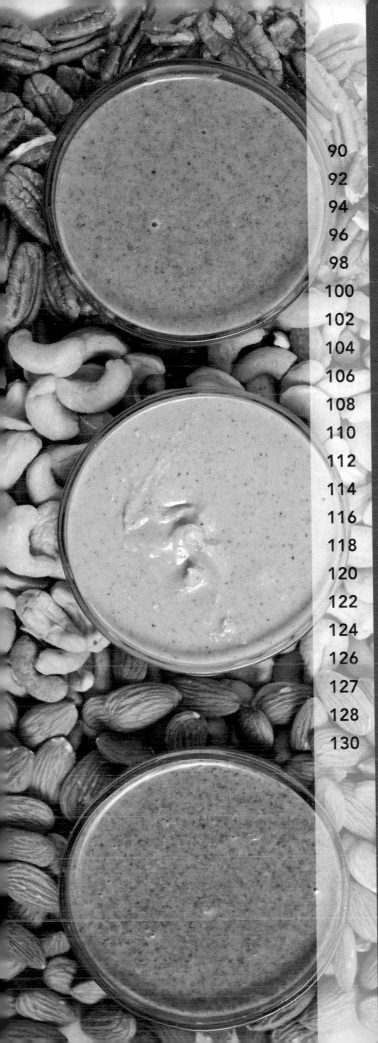

# sauces and staples

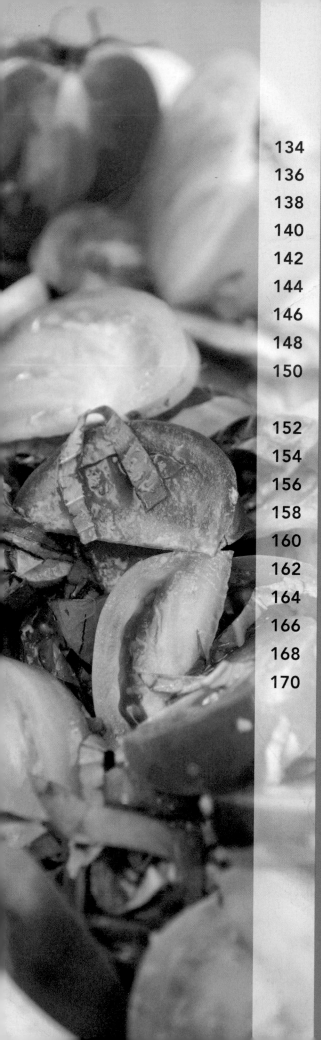

# soups and salads

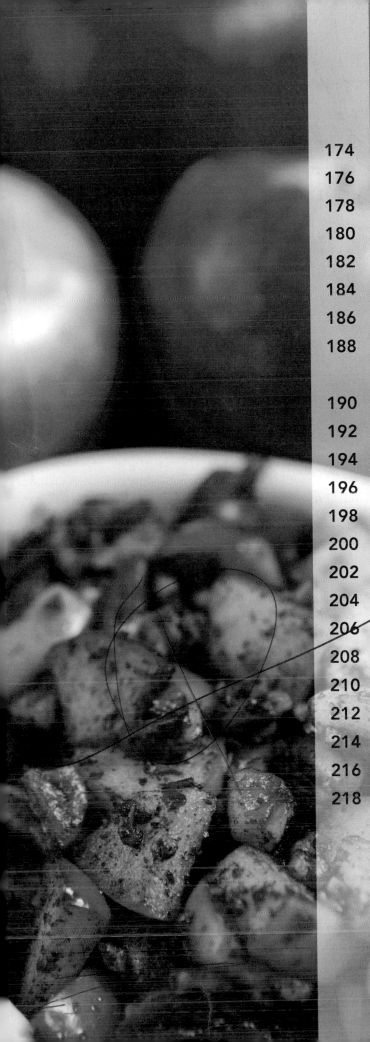

# on the side

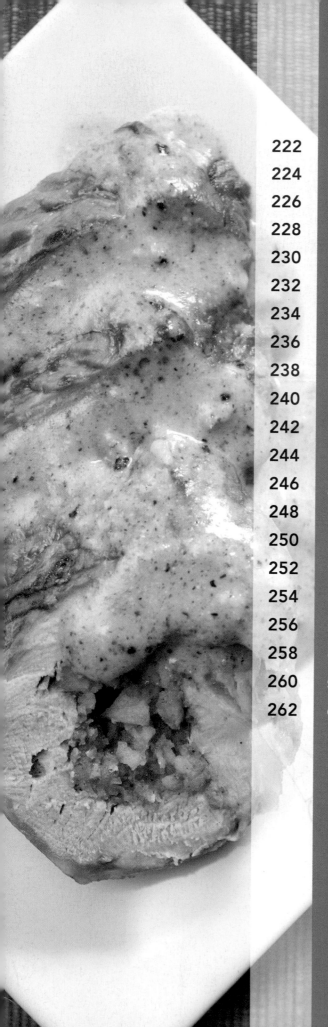

# main dishes

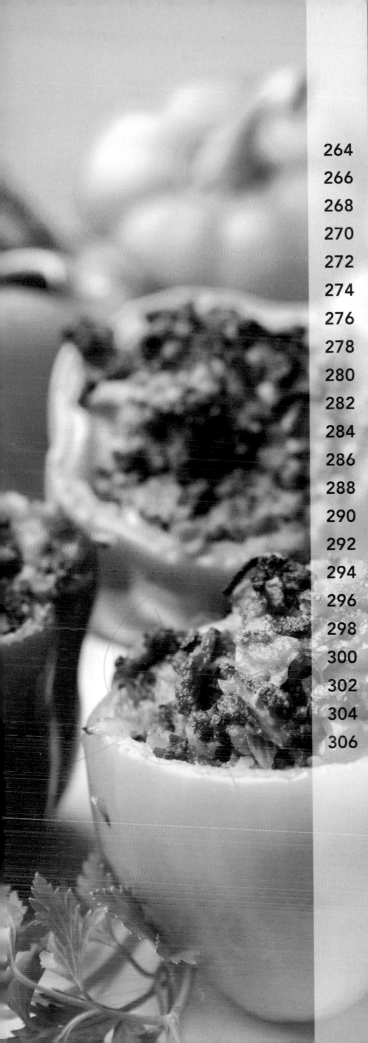

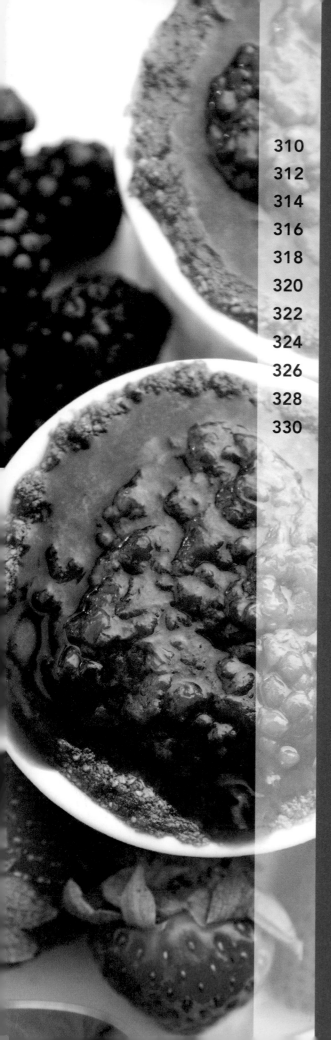

# desserts

# foreword

## by Robb Wolf
### *New York Times Best-selling Author of The Paleo Solution*

I had an idea for a cookbook. Once. Then a set of circumstances proved to me that my cookbook would not be as unique, good, or snazzy as I'd like . . . so I scuttled the whole idea. To understand why the idea of writing my own cookbook seemed silly requires a little backstory. You see, I wrote the *New York Times* best-selling book *The Paleo Solution*, and apparently after you write a successful nutrition/diet-oriented book you produce a follow-up cookbook.

Ducks quack, cats purr, and apparently nutrition gurus write (or subcontract) cookbooks.

So, I was mulling over this idea of a cookbook while on a trip to Atlanta, Georgia. Some of my very dearest friends (who are serious foodies) live in Atlanta, so I was pretty excited about this trip. My wife, Nicki, and I were scheduled to have dinner with two sets of friends: Jeff and Melissa Hayes (owners of one branch of the best gym in Atlanta, BTB Fitness) and Charles and Jules Mayfield (owners of the *other* branch of Atlanta's best gym, BTB Fitness). These folks know good food and good booze, and they are great athletes and outstanding coaches. Dinner was a Thai theme with paleo ingredients that included grilled chicken, a green curry, and cauliflower "rice." It's tough to describe how amazing this food was without using enough four-letter explicative's to give this book an NC-17 rating.

It was amazing.

Every time I've been in Atlanta I've had a meal or two with these folks, and the food that Charles and Jules make is just second to none. I was reflecting on the previous meals I've shared with the Atlanta crew, and right before I lost consciousness from a Curry Coma I mumbled, "you guys need to make a cookbook."

With Southern-tipped drawls, Charles and Jules simultaneously said, "Excuse me?" I repeated myself, all while ladling another helping of four-alarm curry into my bowl.

"Really?" they asked.

"Yesfg," was the closest affirmative I could muster while still shoveling curry and leaving the teensiest respiratory passageway for that silly stuff "air."

Charles and Jules have fed me paleo interpretations of: Greek, Italian, Indian, Mexican, and several other ethnic cuisines, and their food is amazing. Perhaps most impressive for me, however, was Charles & Jules's Paleo spin on Southern U.S. cooking. My family (on my mom's side) is from Appleton, Arkansas, so I grew up with biscuits and gravy, fried okra, berry cobblers, and food so good that you could just weep eating it. Or, you could weep when you (or me in this case) discover you are gluten intolerant and many of the old standards are simply not options anymore if you want to be healthy.

I consider myself an athlete, I work to squeak as much performance out of my body as I can, and good-quality food is central to my quest to stay healthy, lean, and strong. That's all great, but food is much more than "fuel." Food should be about traditions, holidays, family gatherings, and nights on the town with friends and loved ones. This is what *Paleo Comfort Foods* is all about. The best food you have ever eaten, made with ingredients that will not create those other fun social gatherings—the funeral.

As I'm writing this foreword I realize that this book was born of everything that food should be about: People you love, good times, fond memories, and food that is worth a second or third helping. It was a dinner party in Atlanta that convinced me that my cookbook would be an infantile attempt compared to what Charles and Jules make every single day. I make good food, but Paleo Comfort Foods is *great* food. So, in many ways, this is "my" cookbook in that it shows you how to cook the type of food I'd want to eat every day, especially if I have great people to share it with. These recipes are easy and time-efficient, and, as I mentioned, they span the world of culinary offerings. If you or someone you know had reservations about eating "Paleo" because you'd be missing out on some old favorites, you will find help in this book.

Robb Wolf

# acknowledgments

This may be the most challenging part of the book for us. So many people have influenced us over the years, and led us to where we are today. Quite honestly there are too many to mention, but here goes with a short list of people who have made this book possible.

### Charles would like to thank:

The two best parents a man could ask for, Scottie and Lisa Mayfield. You have always given me the love, support, and encouragement I needed. You believed in me when I didn't believe in myself, and showed me that hard work and honesty can take you as far as you want to go. To my amazing sister, Mariah, you have always supported me and were willing to help clean up the messes I've made over the years. Michael, you are such an amazing brother. I can always count on you for a straight answer and feedback on just about anything. My son, Dylan, for having an amazing heart and always being willing to try new things.

Buzz and Phoenix. How would we keep our floors clean without you there to clean up all the spills? You're always willing to hop up in my lap and discuss the trials of the day.

The real talent behind this amazing book: My 'sunshine', loving wife, gardening buddy, and culinary queen, Julie. Do I hear Barry White playing?

### Julie would like to thank:

My mom, Lynn, for fielding all those phone calls while you were at work from your inquisitive daughter who needed to know what temperature to set the oven to, for Sullivan's Apple Pie, and for your constant love and support over the years. My brother, Andy;

sister-in-law, Shada; and, of course, Becket and Aurelia: you always show us some of the best places to eat in Philadelphia, and have introduced us to such culinary delights over the years. You also share in our passion for great, homemade meals. My sister, Kerry; brother-in-law, Gregg; and Chloe; Paige; Grant; and Lowen: You all remind me that when our plates seem really crazy and really full, we never have more than we can handle.

All the BTB Freedomites over the years and, most especially, Erin Elizabeth Evans. . . . It's pretty certain we were meant to be friends, and I am so grateful for you every day!

My California friends, who are too many to name, please know how appreciative I am for the many years of love, support, adventures, and guidance.

Finally, my coauthor, business partner, love of my life, amazing husband. You are my first, my last, my everything.

Julie and Charles would like to thank:

Mark Adams, aka "the Grizz"—where in the world would we be without your amazing talents, patience, and complete support? We know our food tastes great; you make it look even better. You have been in the trenches with us from the beginning. Truly, we will never be able to thank you enough for your influence on this book.

Robb Wolf and Nicki Violetti, you believed in us and got this ship afloat from day one. Our lives changed forever the day we met you in Jacksonville. You welcomed us in as friends, and things have continued to grow. Many tasty dinners, fanny burnings, and cracked coconuts later and here we are.

Thanks for lighting the fire in our culinary bellies to embark on this adventure.

Erich Krauss, our publisher and long-distance tour guide to book writing. When do you sleep? Thanks for your energy, patience, and willingness to be our partner throughout this process. We can't wait to cook for you, sir.

To all the clients, trainers, and friends of BTB Fitness . . . you guys *rock*. We have been so fortunate to have a team of wonderful folks behind us to support us and give us feedback on every aspect of the book.

Lastly, it feels impossible to find words that can truly express our gratitude to Jeff and Melissa Hayes (and Spike and Fuego). Because of you, we are where we are today—yes, even the marriage part. Your passion for eating well and being healthy and fit, and your unconditionally giving yourselves to the community brought us all together; you continue to inspire us professionally and personally on a daily basis. We may never be able to truly express our thanks for your friendship and love, and for steering us clear of bags of all purpose flour, but we'll continue to try. We love you dearly.

# preface

## aka our logical framework for this book

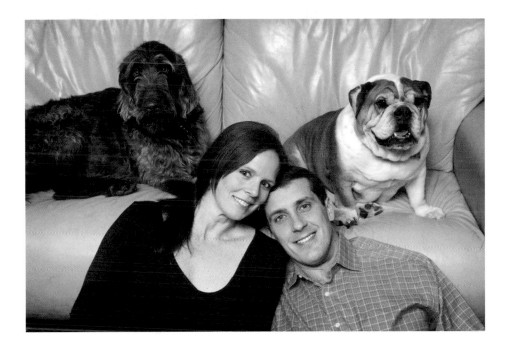

If someone had handed us a fortune cookie early in 2009 that said, "In 2010, you will open a CrossFit gym, get married, and start writing a paleo cookbook," we're pretty sure our cortisol levels would have skyrocketed on the spot and caused us to self-implode, not to mention the gluten in the cookie would have tweaked us out.

Yet, in 2010, that's exactly what happened (the opening of the gym, wedding, and cookbook parts). All that while working our full-time jobs.

When Robb Wolf and Nicki Violetti sug-gested to us that we should write a cookbook, we were excited about the idea, but scared to death about the reality! Yet we've found our-selves enjoying our time in the kitchen togeth-er, laughing at our foibles, eating really well, and having a ton of fun with the project.

Our intention was to create a cookbook that would provide individuals who are eat-ing a paleo-based diet or who are just omit-ting grains, gluten, dairy, and/or legumes from their day-to-day some creative ideas on how to make really tasty meals that are paleo, pri-mal, gluten free, low carb, etc. This book is for everyone: the elite athlete, the grandmoms struggling with arthritis, the busy on-the-go families who are looking for new inspirations for different meals, and people looking to make a paleo meal to bring to their families and friends to show them just how good real food can taste when not laden with chemicals, preservatives, and crap.

If you are picking up this book, chances are you already know what paleo is, or you're living a primal life, or you've been gluten free for a while. There are some phenomenal resources and individuals out there who can explain to you the whys of paleo, what primal really means, and how to implement this way of life into your home with your family. Because there are such great resources out there, we aren't recreating the wheel here. Rather, we've created a cookbook.

We aren't professional chefs by trade, we don't have near the culinary knowledge base that Alton Brown or Shirley Corriher do, nor are we nutritionists, PhDs, or experts on all things paleo. We simply love to cook real foods and love to teach others to cook this way—with real ingredients in new and inventive ways that elicit feelings of comfort and home for us.

There are some recipes or ingredients that will cause some to say, "Well, that's not really paleo!" And our answer to that is best summed up with a quote from Andrew Badenoch over at evolvify.com: "Paleo is a logical framework applied to modern humans, not a historical re-enactment." It seems to us that recently paleo has become kind of like religion—lots of different ways to interpret things, and there really isn't a "right or wrong" interpretation—

just different. Your own paleo compass is what should guide you—not what we say or do, not what some website told you to do. We eat this way (and by this way we mean real foods, with minimally processed ingredients) because it makes sense to us. It tastes good, we feel good, we perform well, and it keeps us healthy. The fact that a caveman did or did not eat something is not what we use here to define what we classify as "paleo"—though the true definition of a "Paleolithic diet" is along those lines. But here's the thing: we're pretty certain cavemen didn't have our Cuisinart food processor, or our Le Creuset assortment, but you'd better believe we're going to use those to cook some tasty food. We particularly like how the folks at Whole 9 position foods and meals: it either makes you more healthy, or less healthy. That's a pretty good measuring stick to gauge your meals.

There is one thing we feel we need to state very clearly too: there are some recipes in life that you cannot apply a paleo framework to. While, yes, there may be some consummate comfort foods that you're able to make without gluten, dairy, and added sugars, there are a lot of recipes that you just can't create while keeping true to paleo guidelines. Macaroni and cheese is nothing without the cheese. There is absolutely no way to make a tasty bourbon caramel sauce without a cup of sugar. Certain chemistry feats in baking cannot be accomplished without some gluten and/or sugar—or if they could, it wouldn't be nearly as worth the cheat for the "real thing." A paleo hoagie roll is something we will never want or ever attempt to make. If we ever want a hoagie roll, cheat it is; our insides will not be happy, and it will be Amorosos (anyone from Philly knows what we are talking about).

Let it be said that dependent upon your overall goals—whether it's to lose weight, gain muscle mass, or avoid some intestinal inflammation—it may be that not every single recipe in this book is a good idea for you. Some of the recipes in here shouldn't be eaten every single day. Some aren't appropriate for those going super strict, say on a Whole 30 plan. Some aren't wise if you are trying to lean out or bulk up, and some may not appeal to everyone. Less than 10 percent of the recipes in here are desserts, because sugar spikes after every meal will do nothing to keep your insulin levels in those nice happy middle ranges.

These recipes can and should all be tweaked as you see fit to make them your own. The hope is that there are some recipes, tricks, and tips that might help you eat a little cleaner, improve your health, or learn something new. If any of those things happen—even for one person—then we will have achieved our goals with writing this book.

Here is our cookbook!

# introduction

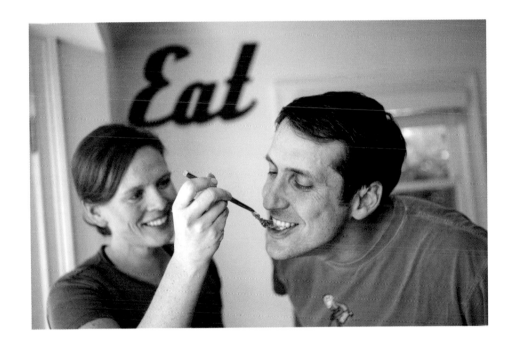

## Charles' History

If I had to put my finger on it, my first memories of the joy of cooking were around six or seven years old. My father was the scoutmaster of our local troop. Despite my age (you're not supposed to be a scout until you're ten) I got to tag along on camping trips and the annual scout jamboree. Jamborees were nice because you drove to your campsite. A loaded-up van and trailer come in really handy when you're hauling twenty-five-pound Dutch ovens, spits, and griddles around. Dad was pretty famous for his cobblers. The cherry was good, but the cherries usually came from a can. If the troop was fortunate enough to have blackberries in season, things stepped up a few notches.

The thing I really enjoyed was each morning after breakfast, Dad would spread the coals out from the fire, which had likely been burning all night, and prop a griddle up on two logs. He would cook pancakes for the troop, and there would invariably be a cup or two of batter left over. Dad would carefully pour out a pancake the size of a large pizza. The trick was flipping it over, and everyone gathered around to see if it would stay together. So, my first culinary quest was pancake flipping. Hey, you have to start somewhere, right?

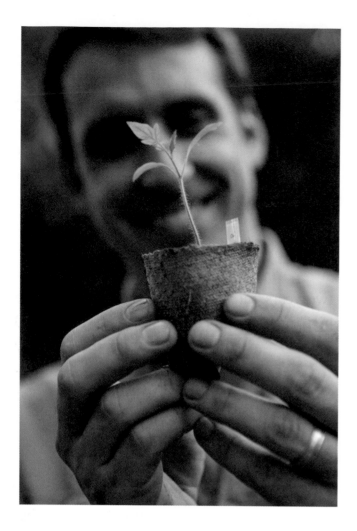

I had it pretty good at home also. My mother hails from Mobile, Alabama, and grew up with all the rich foods and cooking traditions of the Gulf Coast. She left none of them behind when my parents moved to Athens, Tennessee, in the early 1970s. We could always count on the most aromatic house when we got home from school. Mom was always cooking up something delicious. Much of my upbringing centered on the family meal. We had breakfast together most mornings, and dinner was a must. Everyone holding hands, my father would say the blessing and we would finally get to enjoy all the goodness we had been salivating over since we got home from school. This was our time together. Mom and Dad would ask us about our day. Our job was to fill them in on the events of the day without talking with food in our mouths or putting our elbows on the table. I was so fortunate that our table was always loaded up. We were encouraged to try everything, and dessert was only a clean plate away.

My summers were full of activity. We grew up in the country. There was a natural spring in our backyard that fed a creek that flowed into a pond. There were flower gardens all around, a big lawn to mow, and a fort overlooking a pond in the backyard. When I wasn't at soccer, scouts, or summer camp, you could find me home doing any number of outdoor activities. My mother and father had the greenest of thumbs. We had about a half acre (that's pretty big by most standards) garden that was bulging at the seams with a countless variety of vegetables and herbs all season long. Honestly, I grew to dread the garden at an early age. If you've never come home from two hours of soccer practice to hear "please go pick the beans," you may not be able to relate.

Despite my distaste for the constant attention and upkeep required by a garden that large, I learned to appreciate the entire process of planting and harvesting produce. It was not uncommon for dinner to have been picked only moments before it went into a pot to cook. In the summer and fall, my mother would always can a ton of beans, tomatoes, and squash. We would have jars upon jars of tasty goodness all winter long. When spring rolled around, we'd till up the ground and do it all over again.

Some of you might be forming this picture that I was snacking on fresh veggies and fruits to my little tummy's content all year long as a kid. I can't lie. There were plenty of afternoons after a long day of school that I would motor through some less-than-desirable food choices. My "go-to" snack of choice was the following: ½ box of vanilla wafers, ½ jar of peanut butter, and several glasses of whole milk. Those were indeed the days. I would also be remiss if I didn't tell you that my true passion for cooking and food didn't really develop until after I got out of college. For some reason, basketball, soccer, golf, and football seemed much more appealing to me in my younger years; so let's skip to college so as to avoid your complete boredom with my recollections of Mom feeding and me eating.

In high school and college I ate like most folks do. It was cafeteria style. In both instances, I was afforded the ability to go back for seconds (sometimes thirds) of whatever the day's offerings were. Over the years the quality of the offerings became less and less. I recall looking forward to fried day in college. That was the day that Ms. Claire (our fraternity house cook) would break out an endless supply of chicken tenders, cheese sticks, and anything else you could stick in a deep fryer. I'm not sure how many pounds of trans fats have passed my lips, but from 1992 to 1997, it would fill an airport hangar. Throw on top of

that the endless flow of beer and liquor, and you had yourself one potential cow of a man just waiting to burst out of his trousers.

I've always had a pretty athletic build and have been extremely active. This is important to note, since my food intake would have likely ballooned me well beyond the limits of human existence. There have only been two instances in my past that I ever looked in the mirror and felt like the person looking back at me was fat. The first time happened about two years out from college. My weight (since high school) had always hovered around 200 pounds. A few years after I had hung up my intramurals uniforms and had taken up riding in a golf cart as a typical workout, I was weighing in around 235, which did not sit well with me. I joined your run-of-the-mill Globo Gym and started trying to exercise on a regular basis. Lean Cuisine became the meal of choice. The package said "lean" on it . . . that must mean it's good for me. On occasion, I would rifle through four or five of them a day to try and keep a grip on feeling full. Within a few months, I was down twenty pounds and feeling a bit better about myself.

My second "look how fat I am" moment" really marked the beginning of my quest for

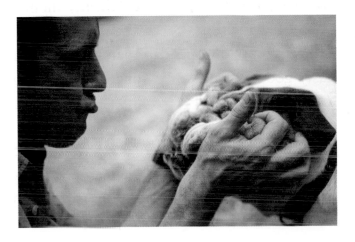

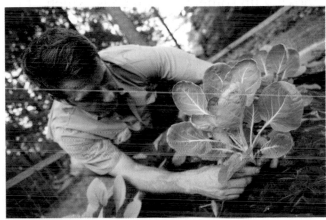

nutritional enlightenment. From 2003 to 2007, I moved four times, got married, got divorced, and started my own financial planning practice. To say that stress was high during those years would be a slight understatement. My exercise regimen consisted of daily trips to my Globo Gym at 5:30 in the morning. Treadmills, elliptical machines, and the assortment of exercise gear made up my entire workout. Instant meals were still a heavy staple in my daily food intake. They were easy and didn't taste awful.

I lined up an appointment with a hydrostatic dunk tank in April 2006 to have my body fat measured. 18.9 percent! I'll never forget that number. The following day I hired a personal trainer. We worked out three to four times a week for the next year. Our sessions were pretty regimented. Monday was legs, Wednesday was back and biceps, and Friday was chest and triceps. I'd try and squeeze an extra day in each week to go through some plyometrics and body-weight stuff. After all, I was extremely motivated to make positive changes in my health.

Fast forward a year later. I was divorced, living with a friend while I renovated my new house, and really looking forward to seeing all the incredible progress I had made with my trainer. I was at 18.3 percent body fat. How could this be? Hydrostatic weighing is the gold standard in body fat calculations, so I had him run the test one more time. All those machines, curls, and big fluffy balls had done me little good. Needless to say, the trainer got the boot. I wasn't going to pay $300 a month for results like that.

The friend I was living with at the time had seen some pretty measurable results with Nutri-system. The year was 2007, I was thirty-three years old and about to begin my first "diet." Everything I read said that fat was the enemy. Nutri-system had their low fat "rib sticking" meals, and I bought my first few months of food. The meals weren't horrible. A microwave away from eating was a great place for me to be, given my busy schedule of working out in the mornings, working all day, followed by a few hours working on my house.

In June, I was finally moved into my new house. I thumbed through the boxes and located the coupon for an outdoor fitness program I had bought earlier that year at a charity auction. It was for one month of "BootCamp." July 9 was my first day, and I couldn't have been more excited to try something new. All of my previous efforts didn't seem to work. Maybe this would do the trick.

My hunger for information now had a teacher to point me in the right direction. The eating philosophy that I adopted thanks to BTB Fitness was a program based on Dr. Barry Sears's Zone. It was obviously a step in the right direction. My body just kept leaning out. My performance numbers at BootCamp and the BTB CrossFit gym were steadily improving. Six months into my relationship with BTB, I took a trip to the "Fat Van," as they called it. The owner of the hydrostatic Body Fat Testing unit (the Fat Van) was a gentleman named Bali. He and I were getting to know one another pretty well. We were both really amazed and excited to see my 12.2 percent body fat come through on the computer. That worked out to around 1 percent of body fat per month. Excuse me waiter, may I have another serving?

Here we go down the rabbit hole. Hold on folks.

By the time the clock rolled over to 2008, I was signed up for my first marathon, ate my Zoned meals and snacks six times a day, and enjoyed every minute of it. I was in the best shape of my life. Finishing the marathon in less than four hours was a big milestone for me.

The summer and fall of 2008 would ultimately be when everything got turned upside down (for all the right reasons). By now, I was becoming good friends with Jeff and Melissa Hayes, the owners of BTB Fitness. My brother, Michael, had turned our family farm into an agricultural tourism center. He was growing fresh vegetables and selling them at local markets and restaurants. I was home in July for our annual Fourth of July party and mentioned to him that I thought it would be fun to load up my car with a ton of his produce and go sell it at the gym one weekend. I'm not sure how much food you thought you could fit in an SUV, but I assure you, it is a bundle.

Several weeks later in early August, I met Michael in Chattanooga and we loaded me up. Boxes of tomatoes, corn, peppers, beans, and squash were loaded up, and I hauled them down to Atlanta for what we affectionately called the "Gym Market". Monday evening I set up several tables in the corner of BTB's CrossFit gym, and laid out my spread. There was a pretty big Zone challenge going on at the time among the clients, and they came in droves to pick out some food. We had only met in passing at this point, and I really didn't know who Julie Sullivan was. But when she walked in the gym that night, I knew I would never forget her. You can always tell a good

foodie by how they meticulously examine their vegetables. Julie carefully picked out some of the heirloom tomatoes Michael had grown and grabbed several other items. We exchanged pleasantries and she was on her way.

The gym market was a success. I made my brother some decent money and got him a stockpile of folks craving his delicious produce. More importantly, I had laid eyes on Julie. In the months to follow, Melissa suggested that we start a food swap. So a handful of select folks began preparing large meals and swapping recipes on the weekends. It was fantastic. I could cook up one big meal and in exchange get several for the week. It was at this point in my life that I found my true joy in cooking.

It was also at this time that Jeff Hayes—co-owner of BTB—had gotten some news that the cancer he had licked a year before was back. He was to go through some pretty harsh treatment and would be on house arrest for a hundred days. Needless to say, Melissa was pretty occupied with caring for her husband and wasn't able to prepare meals for the swap. I began making tons more food each weekend, and would drop off extra meals at their house so they wouldn't have to cook. The joy and fulfillment I got from helping them was really what spurred me to cook even more. Giving is addictive, and I have always had a sense of doing for others. What I didn't know, and Melissa did, was that Julie was also preparing tons of food and bringing it to their house as well. That's when I got the phone call. Melissa called me to ask if I was seeing anyone seriously. She had someone that she thought would be a perfect match for me. "You need

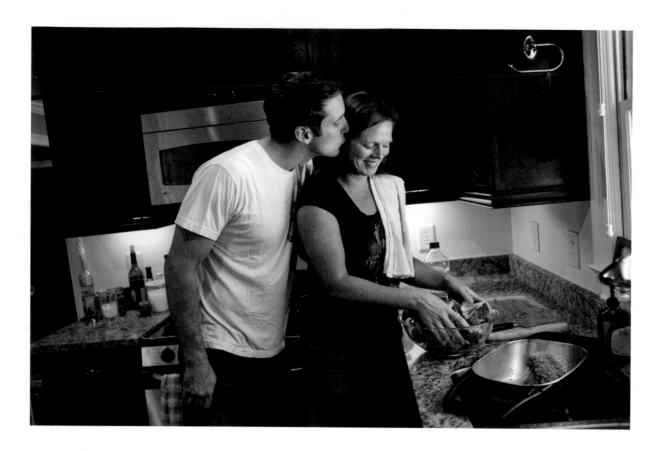

to ask Julie out on a date," she said. I guess Melissa felt like we deserved one another, and she was right.

I'm pretty sure Julie picks up the rest of the story from here. But as they say, the rest was history.

## Julie's History

Motor oil chicken. Swimming. My family. Land of high-speed chases and plastic surgeons.

Sounds like the old Johnny Carson "Carnac the Magnificent" routine. Let's talk about these things and how they influenced where I am today.

Motor oil chicken was the first "meal" I can recall ever creating on my own (come on now, the Easy-Bake Oven chocolate cakes weren't a meal). I'm going to approximate that this was around the time I hit twelve or

so. Quite simple recipe, really: Chicken quarters in a baking pan, Italian dressing drizzled over, and baked in the oven at 375°F. Now that I think about it, the "motor oil" nomenclature for (insert brand name) Italian dressing is about right. Nevertheless, this was the first meal where I can recall turning the oven on and cooking a protein. It was a necessity, really: growing up in a household with a working mom and two siblings, if I wanted to eat before getting back from swim practice at 8 PM, it meant cooking up something besides a Hungry Man dinner. Our accompaniment was usually some Rice-A-Roni and peas (one of the only green vegetables I liked).

After that point, cooking—and food in general—always interested me, though I was far from an adventurous eater. My mom and sister would eat the iceberg lettuce salad, which I always thought was nasty (especially

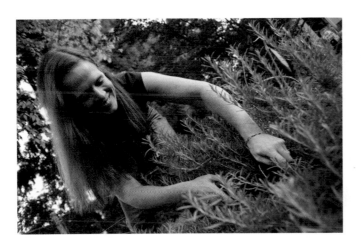
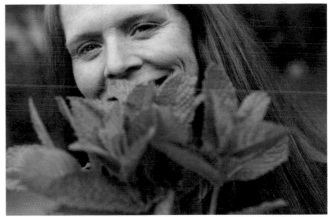

salad dressing). Raw tomatoes would elicit a gag reflex from me, and broccoli, cauliflower, and any cruciferous vegetables were never something I chose to eat. Now baking, that was something I loved, and you could count on me for some awesome brownies-from-a-box.

And then it was off to college. I love my family, loved the small town outside Philadelphia I grew up in, but I wanted to see what else was in the world. So I hoped my financial aid package would be adequate, packed my bags, and headed to Emory University for school.

To help pay for my college tuition after my move to Atlanta, I took a job at a local golf club. It started off as swim coaching, and morphed after the summer into waiting on tables. I do think anyone and everyone should have the experience of waiting tables at some point in their lives. You learn that "a server's role is to make the customer happy" and that the way that a gluten sensitive customer shares with that server 312 requests for modifications can make all the difference in the world. (Go eat at a restaurant with Robb Wolf and you'll see how it's done right).

My experience of waiting tables bolstered my interest in cooking that much more, as I was selected as one of the "fine dining" servers—which is laughable because anyone who knows me knows I'm antiformality incarnate. The fine dining experience, and working the front side of the house while observing the chefs working in the back, exposed me to all sorts of great foods and preparation ideas. I loved taking the knowledge I learned from these talented chefs, then going off and cooking these delectable items for friends in college. Basically, I'd invite myself over to people's apartments so I could escape the dorm and play in their kitchens.

## Swimming

It was also during this period in life that I really focused on "healthy" eating and cooking. Not that I wasn't "healthy" before (okay, maybe the bowl of Lucky Charms in the morning wasn't the best thing for me), but in college you become responsible (for the most part) for every meal you ingest. I came to college as a walk-on for the swim team, and anyone who has been a competitive swimmer knows these are grueling and long workouts and take a lot out of you. I had to keep myself properly fueled.

I remember hitting our 6 AM workouts after something like three to six hours of sleep; going to the University center for breakfast; downing a bagel, some fruit, and some juice; and then heading to class and struggling to keep my eyes open. I just figured I was tired from the workout. Lunches were often some pasta (hey—it's low fat!), some marinara or some pesto for flavor, maybe a little veggies, and some garlic bread or a roll of sorts. Then it was afternoon practice, off to the golf club to wait tables, and get the "family meal" served to the staff.

Nights before swim meets were all about carb loading; pasta, pasta, pasta; and baskets of garlic bread devoured by our team. It was all good though—we were eating low fat! I downed PowerBars at meets because they were fuel for me, the athlete. I was physically active for way more hours per week than the average person, eating low fat and not too many calories, and yet, when you looked at me, someone who was swimming sometimes 10,000 yards or more a day, I looked puffy. I was puffy. I cringe looking back at those pictures now. My theory during that period of life was that it was my body holding onto insulation from the cold pool water temps. Or that I had my dad's genes.

## My family

My dad's genes, my mom's genes . . . indeed, genetics are a large part of who we are, which in my case, is kind of scary. My dad was overweight, and passed away nearly twenty-five years ago of lung cancer. My mom is now a twelve-year breast cancer survivor. Need-less to say, there may be some things, genetically, that I have no control over. However, I strongly believe that much of disease is due to gene-environment interactions. Which is why I want to do, and choose to do, as much as I can to combat those things that I don't have immediate control over, and strive to keep my environment the best that I can.

## Land of high-speed chases and plastic surgeons

In 1998, I moved to Los Angeles for a job in the nonprofit sector (yes, the nonprofit sector exists in Los Angeles. Crazy, I know). Because choosing to work in the nonprofit sector in Los Angeles is not exactly the wisest economic move, I had to be resourceful with my pennies. It was at this time that a dear friend told me that she was going to be volunteering to help out with some cooking classes at Sur La Table (a great cooking supply store – surlatable.com)—they needed folks to set up the kitchen and clean up after class—and in return we received free access to the information being shared, recipes, and store discounts. Of course I signed right up. This may have been one of the smartest moves I've ever made (aside from saying yes to marrying Charles).

While at Sur La Table, I met the fabulous duo of Melanie Barsuk and Taji Marie, the ladies who run Simple Gourmet, as well as the incredibly talented Jet Tila, chef extraordinaire. I was fortunate enough to be asked to help them with many of their private catered affairs, team-building events, and other culinary adventures. Melanie always amazed me in her ability to balance her busy life with two awesome kids and her "lovey" husband, while teaching and putting on amazing catered events. Taji has this amazing creativity when it comes to the artistry involved with food, as well as more passion for cooking than most I've met. It's rare that she does not have a smile on her face too! Jet, well he is like the Dude from *The Big Lebowski*, only even cooler. Pretty much any and every cooking class concerning Thai foods in Los Angeles circa 2000–2007 was taught by Jet, and he honestly taught me all I know about Asian-inspired cooking. I still laugh thinking about a private catered event we did together, as it was Jet (who is Thai-Chinese), Arianna (who is Mexican), and me (the Irish lass), cooking up and serving food for a Passover seder. Random, I know.

Along with the catering gigs with Melanie, Taji, and Jet, which helped me supplement my nonprofit income, I still volunteered at Sur La Table (as we received those discounts!) and learned all sorts of things from chefs along the way. One story I'll never forget: Chef Mark Peel once worked in a kitchen with another really well-known celebrity chef, and he told us a story of how someone had ordered seared scallops, and so Peel tossed the skillet on the burner, turned it on, and immediately put the oil and scallops in the pan. The well-known chef came over, grabbed the pan, and threw it and the scallops on the kitchen floor, yelling that you never put your protein into a cold pan. Lesson learned!

L.A. is indeed a foodies' paradise, and living out there exposed me to all kinds of great foods—many that I never liked or would have tried otherwise. The sushi is outstanding (at many places) due to the access to fresh fish from Asia and the Pacific; fresh farmer's markets are available year-round on numerous days of the week with so much great local produce; Korean, Oaxacan, Vietnamese, Thai, and other ethnic restaurants and grocery stores are scattered about the huge city, and you'd be hard-pressed to find such diversity elsewhere. I know New Yorkers swear by what's available there; however, New York can't really claim the same year-round produce availability (somewhat local, at least) that Los Angeles can.

While I loved the weather in California, my spinning class, amazing friends, and of course the access to beaches, mountains, desert, and great food…the traffic, cost of living, and distance from family wasn't really cutting it for me anymore. I had recently reconnected with friends of mine back in Atlanta, and was offered a position with the American Cancer Society at our National Home Office.

All this brings us to a few years ago, here in Atlanta. I'd been here for about eighteen months, and I'd been running and working out with a personal trainer, but I wasn't seeing the results I wanted. So I did some online searching, and came across BTB CrossFit and Boot-Camp. I could pretty much end this introduction there, as just about everything in my life today is because of BTB Fitness and its owners, Jeff and Melissa Hayes. Seriously. I met Charles through BTB Fitness, began my paleo path because of BTB fitness, we are writing this book because of BTB Fitness. Not only are Jeff and Melissa dear friends of ours, business partners, and all-around great people, but they also inspired us to start this paleo journey. Oh, and their doggy Fuego is my dog-

Godchild.

Let me back up: when I first started with BTB Fitness, it was 2008, and we began a Zone challenge soon after I joined. Two of the best things that came from that: a meal swap with other members from the gym, and me being introduced to the other writer of this book, my amazing husband. I still have an e-mail from August of 2008 from Melissa (she actually framed it for me) that alluded to Charles asking me out: "someone will be asking you out soon. I can't say who. But I wanted you to be prepared with two answers. One: Yes, I'd love to. And Two: I have actually just started seeing someone. . . . That way you are ready . . . just in case you don't like him! I can tell you he is handsome, fit, old enough, taller than you, and moderately well adjusted." Still makes me giggle, especially because at the time I really had no idea who she was talking about. All that aside, I encourage any and all individuals on a paleo path to start a meal swap—as it expands your meal diversity exponentially, and you get to meet a potential partner. Not bad!

Charles did in fact ask me out by way of losing a bet regarding a BTB BootCamp challenge. Since he lost the bet, he had to cook me dinner—and boy did he make an amazing one. Grilled lamb chops, stuffed peppers, and some other delicious food items. We made a similar bet a few weeks later, and I lost this time, so I was to cook him dinner. We made the bet a little more "interesting" this time, and said that the winner got to choose one thing about the dinner. Charles' choice? That I would come with him to Tennessee, and make him dinner . . . and cook dinner for his mom, dad, brother, sister, cousins, aunt . . . it came

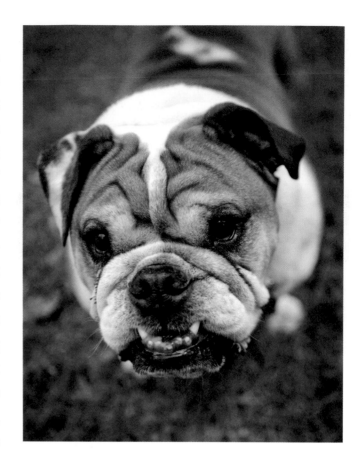

out to be about twelve people that I had never met. The good news is that I think I held my own in the kitchen, and one thing's for sure: I immediately fell in love with the family.

A few months later, after our Zone time of weighing, measuring, and counting everything (Zone is very much focused on the quantities of macronutrients, with food quality being secondary), Melissa mentioned some guy named Robb Wolf, and that she attended his Nutrition "cert" and had some great new information and a slightly different way of eating that didn't involve the kitchen scale, measuring cups, and counting almonds. It was all about this "paleo" concept and eating clean, and Melissa's words were that it made a ton of sense (Melissa's background is in nutrition science).

Wanting to expand our knowledge on all

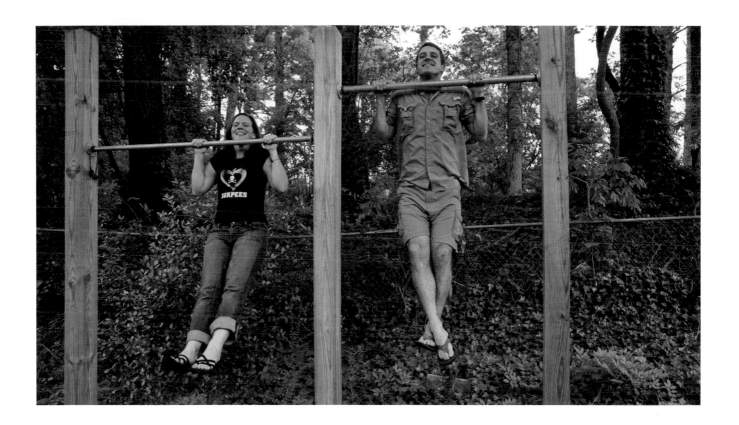

things related to this, Charles and I decided to sign up for one of these "certs" in Jacksonville, Florida. This was a pivotal, life-changing moment, as Robb pretty much convinced us to ditch the weighing/measuring gig (thank you, Robb), and just eat real foods and ditch the crap—except for the occasional tequila.

I remember my first few weeks eating paleo vs. Zone and the difference it made. In my Zone life, my three block breakfasts had typically been: ⅔ cup steel-cut oatmeal, 1 cup strawberries, ¾ cup cottage cheese, and 1½ teaspoons of peanut butter. I loved my breakfast. I did not love the hunger pangs that set in about two hours later, with me about to gnaw my hand off, searching for my next string cheese piece, apple, and almonds. When I switched to eating real, clean foods, eliminating dairy, grains, and legumes, I'd eat a breakfast full of eggs and sautéed veggies, and I'd feel full for hours. And I just felt great

in general. I dabbled in doing Zone portions of paleo-quality foods, but I find I'm just happier eating until I'm full of these tasty, real foods. Since then, I really haven't turned back, and have counted Melissa, Jeff, Nicki, Robb, and Charles among some of the most influential people in my life over these last few years.

## From Both of Us

We love eating this way, cooking this way, and sharing what we know/have learned/experienced with others. We believe that no matter how hard you workout, you cannot "work off" a crappy diet—it will catch up with you internally or externally at some point.

What is our definition of paleo? We eat meats (predominantly grass-fed), poultry (pastured), game (Charles is an avid hunter), fresh seafood, and any other high-quality proteins we can get our hands on. We eat vegetables of all colors of the rainbow. We eat little

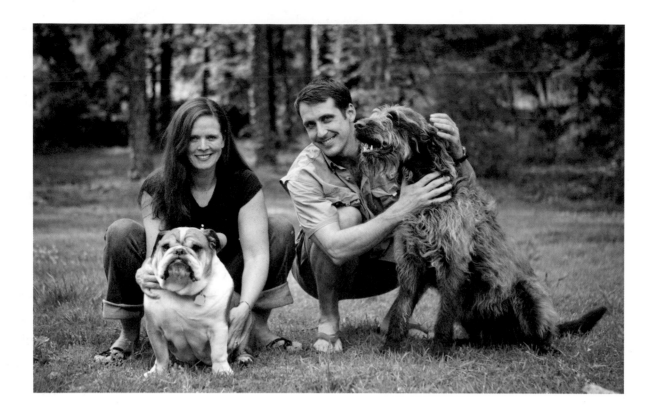

bits of fruit here and there—especially when in season, and picked fresh from our garden. We consume fat without the fear of fat making us fat. When we allow ourselves a cheat, it's because we're choosing to eat something off the paleo path, not because we just cannot manage to do this all the time! We are conscientious in our choices, as everyone should be. No one makes you eat a Twinkie. No one. No one made us eat cheesesteaks in Philadelphia—we chose to eat those. We know how our bodies feel after eating gluten, and it is not pretty.

We eat this way because we look, feel, and perform better eating this way. We sleep better. We hardly ever get sick. We have sustained energy levels throughout the day. We've seen incredible results for us and stunning results for family members, friends, and clients. We've heard hundreds, if not thousands, of anecdotal stories of people whose lives have been changed for the better by sticking to these real,

unprocessed foods. People reversing autoimmune issues, reversing fertility issues, and just plain looking good naked.

In our minds, we are all an experiment of one in this life. There are some people who can function great on a vegan diet. Power to them! There are some folks who function great on a Slim Fast diet. Power to them! For us, eating this way isn't a diet, isn't a phase, isn't something we'll do for thirty days and stop. We've been eating this way for the better part of three years (with cheats now and then), and this is how we choose to live our lives.

How exactly do we incorporate all of this into our lives? Sleep is critical for us, the holy grail if you will, and we both try *really* hard to ensure that we get our eight hours of sleep a night. We eat really clean. Our freezer is stocked full of locally sourced, grass-fed and finished beef and venison cuts Charles procured. We seek out local farmers' markets and CSAs to source our vegetables, fruits and poultry; while Trader Joe's is about twenty minutes away, thank goodness there *is* a Trader Joe's here. In the summertime, our garden typically overflows with tomatoes, lemon cucumbers, zucchini, yellow squash, spaghetti squash, peppers, okra, Italian basil, Thai basil, rosemary, cilantro, Italian parsley, chives, and whatever else we can grow. We can a bunch of our own tomatoes, and Charles' mom also has a pantry full of home-canned goods that she's more than willing to share. Sundays are typically our cooking day, where we make our meals for the week—or as many as we can—and enjoy our time with one another. This is a *critical* step in making sure we (two people, two full-time jobs, two-part time jobs, and writing this book) have meals throughout the week and don't have to eat out all the time.

We work out about three times a week, coach a bunch more, work full-time jobs, and love our BTB CrossFit family and helping members to achieve their goals. That's how we live our lives. It does not mean it's how you should live your life (though we think getting adequate sleep and sourcing with high-quality protein should be nonnegotiable for everyone!).

There are tons—and we mean *tons*—of resources out there that can explain to you the whys of all this: why no grains, why no legumes, why no dairy. Bottom line for us is this: We feel better eating these real, unprocessed foods that really are what our ancestors ate, and we know we're getting the vitamins and nutrients we need.

All that being said, "eating paleo" is a loose framework that is subject to loads of interpretations. Go search some paleo recipes,

and you'll see what we mean. There will be some readers who will curse us out for using red wine in a recipe, others will lament the use of certain vinegars, while others still will be mad we don't use agave nectar (no thanks!). Our advice: Go read up on substitutes for these items, and find ones that suit you. Same goes for an ingredient you don't like. Skip it or find a substitute. Just be smart about your choices. If you are replacing coconut milk with almond milk, you had better make darn sure the almond milk is all natural without added sugar!

This cookbook is not intended to be all things to all people. Rather, it is intended for those who want to expand their "real foods" cooking repertoire, learn a few bits here and there, and maybe get some creative ideas on adapting recipes to these frameworks. Perhaps this book will give you some paleo-friendly desserts you can bring to that next social gathering, or an appetizer that lets other people see that eating this way can be fresh, tasty, and delicious.

If you are new to paleo or primal life, and want to get into the whys, we have some great resources to get you started:

• www.robbwolf.com—forums, podcasts, blogs . . . egad, there is a ton of info here! We could spend days reading his stuff. Oh wait, I do. Also, Robb's *New York Times* best-seller, *The Paleo Solution*. Robb has done an exceptional job of bringing the paleo way of life into the mainstream. We're still hoping that Jon Stewart will interview him someday. A dear friend and inspiration to thousands—including us—Robb presents paleo information in a very palatable way (pun intended).

- www.everydaypaleo.com—Sarah Fragoso is that busy mom of three who does it all—and wrote a book about it, too. *Everyday Paleo* takes the paleo lifestyle and provides you with how to integrate this way of life into your family, making the whole family healthier.

- www.whole9life.com—Melissa and Dallas Hartwig have done their homework, and they live, eat (literally), and breathe this stuff. They have a super helpful Whole 30 program to get your paleo party started (meaning, eating real stuff—being super strict—to reset your body).

- www.thepaleodiet.com—Professor Loren Cordain's site (Robb Wolf's mentor), with a book of the same name. Lots of great resources there—especially the FAQs, so that the next time someone asks you why quinoa isn't a good idea on paleo, you can have some nice science behind your answer.

- www.archevore.com (fka panu.com)—Dr. Kurt Harris has adopted what he calls a Paleo 2.0 approach and has a great thing going over there on his site, with boatloads of info, getting really science-y at times.

- www.marksdailyapple.com—Mark Sisson is the primal man, and has a great site, some fantastic books, and a very active forum to help you in your primal journey.

Gary Taubes, Drs. Michael and Mary Eades, Art DeVany—we could list hundreds of resources for you, but trust us: these initial ones will be plenty for you to chew on for a while.

Want more info? Type in "paleo diet," "primal eating," or "paleo 2.0" into the Google machine, and you'll have lots more to choose from, everything from busy moms cooking paleo for their family, to recipes, to the ever-popular "Paleo Hacks" where folks ask questions and the paleo community responds.

Now that you've gotten your paleo education by reading all those books, blogs, and more, here's how to implement this book:

These recipes are filled with ingredients and foods (for the most part) that your grandmother would recognize. However, here's what you won't find in these recipes: grains or gluten, legumes (with the exception of two recipes using green beans, in which you're eating mostly the bean pod, and they don't have near the lectin load as dry beans), and the only bit of dairy is with a few recipes that really do need the milk solids in non-clarified, but still grass-fed butter. Let it be said that there are tons of ways you can tweak certain recipes to add in some dairy, or whatever your fancy might be. These recipes aren't only for those people living a paleo lifestyle…if you're a gluten-free household, following a primal diet, or just wanting to eat real whole foods, this book is for you. However, since we personally live a paleo lifestyle, these recipes all work in the way we choose to live our lives. Many people who are gluten-free still have a lot of processed foods in their lives. These recipes eliminate most of that, and provide you and your family with real, nutritious foods.

For us, eating paleo isn't a diet. It's a way of life. It's a clean way of life. It's a tasty way of life that helps us to look, feel, and perform better. We hope you enjoy these recipes and that this book helps you and your family live the healthiest life possible.

# kitchen foods
## the basics

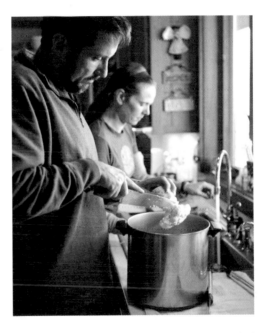

Making sure you have good proteins, carbohydrates, fats, and a bunch of pantry staples will make your life infinitely easier. Seriously. You will be way more tempted to call for pizza delivery if you find yourself with nothing to eat at home. Oprah may have her favorite things, and these are some of our most favorite things that we typically keep on hand at home:

protein: Let's start with the basics. When we set our household budget for the year, and try to figure out where to save money/cut costs,

we both wholeheartedly agree that we will not and do not skimp on good quality proteins. There are just too many great things about grass-fed, locally raised beef, shaking the hand of the farmer who raises chickens on pasture, in a humane way, and knowing that your fish supply isn't full of all kinds of contaminants from being farm raised. Go and find farmers in your area where you can buy directly from them, ask about their animal husbandry practices. Try to visit a feedlot, and you'll likely be scarred for life—it is not pretty. Support your local farmers, pay a little extra to get

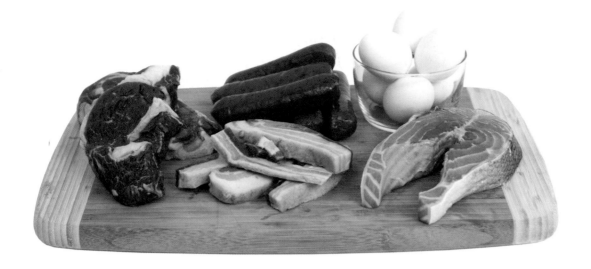

the amazing grass-fed stuff. We don't specify "grass-fed beef" or "pastured chicken" or "wild-caught fish" in every recipe, as those are principles that are assumed in our house. Making the choice to stick to higher standards with these products does make a difference, both for your health and the local economy www.eatwild.com is a fantastic resource to help you find local farmers raising their animals humanely. Keep in mind that our cooking instructions (when it regards beef) is for grass-fed beef. Grass-fed beef tends to cook faster than the grain-fed beef. If you can only get the latter, pay attention to your cooking times as you may need to cook things longer. Proteins we almost always have on hand:

- Grass-fed ground beef
- Grass-fed roasts & steaks
- Salmon (wild-caught)
- Chicken (pastured, organic)
- Bacon (nitrite and nitrate free, from local farms who treat the animals right)
- Eggs (pastured—we use large-sized eggs in all our recipes)
- Frozen deer meat of various cuts (hunted by Charles)
- Ground turkey
- Canned salmon
- Deer jerky

carbohydrates: Yes, Virginia, vegetables and fruits are carbohydrates. They may not be as carb-dense as, say, a bag of flour, but veggies and fruits have all kinds of great vitamins and minerals going for them—in addition to containing carbs. We really like buying what is fresh and in season, sourcing locally when possible, and hitting the farmers' markets for our bounty (when not procuring things from our own garden). Some people get all wound up about organic, saying 100 percent of all fruits and vegetables should be organic. Here's our take on that: for starters, buying an organic piece of fruit that was grown 5,000 miles away doesn't make all that much sense to us, when there may be options right in your own vicinity. However, everyone

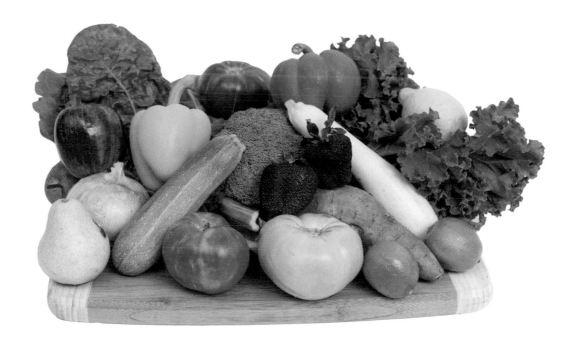

has their own standards, and you are free to choose what makes you happy, of course. The folks at Whole 9 put out a pretty good guide as to which fruits and vegetables are "dirtiest" and might make more sense to buy organically. Buy vegetables and fruits that you know you like, and try some new ones too. Look for things like canned tomatoes without a bunch of additives, and frozen vegetables are always wise to have on hand. Vegetables/fruits we almost always have on hand (not counting those items that are seasonal):

- onions
- garlic***
- broccoli
- cauliflower
- carrots
- apples
- celery
- greens (leafy winter greens, salad greens)
- cucumbers
- green onions

- berries (when in season)
- spaghetti squash
- lemons
- limes

***Garlic gets used a ton in our recipes, as we love fresh garlic. To that end, we need you to repeat after us: "I will never (you: I will never) ever (ever) not *ever* (not *ever*) buy garlic (buy garlic) that comes in a jar (that comes in a jar)." Yes, I know, you're busy. So are we! The taste of fresh garlic is so far superior to that stuff in a jar, and that stuff is just plain nasty. If you simply *must* have a shortcut, buy those cloves of garlic that are already peeled and vacuum sealed. If you must. But if we ever catch you using stuff from the jar, just know that the only person who will suffer is you, and whomever you are serving a less-than-stellar dish to . . . just saying.

fats: You will need to find a variety of fats in your paleo kitchen. Variety is the spice of life,

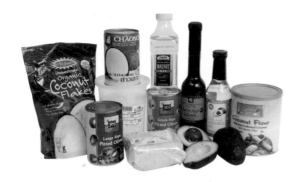

and these are hugely important for your cooking needs and for helping you reach satiety at meals. Arm yourself with these at all times, and purge your house of the canola, safflower, Crisco, etc. Here is what we keep on hand:

- olives
- good-quality olive oil
- coconut oil
- coconut milk
- unsweetened coconut flakes
- coconut butter (yum!)
- almonds
- walnuts
- hazelnuts
- macadamia nuts
- grassfed butter (clarified for most recipes)
- avocados
- avocado oil

pantry items, herbs, and spices: Having a well-stocked pantry with the items and spices you may need for just about any recipe will make a world of difference for you.

- cans or jars of tomatoes
- aged balsamic vinegar (look for the brands without added caramel coloring that list just "aged balsamic vinegar" as the ingredient)
- apple cider vinegar
- red wine vinegar
- tomato paste
- curry pastes (we like Maesri or Mae Ploy brands for Panang, Green, Yellow, and Red curry pastes—read the labels though, as some may contain mung beans or soy, which could negatively affect those with celiac or other very sensitive conditions)
- tamari (wheat-free soy sauce) and/or coconut aminos
- mustard (Dijon, powdered, you name it)
- chicken stock
- beef stock
- anchovies
- chipotles in adobo
- blanched almond flour (we like the Honeyville blanched almond flour for baking, and Trader Joe's almond meal)
- coconut flour
- sea salt
- pepper
- Any spices you particularly like. We suggest: turmeric, curry powder, chipotle powder, cayenne pepper, cinnamon, red chili flakes, dried thyme, dried rosemary, dried sage, garlic powder, onion powder, the list goes on and on…
- Fresh herbs that we like to grow and/or have on hand: flat-leaf (Italian) parsley, cilantro, basil, rosemary, thyme, and oregano.

# cooking tools
## the basics

**Cooking awesome food is a lot like going on a trip. There are some bare essentials that one must pack, a few items you would certainly like to take, and those items that if you can fit in your bag would be awesome. You're making an investment in your health, longevity, and sheer enjoyment of food; you will want the equipment necessary to pull this journey off.**

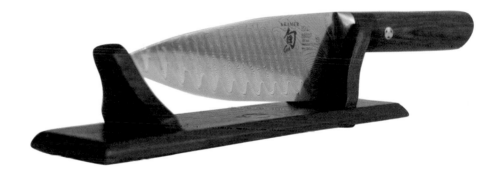

### chef's knife

There really is not a need to buy a block of knives for paring, slicing, and dicing. You can do most anything you require with a quality chef's knife. A chef's knife is kind of like a car—everyone has their own particular taste and feel that they like. Julie is a tried-and-true Shun girl. I'm warming to the Shun, but have always loved my Wüsthof. We now own four chef's knives, including a travel version. On nights when we are cranking up several dishes, they are in heavy use. A good chef's knife will be with you for years to come. We recommend visiting your local kitchen supply store (Williams-Sonoma, Sur La Table, etc.) and try out quite a few knives. Buy the knife that feels the best in your hand, and the length that works for you. We don't care what it looks like—you want to buy one that you are comfortable with. We recommend sharpening twice a year, and honing (with a kitchen steel) before every use. The longevity of your blade will depend on the quality of the steel/knife, the surfaces you cut on, and how safely you store it. The least safe knife in your kitchen is your dullest one. We absolutely suggest taking a basic knife skills class at your local cooking store to make you more comfortable with slicing and dicing things, as it really will make you more confident in the kitchen and may save you a trip to the emergency room for stitches to a finger!

## paring knife

These are perfect for those little jobs—hulling strawberries, slicing an apple, or peeling things by knife. Again, find one you like the feel of in your hand.

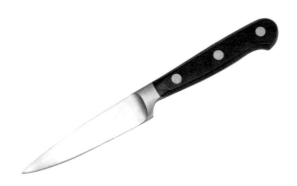

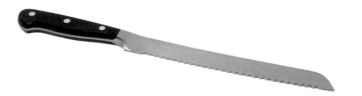

## serrated knife (aka "bread" knife)

Don't throw this away just because you are no longer baking loaves of bread. Serrated knives are wonderful in slicing tomatoes, and we use ours all the time.

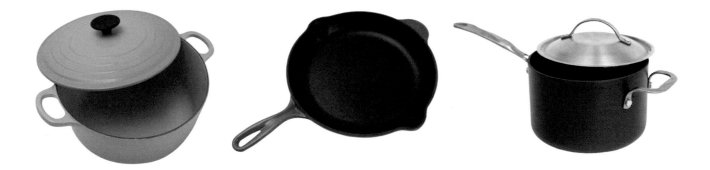

## cookware

We find that three essential pieces will cover most, if not all, cooking jobs: 1.) A Dutch oven of sorts is a must in our house. Try and get something that is heavy and deep. Julie turned me on to Le Crueset when she got me the most wonderful round French oven (Dutch oven as it's most commonly called) for our first Christmas as a couple. They distribute heat evenly and are very beautiful pieces. And while, yes, they are heavy, that is also a selling point, as this helps the piece retain and evenly distribute the heat. These enameled cast-iron pieces are so versatile—good for everything from boiling water to simmering a tomato sauce to braising short ribs in the oven for a few hours—The beauty of these pieces is that you can use them on the stove, in the oven, in the fridge, or even freezer. Better yet, a good Dutch oven will last for decades—and brands like Le Creuset come with a lifetime warranty. A good all-around size to start with is a 5.5 quart (4.3 liter) one.

2.) A good frying pan or skillet is also an essential piece in our home. At least a 10-inch (24 cm) diameter is a good start, and heavier is better for distributing heat and holding up to the rigors of cooking. We're fans of the Le Creuset enameled cast-iron skillet; it's not Anolon or Teflon, but rather' a porcelain enamel that makes it a great cooking surface that does not need seasoning. We also have an All-Clad stainless steel skillet and sauté' pan, as they also come in very handy with all that we make.

3.) Our third most commonly used piece for the stove is a decent sauce pan. Anywhere in the range of 1–3 quarts (1–2.9 liters) should do it.

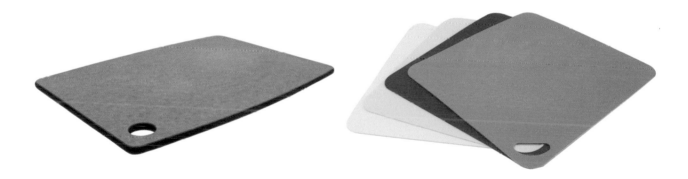

## cutting board

A good wooden cutting board will go miles to help you keep those knives sharp. They also allow for easy transport from counter to pot when dicing and slicing. We recommend, while you're shopping, to go ahead and pick up a few cutting mats. These are usually very thin and can be washed in the dishwasher. They make it really easy to go from trimming raw meat to slicing up vegetables without having to rinse the cutting service.

## measuring tools

A set of measuring cups and spoons are extremely useful. These most certainly come in sets, and you'll want to buy at least one set of cups and a set of spoons. A Pyrex measuring cup is also ideal for measuring liquids.

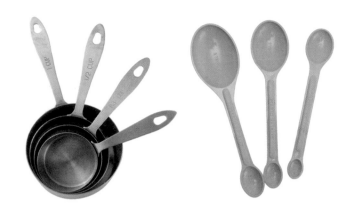

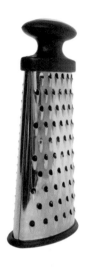
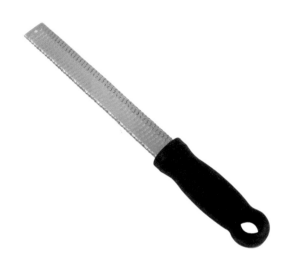

## grating utensils

A box grater and microplane are fantastic tools to have, for everything from getting that fresh lemon zest to grating some zucchini, cabbage, or cauliflower (key for riced cauliflower). We would say these are critical, especially if you don't have a food processor.

## utensils

Several spatulas (the rubber head kind are fine, or wooden) are inexpensive and used all the time in our kitchen. If your cookware involves enameled cast iron or another more sensitive surface, you'll want to be certain to use these, not metal spoons. A set of tongs is great to have on hand too, as nothing flips that big seared pot roast better than a set of tongs. Don't forget a few slotted spoons and a whisk to complete your beginner's list of requirements.

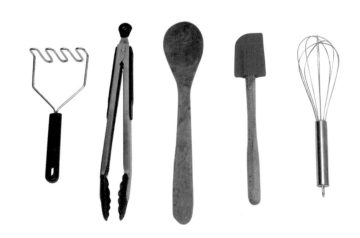

## thermometer

Go into any restaurant kitchen, and every single chef will have an instant-read thermometer in his or her chef's coat. It's quite honestly the only foolproof way to know the internal temperature of your meat/chicken/pork.

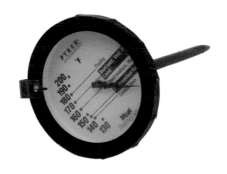

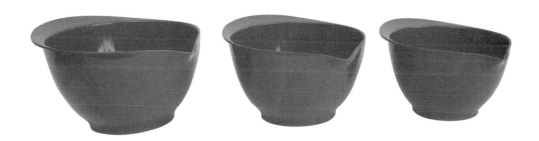

## mixing and prep bowls

Buy a set of these to arm yourself with three or four. When you are frantically throwing several dishes together, it's nice to have all your chopped ingredients in one place. A set of small glass prep bowls is inexpensive and really important for your "mise en place" (translation: everything in its place—getting all your ingredients ready for some fast cooking) which is really useful when doing such things as a quick scramble or a sauce at the very end of cooking your meat.

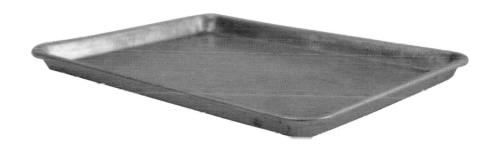

## sheet pans (aka cookie sheets)

Pick up a few of these for oven roasting, finishing things in the oven, or even just letting things marinade. We suggest the half-sheet pan size and ones that have a slight lip around the edge, so if you have liquid involved, you don't make a mess in your oven.

## garlic press

You already promised us you were going to never buy garlic from a jar. Having a garlic press will make you forget about the jar, as mincing garlic takes one squeeze and you're done. The Rosle press is like the Lamborghini of garlic presses, and it cleans easily.

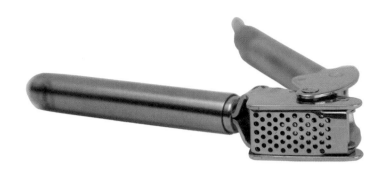

## these would be nice

You may want to throw a chef's hat in this list, because you are stepping up to the plate big time. These next few items are really nice to have around when it comes time to get cooking in your house. Though they aren't essentials, once you have experienced life with some of these pieces of equipment, chances are you won't remember life before them!

## the mighty food processor

Nut butters, cauliflower rice, and salsas . . . oh my! Chopping, slicing, and blending things by hand is cool. However, it can sometimes take a long time. If you're looking to purchase a food processor, we suggest getting at least a 9-cup (2-liter) work bowl size. Cuisinart is a fantastic brand, and they have really come out with some amazing products in the last few years. Their newest food processor—the Elite—comes with three work bowls of various sizes. It's awesome.

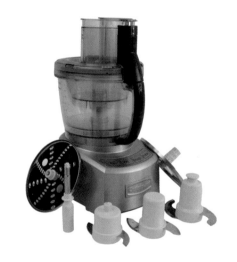

## the magic bullet

Some of those infomercials are worth every penny. There has been a Magic Bullet on my kitchen counter for as long as I can remember. This is a mini version of a food processor, with less parts and even easier cleaning. For less than $50 you can make quick salsas, chop nuts, and grind spices, and clean up is a snap. You can mix up dressings in minutes and easily store them in the refrigerator until it's time to eat.

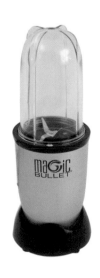

## a large wok

These are super handy if you are in the mood to just throw a bunch of stuff together and let it cook (like a quick and easy stir-fry). They are also considerably lighter than heavy Dutch ovens and clean up very easily.

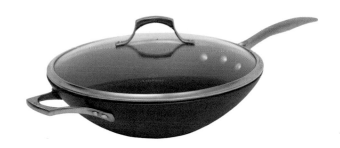

## drying rack (aka baking rack)

A metal drying rack can be used to cool things off or heat them up without having to worry about them getting drenched in their own fluids. We use our rack to oven-bake bacon all the time. It frees up your frying pan for other use and saves you from the grease splatter. Just make sure your racks are oven safe.

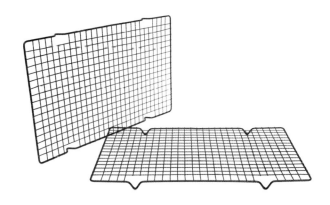

## lemon or lime squeezer

A handheld citrus juicer is extremely handy for getting every last drop of goodness out of a lemon or lime. You can do the same thing with a reamer, except you might have to pick out a seed or two. NorCal margarita, anyone?

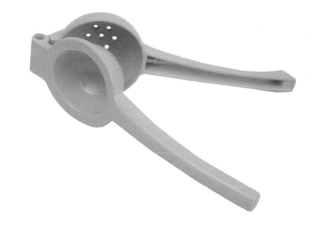

## meat mallet

There are plenty of ways to pound meat. Having a tool specifically designed to do the work that has heavy weight evenly distributed is ideal.

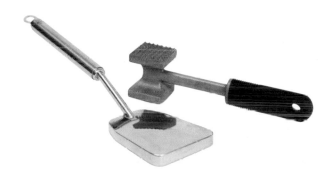

## baking dishes

Simplicity rules the day here. You can usually get a set that includes three various sizes to start, and build on your collection as time goes on. Glass or ceramic are fine.

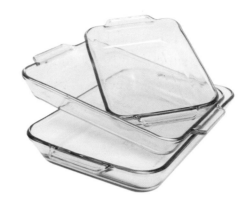

**In a "Perfect World"**
**The kitchen could turn into your ultimate hobby. We know how expensive hobbies can be. That said, here are just a few items that warrant mentioning. They get regular use in our household, but may be a step or two away for most folks.**

## an outdoor grill and/or smoker

You can grill most anything on a stove-top grill pan. You can make something taste like it was smoked in an oven. That said, an outdoor grill is a really nice thing to have on the patio. Why not go for the gusto? I've had a Big Green Egg on my porch for years. They are the Swiss Army Knife of outdoor cooking and give you options for all sorts of smoking and grilling techniques. Save your pennies and bring one home someday. If the Egg just isn't in your budget, there are plenty of gas and charcoal options that don't carry quite the price tag and still produce that great outdoor-grill flavor.

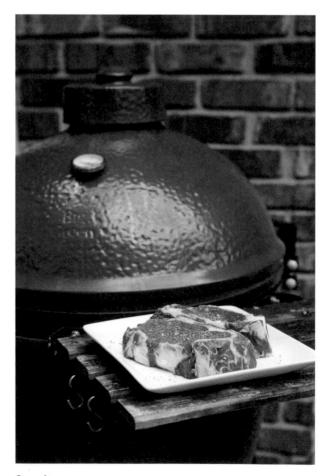

### immersion (stick) blender

Having the ability to blend things in the pot is nice. Immersion blenders are super handy for making bisques, cauliflower mash, and whipping up sweet potatoes in a snap. They are really easy to clean and store. A handheld mixer can accomplish the same thing.

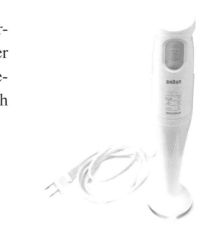

### vacuum sealer

We call ours the Food Saver 1000. I'm not really sure what version it is, but 1000 sounds cool. Vacuum sealing can increase the freezer life of anything you throw together. We are always cooking extra food with the intent of freezing some. You'll be amazed at how well flavor and the integrity of meat is maintained when you vacuum it up and place in the freezer. We've done this with ribs, pulled pork, burgers, and all have tasted exceptional when defrosted and reheated—still super moist and tender. Having a stash of frozen (cooked) meats and chicken breasts ready to be thawed on a moment's notice will ensure that you always have something on hand to eat.

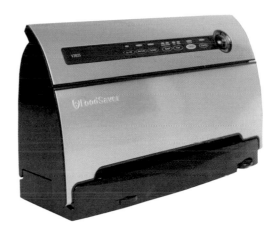

### extra freezer space

Now you can't go freezing every leftover in sight without a place to put them, and while most refrigerator/freezer combinations offer a good amount of freezer space, sometimes you need more. You can get a reasonably sized freezer for a few hundred dollars. These come in really handy when it comes time to store lots of leftover cooked food. We love using my dad's smoker and cooking up a bunch of lamb, ribs, chicken, and fish, then freezing those for future consumption. Having extra space also allows you to buy protein in bulk, which can help you realize a significant cost savings on grass-fed beef. We went in on a grass fed cow last year with several friends. We saved a boatload of money on the meat, but would never have been able to pull that off without somewhere to keep 62 pounds of meat. A worthy investment, in our opinion.

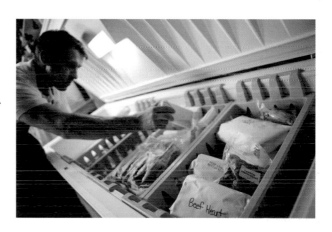

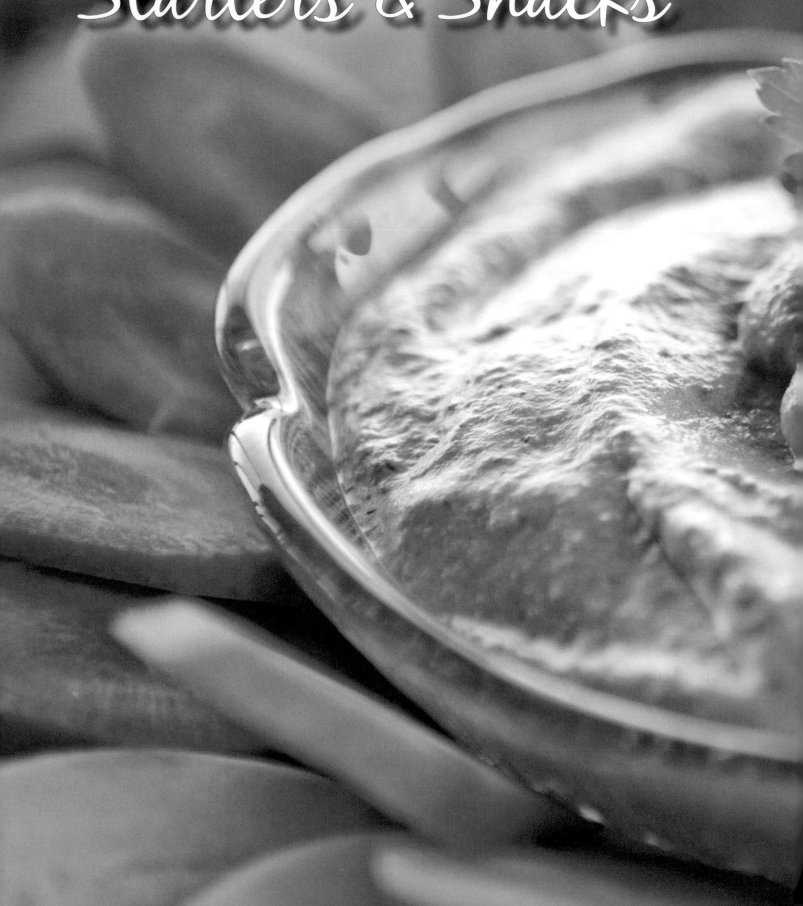

# Starters & Snacks

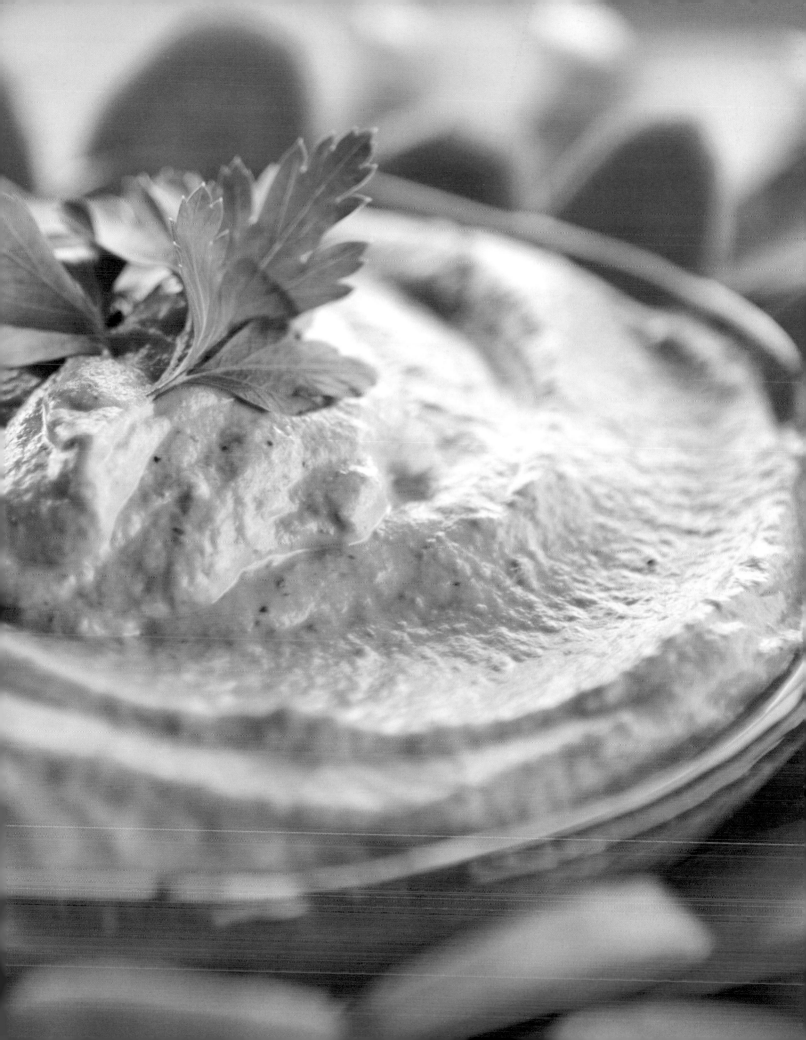

# pickled shrimp

*You can bet that if my mom, Lisa Mayfield, is hosting a large gathering, Pickled Shrimp will be served. My problem is that I'm usually full before dinner whenever she decides to throw this recipe together. There is no easy way around the labor involved with peeling the shrimp in this recipe. It will be worth the effort. Prepare yourself to be showered with compliments by all those attending your next cocktail function. WARNING: The toughest part of this recipe is giving those delicious shrimp a full day to marinate—but trust me, it's vital to really get the flavors infused properly.*

| | |
|---|---|
| 2 | cups (500 mL) olive oil |
| 1 | cup (250 mL) white vinegar |
| 4 | tablespoons capers, with juice |
| 3 | teaspoons celery seed |
| 2 | teaspoons salt |
| ~ | a few drops Tabasco |
| 3 | pounds (1.5 kg) shrimp, in shells |
| ¾ | cup (75 g) celery tops, chopped |
| ½ | cup (50 g) pickling spice |
| 1 | tablespoon salt |
| 2½ | cups (250 g) onion, sliced |
| 10 | bay leaves |

## Marinade

1. Combine olive oil, vinegar, capers and their juice, celery seeds, 2 teaspoons of salt and Tabasco drops.
2. Mix well.

## Shrimp

1. Cover shrimp with boiling water, add celery tops, pickling spice, and salt. Let simmer for 5 minutes or until shrimp are bright pink.
2. Drain, peel and devein shrimp under cold water. Make alternating layers of shrimp, bay leaves, and onions in a baking dish.
3. Pour marinade over shrimp and onions.
4. Chill for 24 hours, occasionally spooning marinade over shrimp.

**Tips & Tricks**—*Using a large Tupperware dish with a lid instead of a baking dish will allow you to flip the shrimp several times while they marinate. The Tupperware is really nice to avoid spilling in the refrigerator. Serve the shrimp with toothpicks in whatever container you want.*

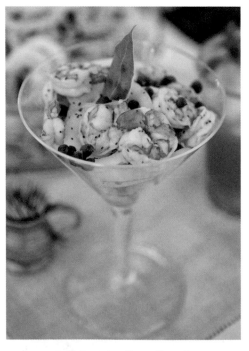

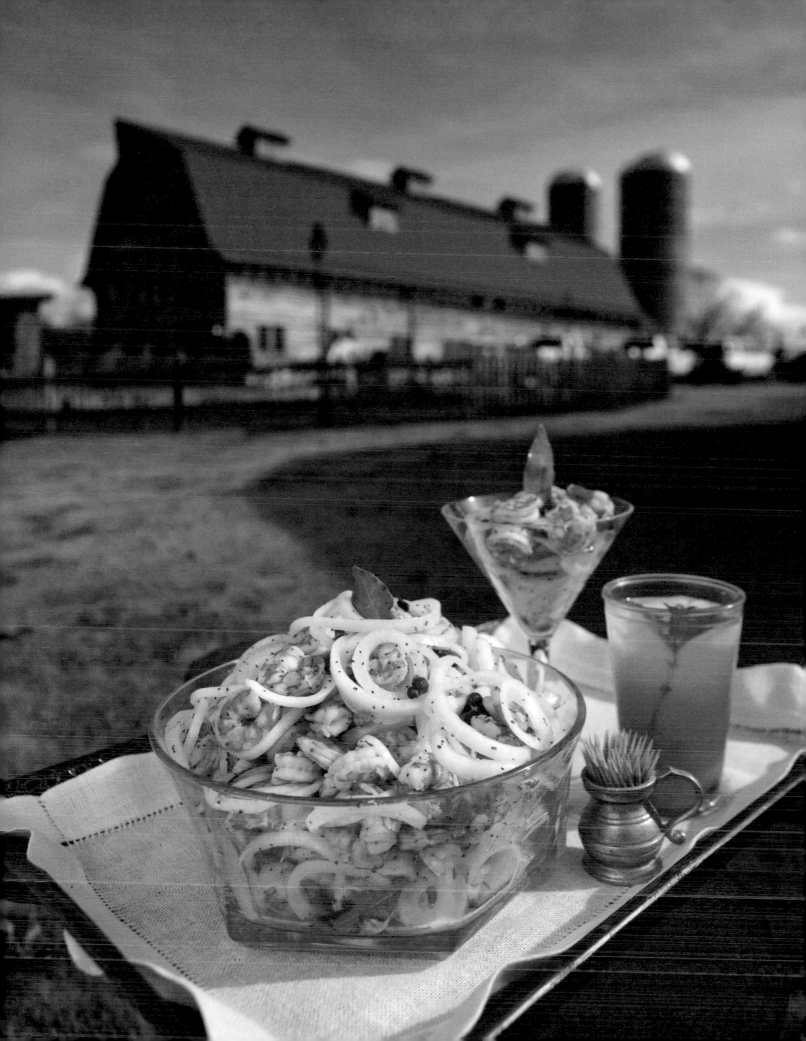

# sheepishly good meatballs

*We certainly love our lamb. It is a relatively lean meat and has such a unique taste and aroma. It also packs a mean punch of vitamin B. This recipe will have your house smelling oh so amazing. We are confident that there won't be any leftovers. If you find that you are left with a few meatballs when the day is done, chop them up and add them to a breakfast scramble to enjoy the next morning.*

| | |
|---|---|
| 1 | tablespoon unsalted butter |
| ½ | cup (75 g) shallots, minced |
| 1 | cup (100 g) mushrooms, finely chopped |
| 2 | pounds (900 g) lamb, ground |
| ¼ | cup (7 g) fresh parsley, chopped |
| 1 | large egg, beaten |
| 2 | tablespoons lemon zest |
| ½ | tablespoon dried oregano |
| 1 | pinch salt & fresh ground pepper, to taste |
| ¼ | cup (60 mL) olive oil |
| ¼ | cup (60 mL) tomato sauce (see recipe page 130) |
| 2 | tablespoons red wine |
| 1 | small garlic clove, minced |
| ¼ | teaspoon ground cinnamon |
| 1 | pinch ground pepper, to taste |

1. Melt butter over medium heat in skillet. Stir in shallots and sauté until tender.

2. Transfer to large bowl and add mushrooms, lamb, parsley, egg, and lemon zest to bowl with shallots.

3. Sprinkle in oregano, salt & pepper as you mix all contents together. Let stand in refrigerator for 1 hour.

4. Form lamb mixture into balls about the size of a ping pong ball (or golf ball if that helps) and set aside.

5. Heat olive oil in same skillet over medium-high heat.

6. Cook meatballs in batches until evenly brown on all sides and place on paper towels to drain. Once they are done, transfer them to a serving dish and keep skillet contents on heat.

7. Mix tomato sauce, wine, garlic, and cinnamon into skillet. Cook until well blended. Season with black pepper to taste, then pour the sauce over the meatballs. Serve with toothpicks and enjoy.

**Variation**—*Try these with nearly any ground meat, but you'll have to change the name.*

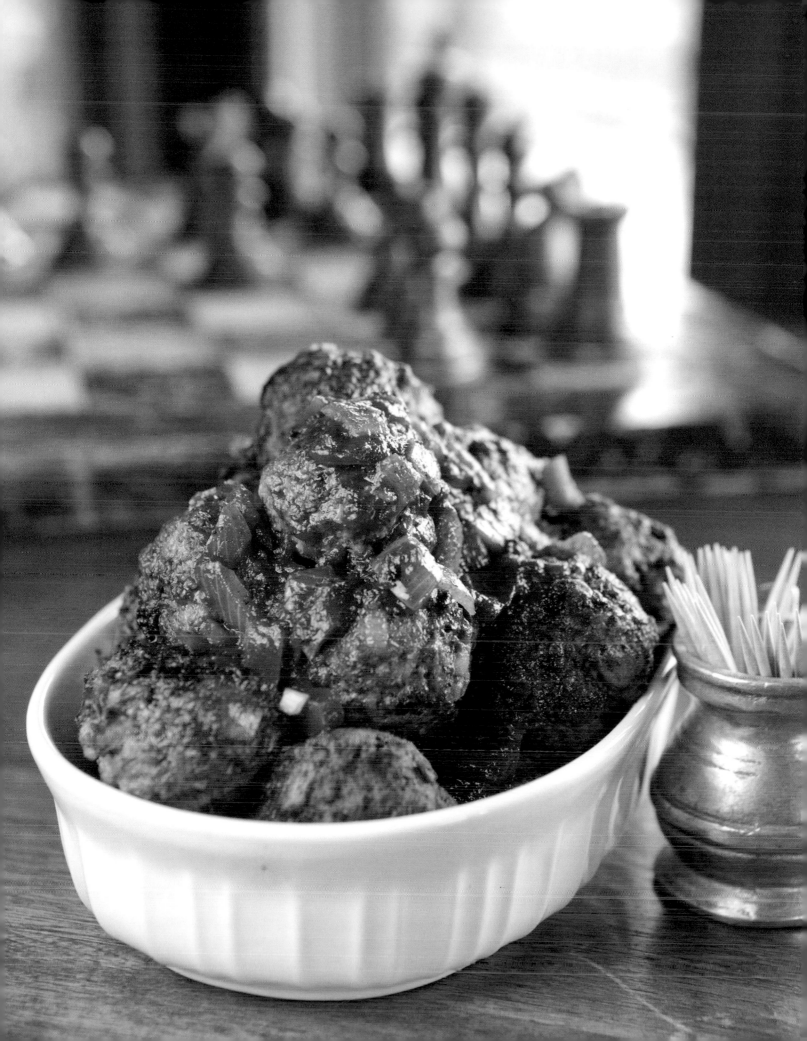

# spicy salmon salad or dip

*This is a recipe that gets its inspiration from my Simple Gourmet days. Except back then it was always made with shrimp, and the avocado was always a key part of the recipe. We also served these on some tasty sesame crackers back in the day—but quite honestly, I love the crunch of the cucumber. I'd say this was probably one of the most popular appetizers we ever served at catering functions. It's a little like spicy tuna, but without the tuna.*

*This version is great served as a dip, where guests can spoon it themselves onto sliced cucumbers, endive or small nori sheets (seaweed sheets – what are commonly used for sushi). However, I like to have it all plated and presented nicely.*

| | |
|---|---|
| 6 | ounces (150 g) cooked (baked or grilled) salmon |
| 2–3 | tablespoons Paleo Mayonnaise (see recipe page 100) |
| ~ | squeeze of Sriracha, or other chili paste, to taste |
| 1 | tablespoon chopped cilantro or chives |
| 1–2 | teaspoons sesame oil |
| 2 | teaspoons black sesame seeds |
| 1 | avocado, diced (optional) |
| 1 | large English cucumber, sliced |

1. Break up cooked salmon into small chunks.
2. With a fork, mix together with the next five ingredients.
3. Taste and season to your liking, adding in more kick via the chili paste if you'd like.
4. Gently mix in avocado (if desired) and spoon onto cucumber rounds. Serve immediately.

**Variation**—*The original Simple Gourmet recipe for this was made with cooked shrimp, which is super tasty too. Feel free to use shrimp if you cannot find good fresh salmon. This dip keeps great in the refrigerator for a day or two, so it's a great do-ahead appetizer for your next dinner party. If making ahead of time, and you'll be using avocado, don't mix in the avocado until you are ready to serve, as the avocados will brown. If you prefer a super-spicy mixture, add in some chili oil to give it some extra kick.*

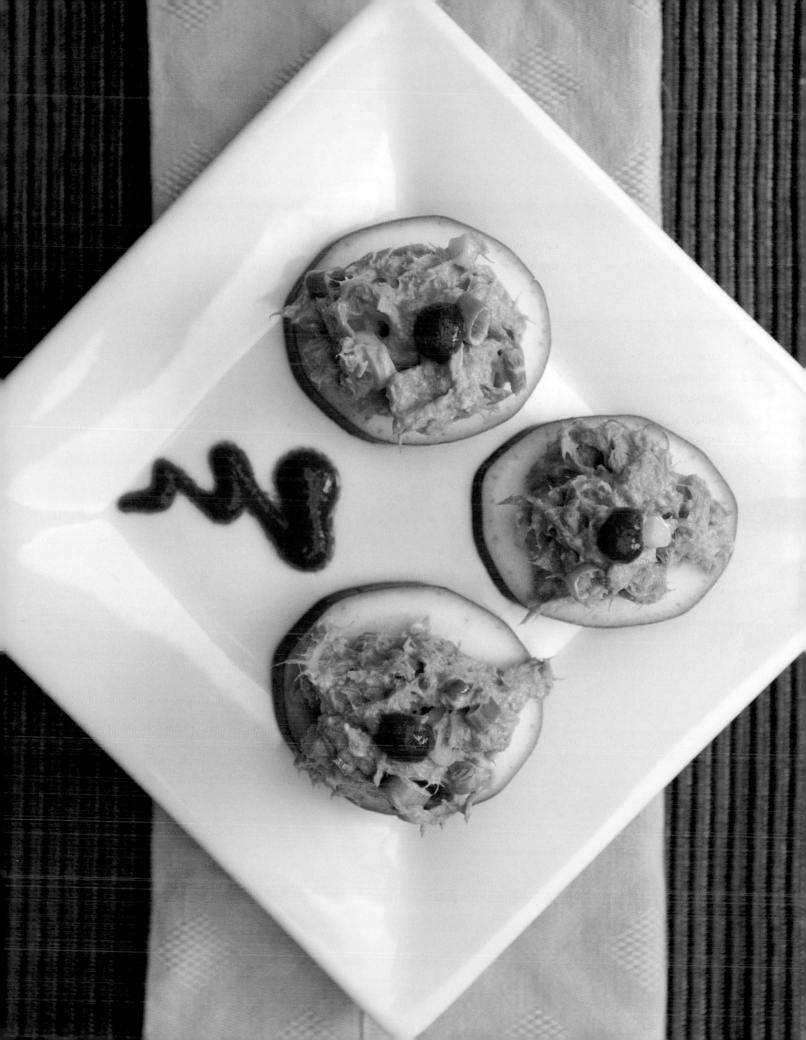

# devilish eggs

*If there was one appetizer that just had to see its way to the picnic table in the South, I would say it would be deviled eggs. The trick to these is getting the eggs just right so they peel easily and don't have any gray/green discoloration in the middle. A quick Internet search will reveal about three dozen methods for getting them just right. If you're having trouble with the eggs, try another method. Make a small batch to start. You don't want to boil a dozen eggs and have them come out hard to peel. Below is the method that seems to work for us.*

| | |
|---|---|
| 1 | dozen large hard-boiled eggs, peeled |
| ½ | cup (125 mL) Paleo Mayonnaise (see recipe page 100) |
| 2 | tablespoons dill pickles, finely chopped |
| 2 | teaspoons prepared mustard |
| ½ | teaspoon black pepper |
| ¼ | teaspoon salt |
| ~ | paprika, to garnish |

1. Cut eggs in half (lengthwise).
2. Empty out yellow yolks into medium bowl.
3. Mash with spoon and add mayonnaise, mustard, chopped pickles, salt, and pepper. Mix/mash all these ingredients well and spoon into a ziplock bag or icing bag.
4. Assemble egg halves on your serving platter and pipe the filling into each egg. Garnish with paprika and enjoy.

## How we hard-boil eggs

- Place eggs in sauce pan large enough to hold them in a single layer.
- Add cold water to cover eggs by 1 inch (2 cm).
- Bring water to boil on high heat and immediately remove from heat and cover.
- Let eggs stand in hot water for 15 minutes (12 for medium, 18 for extra-large).
- Cool eggs completely under running water or an ice bath and refrigerate for later.

**Variation**—*Chop up some fresh dill and add it into the mixture.*

**Plan Ahead**—*Hard-boil the eggs a day or two before just in case.*

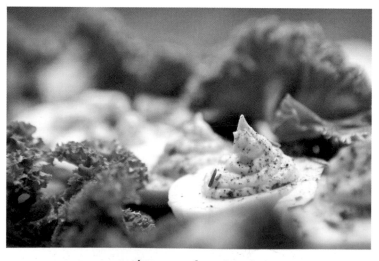

paleo comfort foods

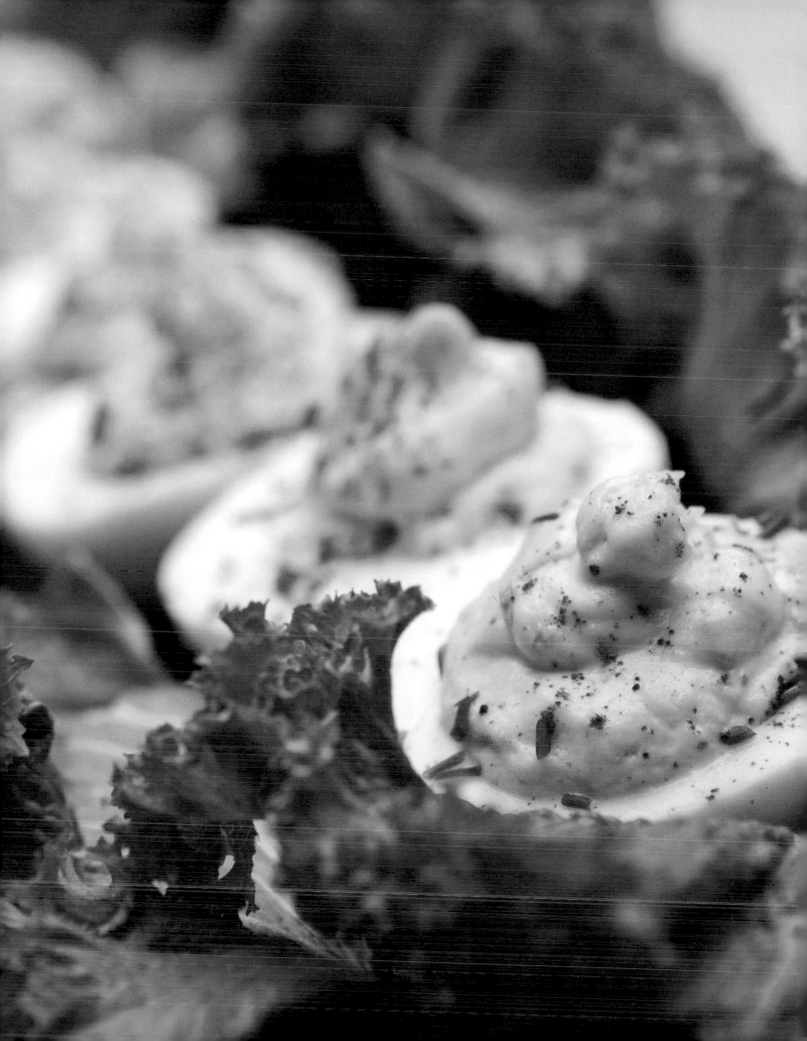

# maryland crab cakes

*Talk to someone from the Mid-Atlantic states, and you'll soon realize that crab cakes are not taken lightly. Nor should they be, as crab meat is something that should be savored, and not masked with a bunch of filler. Yes, it's expensive, but well worth it every once in a while. Any self-respecting person from that part of the country will also tell you that Old Bay seasoning is pretty much a staple in any and all crab cakes. While yes, it is just a blend of existing seasonings that you probably have in your cabinet, there is something nostalgic about Old Bay, and I really do think it makes a difference.*

*I am a firm believer that the right sauce will elevate your crab cakes that much more. My personal choice is often the Remoulade Sauce (page 98) or even the spicy Chipotle Dipping Sauce (page 94). The Pineapple Salsa (page 82) with entrée-sized portions of these will make you think you're dining out on some tropical island!*

| | |
|---|---|
| 1 | large egg |
| 2 | tablespoons Paleo Mayonnaise (see recipe page 100) |
| 1 | teaspoon Dijon mustard |
| ½ | teaspoon Worcestershire sauce |
| ¼ | teaspoon Tabasco |
| ¼ | teaspoon lemon juice |
| 1½ | teaspoons Old Bay seasoning |
| ~ | fresh black pepper, to taste |
| 1 | pound (450 g) fresh jumbo lump crab meat, picked over for shells |
| 1 | tablespoon red pepper, finely diced (optional) |
| 2 | teaspoons sliced green onion |
| 1 | tablespoon fresh chopped parsley |
| ¼ | cup (40 g) almond flour + ⅓ cup (50 g) for dredging |

1. In a small bowl, whisk together egg, mayonnaise, mustard, Worcestershire, Tabasco, lemon juice, Old Bay and pepper.

2. Place crab meat in a separate bowl, trying not to break up too many of the big chunks of crab.

3. Pour the liquid mixture over the crab and, using your hands, gently mix all together. Add in peppers (if desired), green onions, and parsley, as well as ¼ cup (40 g) almond flour, and combine all. Set additional ⅓ cup (50 g) almond flour aside in a separate bowl.

4. Form mixture into crab cakes of desired size (I like to use a ¼-cup [40-gram] measuring cup to create appetizer-sized portions). Dip top and bottom of the crab cakes in the almond flour, and set on greased sheet pan. Refrigerate for at least one hour.

5. Preheat oven to 400°F (205°C). Place crab cakes in oven for 15–20 minutes or until golden brown.

**Variations**—*Feel free to get creative and add in some celery, jalapeños, or other ingredients into the crab cakes as you see fit. Just be forewarned that some folks are purists and may scoff at such additions. Blue crab is very much the favorite crab of choice for those who spend time on the Chesapeake, but Dungeness also works fine for these.*

**Tips & Tricks**—*If you would rather pan fry these, go right ahead! I just find doing a bunch of them in the oven is easier.*

**Ingredient Notes**—*As with any of our recipes that call for Worcestershire, seek out one that does not contain HFCS or any gluten-containing ingredients. The Lea & Perrins reduced sodium brand in the United States does have sugar and molasses, which we are personally okay with, given the minimal amount used in the recipe. If you're going super strict and want to ditch the sauce, go right ahead!*

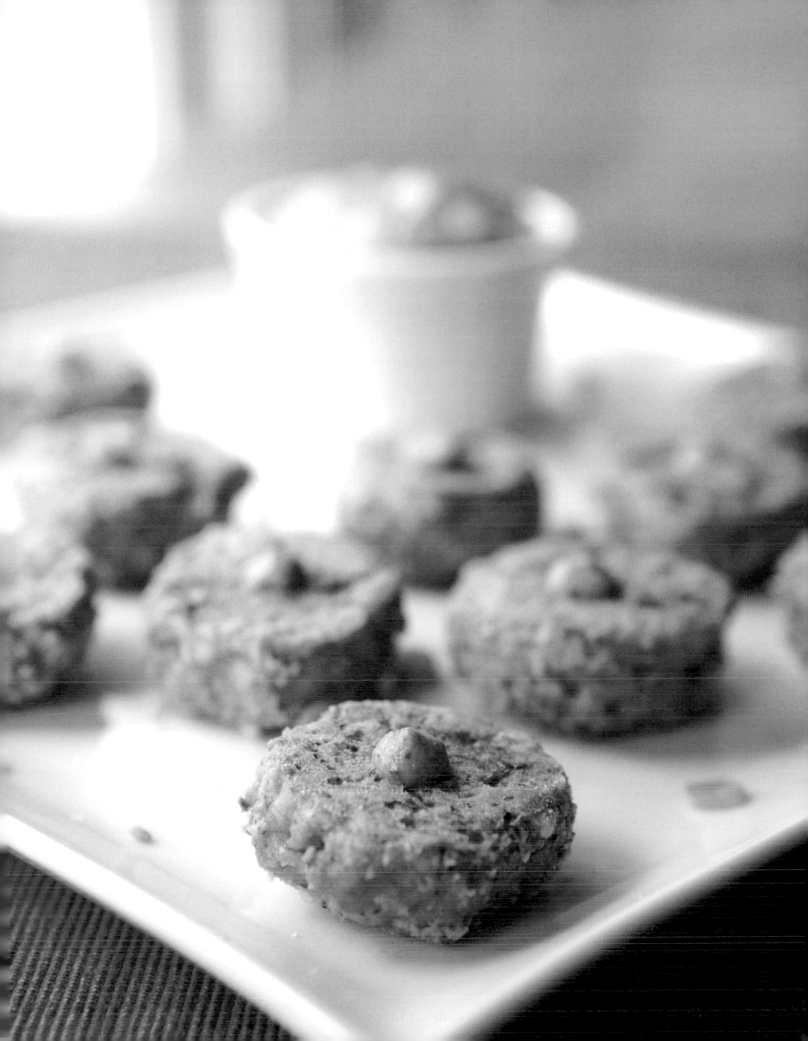

# spicy chicken wings

*Chicken wings are the sport fanatic's ultimate comfort food. They work well as an appetizer or main dish. Chances are your wings won't look like the ones you get at your local watering hole. Don't fret. All of the flavor is there, and you don't have to worry about all the bad ingredients you'd be consuming with commercial fare. If you're planning on hosting a large crew, consider doubling or tripling this recipe. Leftovers can be sent to Charles.*

---

| | |
|---|---|
| 20 | Chicken wings—drums & flats |

*Hot sauce*

| | |
|---|---|
| 2 | tablespoons hot sauce |
| ¼ | cup (60 mL) butter |
| 1 | tablespoon apple cider vinegar |
| ½ | teaspoon paprika |
| ½ | teaspoon cayenne pepper |
| ½ | teaspoon black pepper |
| ¼ | teaspoon garlic powder |
| ⅛ | teaspoon celery seed |

1. Preheat oven to 375°F (190°C) and place wings on greased sheet pan.
2. Bake in oven for 30 minutes, or until cooked through and crispy. While they are cooking, start the sauce.
3. Combine hot sauce, butter, vinegar, paprika, cayenne, black pepper, garlic powder, and celery seed, in a medium saucepan.
4. Set over low heat, mixing until butter is completely melted and combined; simmer for 5 minutes and remove from heat.
5. When wings are baked, dip in sauce to coat well, then shake off excess and return coated wings to baking sheet.
6. Reduce oven temperature to 250°F (120°C) and give wings another 15 minutes. Toss wings in remaining sauce after you remove from oven and serve.

---

**Variations**—*Try grilling or smoking the wings to add a little smoky flavor.*

**Ingredient Notes**—*Check the label on your hot sauce for things you can't pronounce and avoid those that contain ingredients that might scare you.*

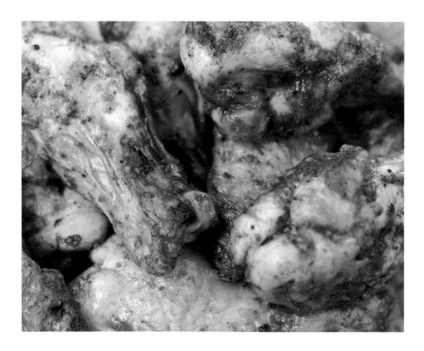

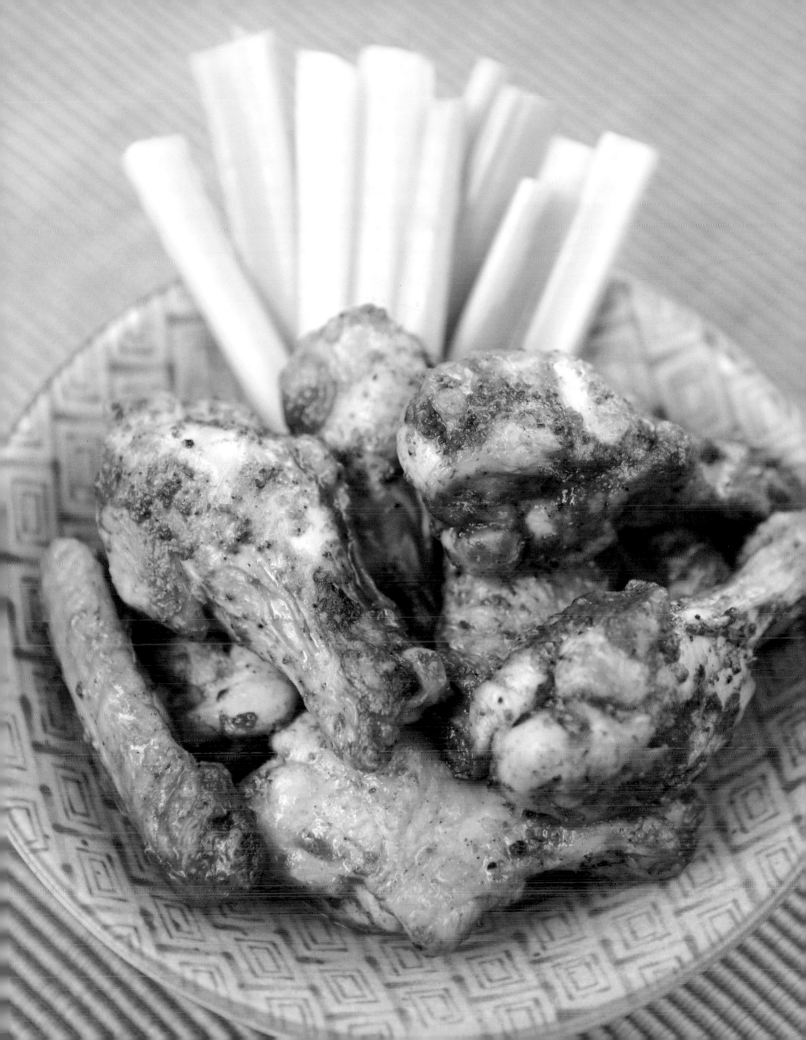

# bacon-wrapped dates

*These are a quick tasty snack for any occasion. Guess what, if they fall apart you still get to eat sweet dates, nutty nuts and bacony bacon!!!*

*It is reported that date palms have been around for well over 50,000 years and are the world's oldest cultivated fruit. Dates have a very strong presence in Middle Eastern and Arabic history and cuisine, and it's not hard to see why—these soft, chewy, sweet fruits are super tasty. They are also super sweet—indeed nature's candy—so if you're working on leaning out, might be best to limit yourself to one or two of these!*

*Feel free to put your favorite nut inside the dates. I think pecan quarters, almonds and macadamia halves work great.*

---

| | |
|---|---|
| 2 | **dozen dates, pitted** |
| 2 | **dozen almonds, blanched** |
| 8 | **strips bacon, cut in thirds** |

1. Preheat oven to 450°F (230°C).
2. Stuff each date with an almond and wrap with piece of bacon.
3. Place on a heat-proof cooling rack set inside a sheet pan. Make sure loose ends of bacon are facing down.
4. Cook them to a crisp on one side (4–6 minutes), flip and cook other side to crisp (another 4–6 minutes).
5. Place on paper towels to soak up excess grease and serve.

---

**Tips & Tricks**—*You may find it challenging to keep the bacon together. If so, run a toothpick through the bacon sideways to hold it.*

**Ingredient Notes**—*Medjool dates are the ideal date, and you can most likely find them in the produce section of your grocery store in the fall season.*

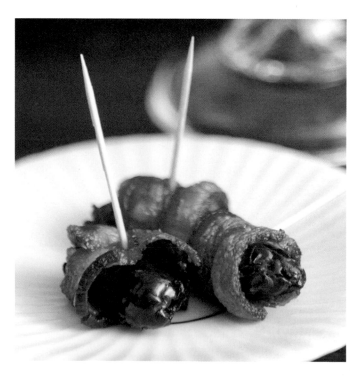

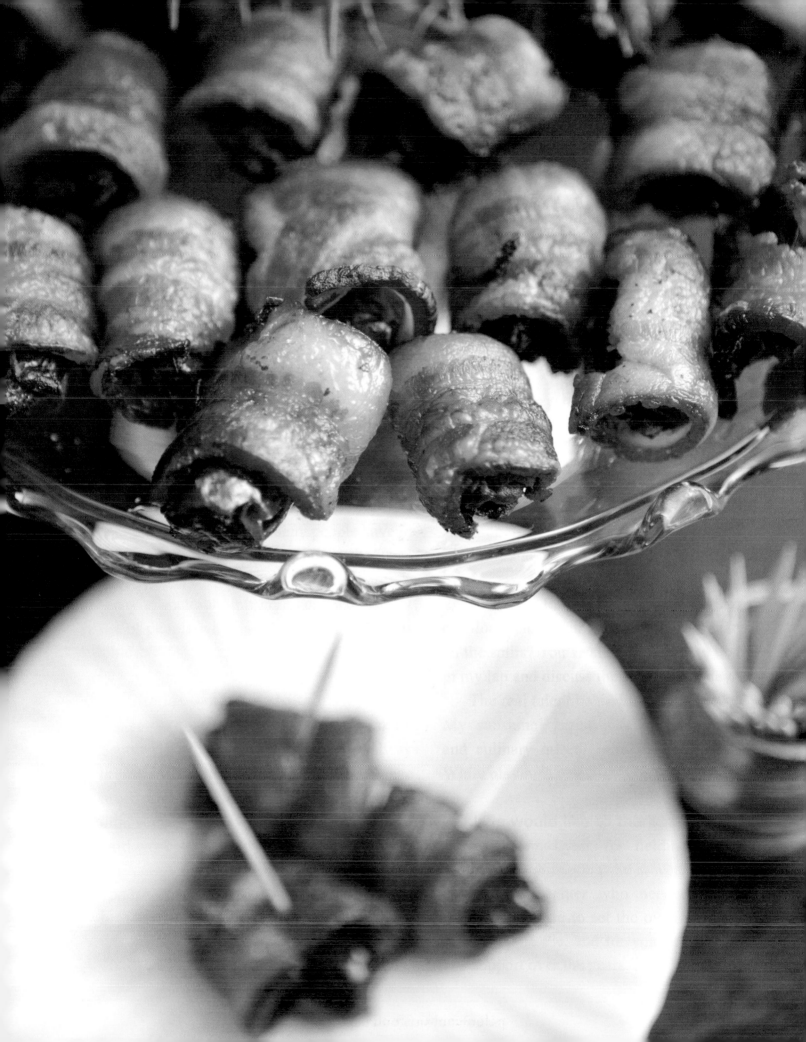

# morning glory muffins

*This recipe wasn't in any cookbook. Mom copied this one off the old sheet of paper that was passed down to her years ago. Obviously I doctored it up a bit to make it gluten free. It has brought smiles to the faces of the Mayfield household for years. I turned the muffins into mini-loaves a few years back and gave them out as Christmas presents to friends and neighbors. The batter for this will be very thick. You may have to use a spoon or spatula to get it all in the muffin pan.*

*Delicious!*

---

| | |
|---|---|
| 2½ | cups (375 g) almond flour |
| 1 | tablespoon cinnamon |
| 2 | teaspoons baking soda |
| ½ | teaspoon salt |
| 2 | cups (100 g) carrots, grated |
| 1 | large apple, peeled, cored and grated |
| 1 | cup (75 g) shredded coconut |
| 1 | cup (150 g) raisins |
| 3 | large eggs |
| 2 | tablespoons honey (optional) |
| ½ | cup (125 mL) coconut or avocado oil |
| 1 | teaspoon vanilla extract |

1. Preheat oven to 350°F (175°C) and grease a standard-sized muffin pan (12 cups).

2. Combine almond flour, cinnamon, baking soda, and salt in large bowl. Add carrot, apple, coconut and raisins and combine well.

3. In separate bowl, whisk eggs, honey, oil and vanilla extract together.

4. Pour this mixture over your dry ingredients and mix well. This batter will be very thick.

5. Spoon out into muffin pan and place on middle or upper rack of your oven for 40-50 minutes for large muffins, 20-30 minutes for smaller muffins.

6. When a toothpick inserted in the top of a muffin comes out clean, they are done.

7. Cool muffins in pan for 8–10 minutes and then remove to a rack to finish cooling.

---

**Variations**—*Add in a teaspoon of orange zest for some extra zing. You can also replace raisins with a cup of chopped dates. This batter can also be used to make a morning glory loaf. This will make one really large loaf, or two smaller loaves. Just increase your baking time to approximately 45–60 minutes.*

**Tips & Tricks**—*The smaller you can grate the carrot/apple the better. These muffins tend to end up a bit moister if you allow the batter to sit for 30–60 minutes before spooning into the muffin pan.*

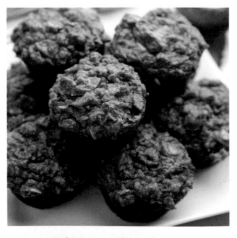

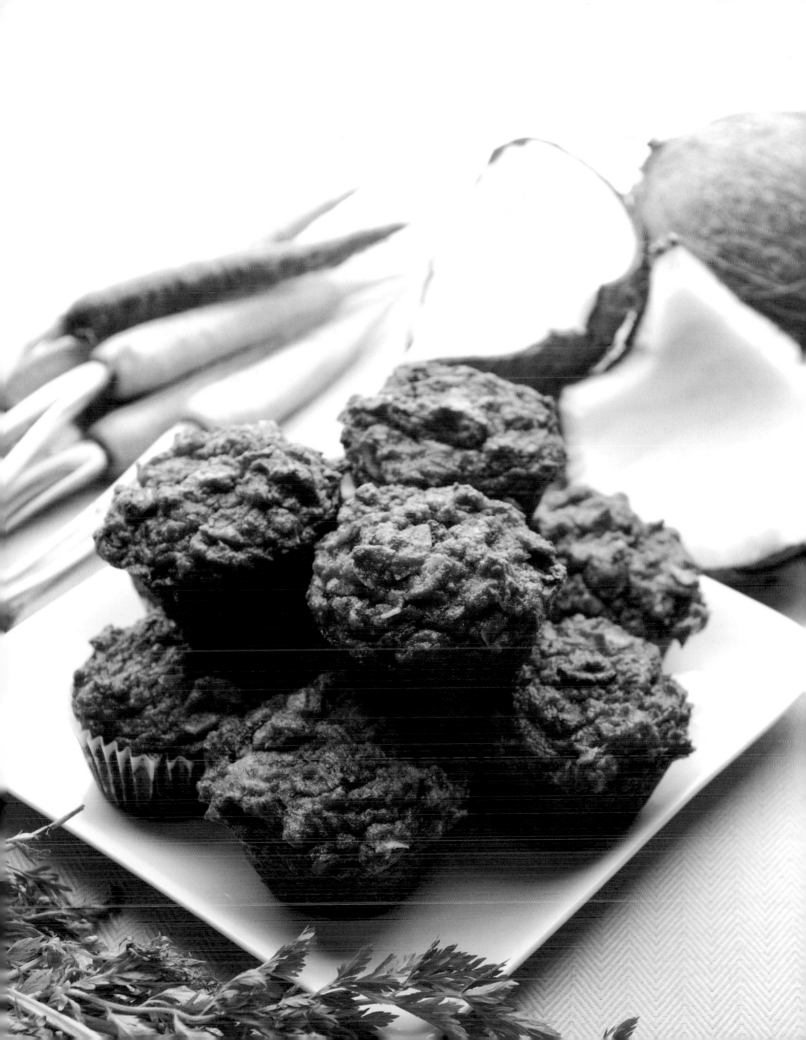

# sausage balls

*Honestly, this is a Lisa Mayfield special. I watched her make these one day to serve at my sister's stationery store for an open house. Making just a small modification to her original recipe has resulted in a paleo dream appetizer just waiting for you. One of the things Mark, our photographer, has enjoyed is sampling just about everything we cook. He commented when trying these that he didn't even like olives and yet had a hard time putting the plate of these down. Speaking of which, where did that plate go?*

*You'll love how easy these tasty sausage balls are to put together. They are well worth the 10 minutes of really messy hands.*

---

| | |
|---|---|
| ½ | teaspoon red pepper flakes |
| 1½ | pounds (750 g) ground pork sausage |
| 6 | ounces (150 g) pitted green olives, from can |

1. Mix pepper flakes with ground pork.

2. Measure out a tablespoon of sausage at a time and press firmly into palms to flatten.

3. Place olive in middle of flattened sausage and fold around the olive to create a ball. Roll the sausage around using fingers to pinch any cracks together. Repeat with remaining sausage and olives.

4. Bring a frying pan to medium-high heat and place the sausage balls into the pan.

5. Turn sausage about every three minutes for 15–20 minutes of cooking. They should be browned on all sides and cooked through. Remove to a clean plate, and repeat the same process for the remaining balls.

6. Serve on a platter with any remaining green olives.

---

**Variation**—*Replace ½ pound (250 g) of pork with ground andouille sausage.*

**Ingredient Notes**—*When it comes to finding good olives, read the label on your olives very carefully. Try to avoid preservatives. Whole Foods has some canned olives without any additives at all.*

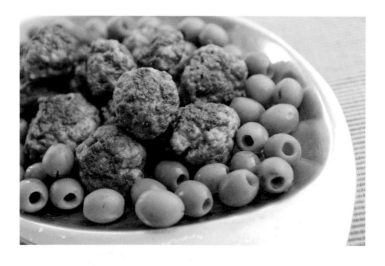

paleo comfort foods

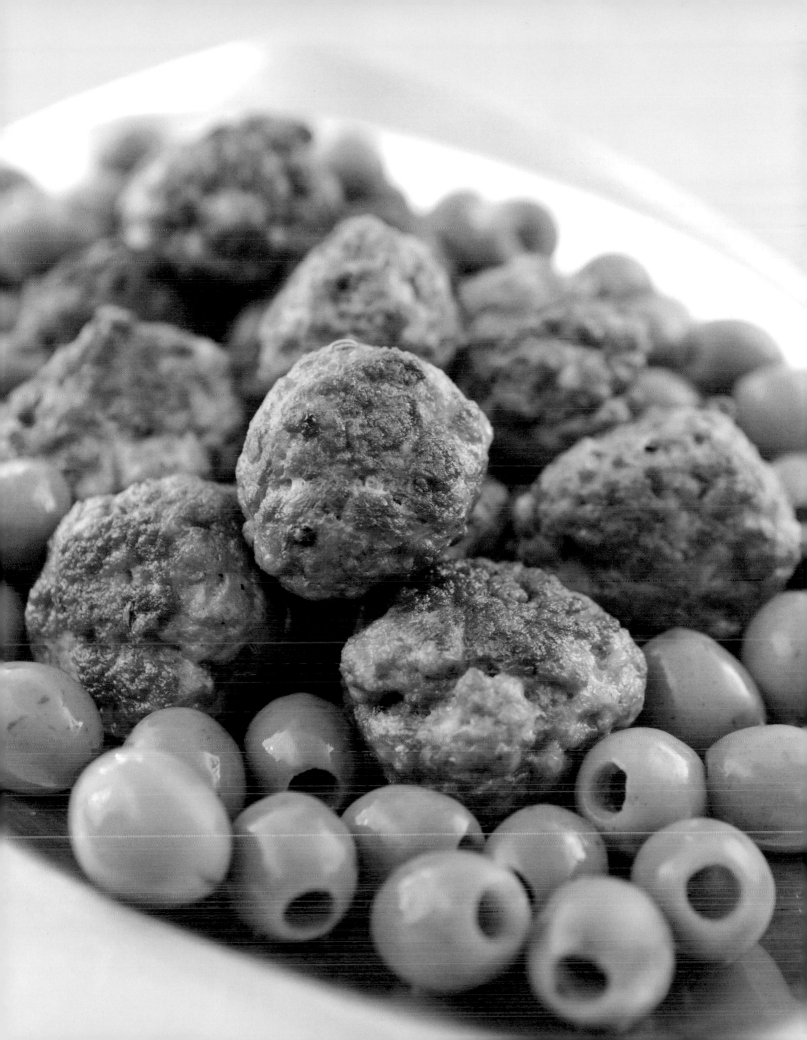

# sliders

*Big things often come in small packages. These sliders pack a flavorful punch that is sure to be enjoyed by all. This recipe can be written dozens of ways, depending on your various condiment preferences. The best thing about these paleo-friendly offerings is that you don't have a doughy soft bun to get in the way of your fresh lettuce and tomatoes.*

*Sliders can be a great appetizer for a big crowd or a meal for a smaller crew. This is also a really fun recipe to get kids involved in the process. Who doesn't remember getting to make burgers as a kid?*

---

| | |
|---|---|
| 1–1½ | pounds (500-750 g) ground beef |
| 1 | large egg |
| 1 | small onion, finely chopped |
| 1 | cup (100 g) mushrooms, finely chopped |
| 1 | teaspoon black pepper |
| ½ | teaspoon garlic salt |
| 1 | each: yellow, red, green bell pepper |
| 1 | small onion, sliced |
| 3 | small tomatoes, sliced |
| 1 | head iceberg lettuce |
| 6–8 | medium portobello mushrooms |

1. Preheat your grill to medium-high heat. Be sure you have a clean grate and wipe it down with a little oil when hot.
2. In a large bowl, mix ground meat, egg, chopped onion and mushrooms. Sprinkle in black pepper and garlic salt as you're mixing the meat.
3. Form small burgers with hands (no need for a fancy slider mold here). The burgers will be about 2 inches in diameter.
4. Slice all three peppers down the sides to form large flat pieces (think like you're cutting the walls off a house).
5. Slice other onion and tomatoes thinly (about ⅛ inch). Pull lettuce apart into individual leaves. Try to keep them whole (as large as possible).
6. Grill burgers 3-5 minutes per side, depending upon your desired doneness. Grill peppers and mushrooms 2-3 minutes per side, or until cooked through.
7. Stack burgers between peppers or mushrooms and wrap with lettuce. Add the onion and tomato slices if you're so inclined.

---

**Variations**—*If you'd like, slice the tomatoes a bit thicker to use as bun—just know they'll be pretty juicy.*

*—With sliders/burgers you can use almost any ground meat you want. We like to occasionally use ground turkey or ground venison.*

*—We always try to have a batch of our homemade Paleo Mayo (page 100), Cave Ketchup (page 102), or Chipotle Dipping Sauce (page 94) ready to serve on top of these.*

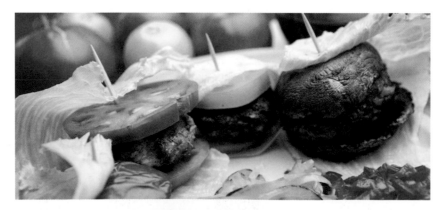

paleo comfort foods

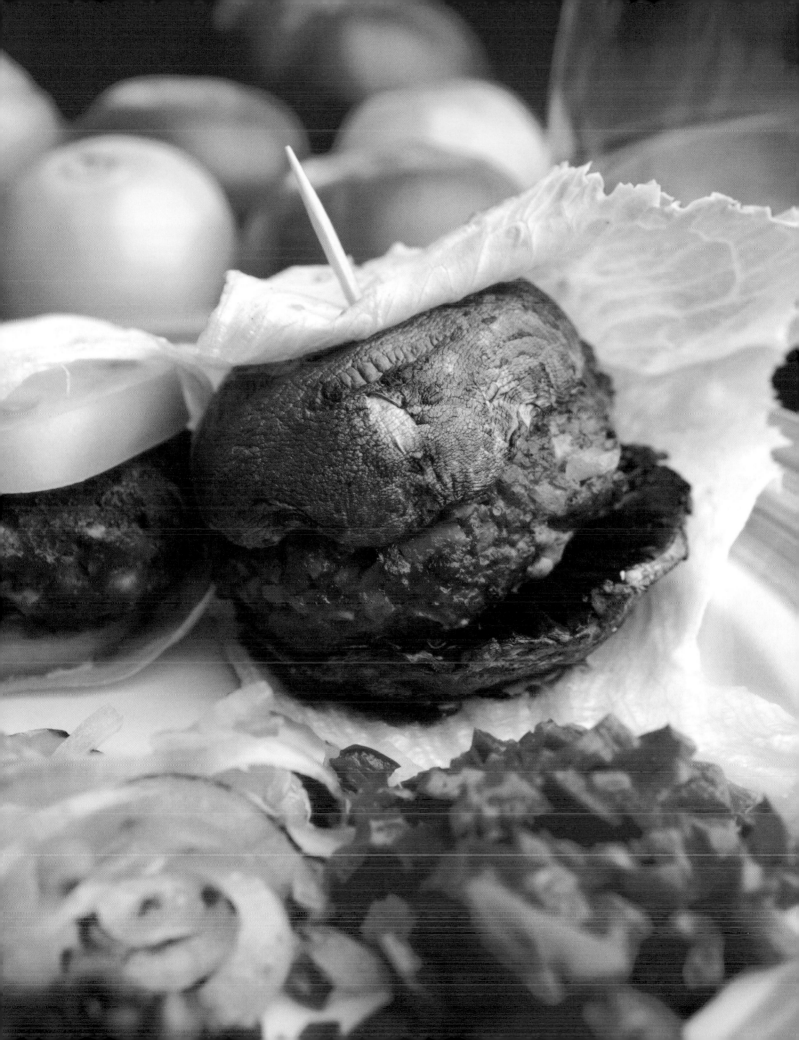

# paleo spiced nuts

*Mark my words: you can never make too much of this recipe. When we host gatherings—such as our annual croquet tournament—we love whipping up some of these spiced nuts for friends to snack on. Not only does the house smell amazing with the aromas of toasted nuts, cinnamon, and vanilla, but served warm out of the oven, pounds of nuts will vanish instantly. Make up a container full of these and bring them as your next host or hostess gift or fill small baggies with this mixture as gifts for friends! These spiced nuts will keep indefinitely in an airtight container—in the refrigerator is best if you won't be eating them for a while.*

| | |
|---|---|
| 1½ | teaspoons cumin |
| ½ | teaspoon chili powder |
| 1½ | teaspoons cinnamon |
| ¼ | teaspoon cayenne pepper |
| 4 | cups (400 g) assorted nuts (pecans, walnuts, cashews, almonds) |
| 1 | teaspoon vanilla extract |
| 1 | tablespoon butter |

1. Mix the cumin, chili powder, cinnamon, and cayenne in a small bowl and set aside.
2. Preheat a large cast-iron skillet or other large skillet over medium heat.
3. Add nuts and toast until slightly browned, being careful not to burn.
4. Add butter and vanilla to coat nuts, then sprinkle spice mixture over nuts and stir until well combined.
5. Spread nuts out on large cookie sheet to dry, or serve warm right out of the pan.

**Variation**—*The cool thing about this recipe is that you can make this mix with any variety of nuts you wish. If you don't like almonds, or you only like pecans, make a mix that suits you.*

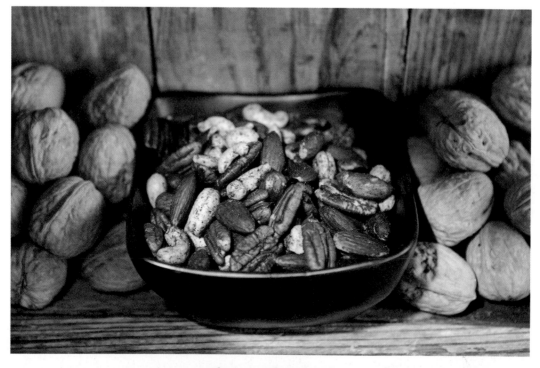

**paleo comfort foods**

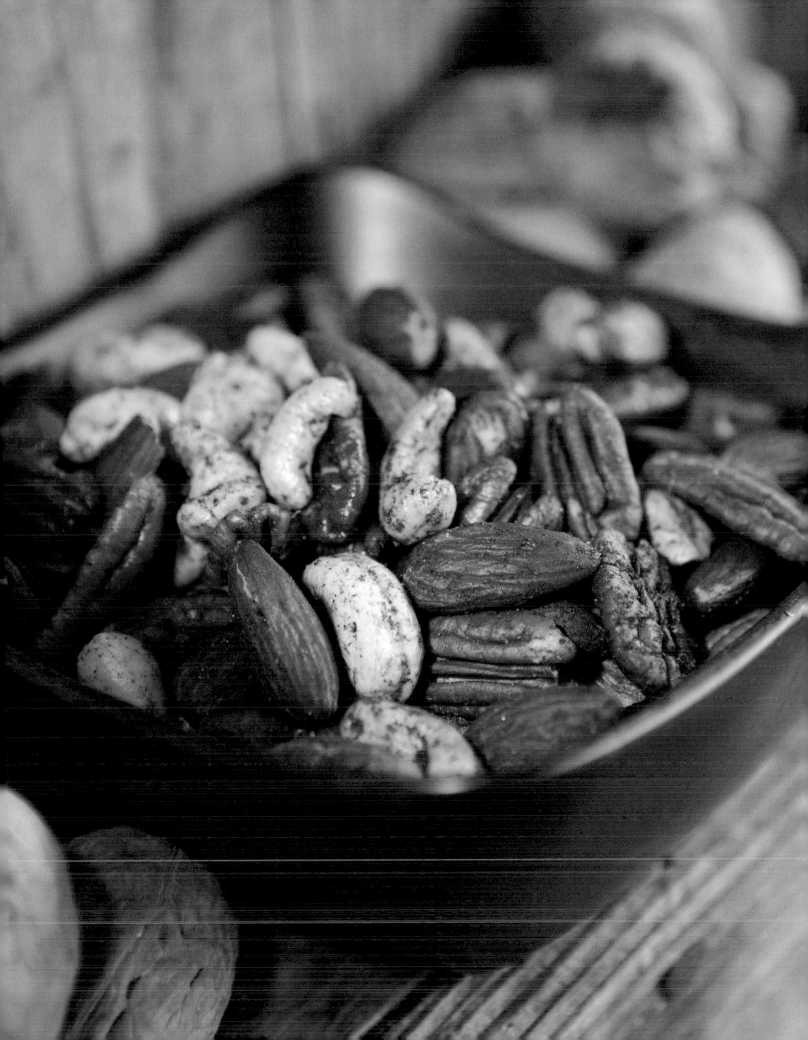

# basic salsa

As a child, my vegetables of choice (meaning the only ones I really ate) were peas, corn, and of course ketchup (or tomato sauce). I remember trying to force myself to eat raw tomatoes once in college, and the consequences were not pretty. Real salsa wasn't part of my childhood for the most part either, since Mexican food for us usually meant Taco Bell, and I wouldn't exactly say their packets of sauce are remotely like a fresh salsa. When I moved to LA after college and would dine at authentic Mexican restaurants, I was exposed to real salsa, and it quickly became my favorite condiment. Nowadays, I will put salsa on anything and everything. Nothing says good morning like eggs with a hefty dose of salsa. As I've never been really big on salad dressing (ranch and bleu cheese make me gag), salsa very often is my go-to salad dressing. And the best part? Salsa is super healthy and good for you. No additives or preservatives, and oh-so-tasty when made with tomatoes picked fresh from your own garden.

| | |
|---|---|
| 6 | Roma tomatoes |
| ½ | bunch cilantro |
| ½ | white or red onion, peeled |
| ~ | juice of 1 lime |
| 1 | jalapeño pepper |
| 1 | habanero (optional—only use if you want an OMG my mouth is on fire salsa) |
| 1 | clove garlic |
| ~ | fresh ground pepper |

## There are two ways to make this salsa

Method #1: Take all ingredients and mix in a food processor. You do not need to chop anything. Just pulse a few times and you are done.

Method #2: Hand chop the tomatoes, cilantro, onion, peppers and garlic, and combine in a bowl with the lime juice.

**Variations**—It really is incredibly easy to make your own salsa, and you can get all kinds of creative with this too. Oven-roast your tomatoes, onions, and peppers first (like in the Fire-Roasted Salsa in this book), and then mix in a food processor. Use some yellow or purple tomatoes and add in chopped bell (sweet) peppers. Try adding in some chipotles or green onions or use lemon if you have no lime, the possibilities are endless! Whatever you make, it typically keeps in the refrigerator for at least one week.

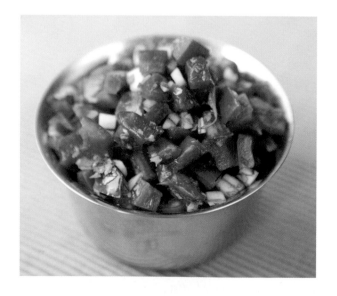

paleo comfort foods

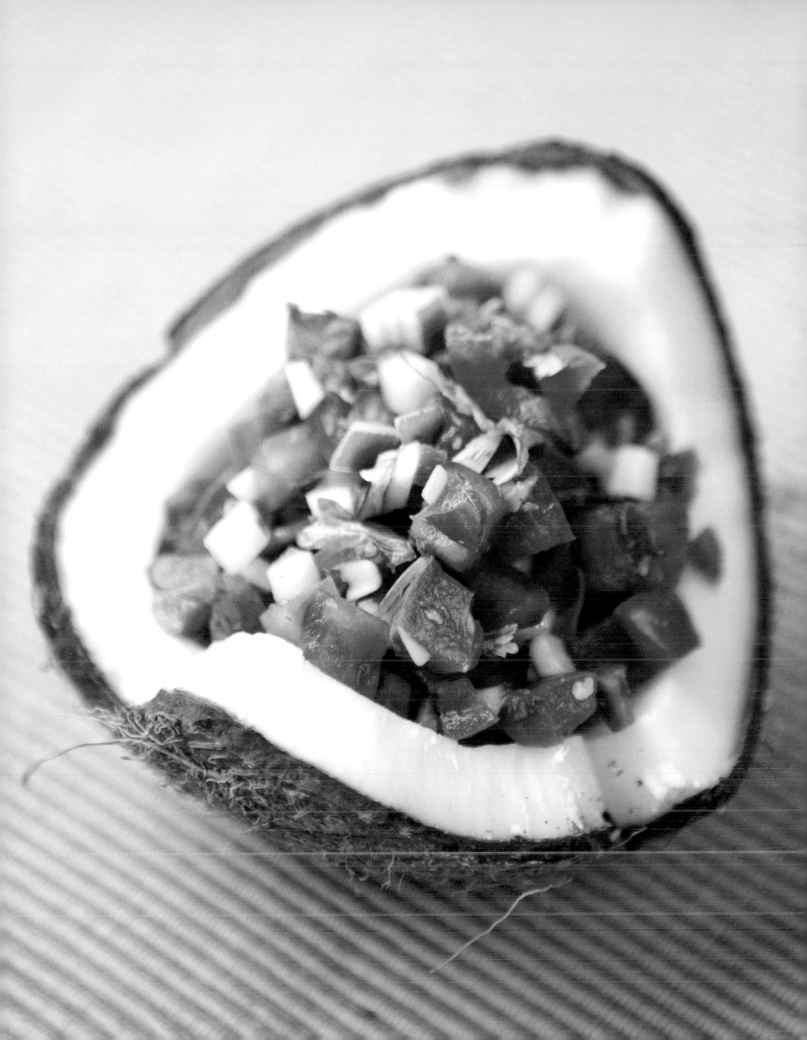

# chunky guacamole

*Yes, I could eat guacamole as a main course all by itself on any day of the week and twice on Sundays. Hard to believe I couldn't stand the stuff growing up! A while back, when I was on vacation with friends in Mazatlan, Mexico (I like to call it the Jersey Shore of Mexico—no offense to anyone), we would devour plates of the most incredible, freshest guacamole. There was one restaurant I think we went to three or four times just to have their huge plate of guacamole. Nothing—not even tequila!—paired as beautifully as guacamole did with our freshly caught and cooked fish. I often think of guacamole as the "perfect fat" for people living the paleo lifestyle. The beauty of guacamole is that if you have already made a salsa or pico de gallo separately, just stir that in with some avocado and you've killed two birds with one salsa recipe!*

| | |
|---|---|
| 2 | ripe Hass avocados |
| ~ | juice of 1 lime |
| 1 | jalapeño or serrano pepper, minced and seeds removed (keep seeds if you want it hotter) |
| ½ | small red or white onion, minced |
| 1 | clove garlic, minced |
| 1 | Roma tomato, seeded and chopped |
| 2 | tablespoons cilantro, chopped |
| ~ | salt and pepper to taste |

1. Scoop out the avocados into a medium bowl or molcajete, removing the pits.
2. Squeeze lime juice over the avocados, then roughly mash with a fork.
3. Add in all other ingredients, and use fork to gently combine.
4. Serve immediately.

**Tips & Tricks**—*The best way to keep avocado (or guacamole) from browning? There is an enzyme in avocados that catalyzes the reaction between oxygen and certain chemicals in the avocado (same is true in apples and potatoes). Contrary to popular belief, the pit in the middle of your fresh batch of guac won't do much except keep the guacamole it is in contact with from browning. Lime juice—and the acid from it (which helps with the pH and provides the vitamin C that binds to the enzyme) is your first step in the right direction. Secondly, if you are looking to make the guacamole early in the day and serve later, place plastic wrap directly on the surface of the guac—really press it in so you have no air pockets—and then place a cover over the whole bowl/container. This should help!*

**Ingredient Notes**—*When it comes to choosing a ripe avocado, look for avocado skin that is dark green to almost a black color, and for it to have a tiny bit of give when you press lightly with your thumb. Too much give and it's likely they are bruised. If you choose the very green, still hard avocados, these aren't ripe yet and you will want to put those in a paper bag along with an apple to speed along the ripening process for a few days. Interesting note: avocados—like bananas—don't actually ripen on the tree, so you'll never see a "tree-ripened" avocado. In order for an avocado to ripen properly, it must be picked when it's mature.*

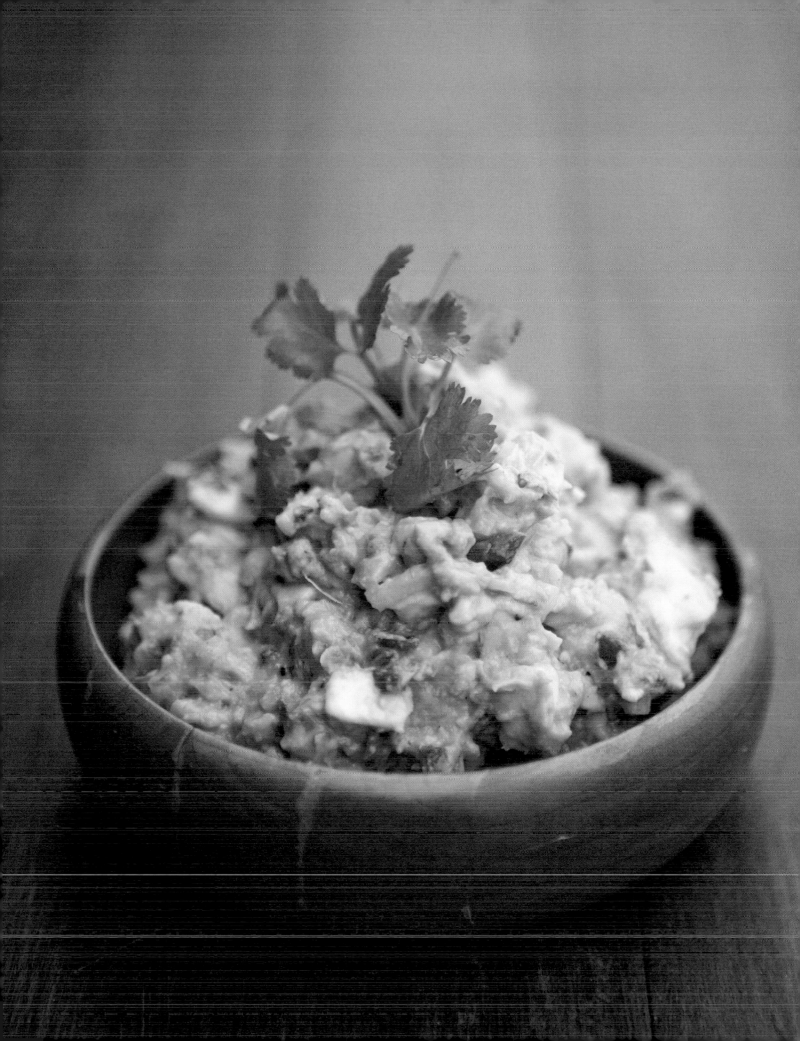

# fire-roasted salsa

*Salsas make me happy. Really good salsas with a kick make me really happy. This is one of those salsas that makes me really happy. Let it be known that our tastes for heat may differ from yours. Meaning: things with a slight kick are very palatable to me. But for some friends of mine it sets off a three-alarm fire in their mouth—as in people cursing my name for several days afterward.*

*Fire-roasting tomatoes adds such a great smoky dimension to salsas. When I first ate at a Baja Fresh restaurant in Los Angeles, I was mesmerized by their smoky salsa and how they made it. I never got the official recipe, but this is my spin on it.*

---

| | |
|---|---|
| 6 | Roma tomatoes, halved lengthwise |
| 1 | small white onion, quartered |
| 1 | clove garlic |
| 1 | jalapeño, roughly chopped |
| ¼ | cup (8 g) cilantro |
| 1 | dried New Mexico, chipotle, or guajillo chili pepper, rehydrated |
| ~ | juice of 1 lime |

1. Preheat oven broiler.

2. Place the tomatoes on a foil-lined sheet pan, and broil to char the skins 13–15 minutes, then flip and char the other side for another 5 minutes.

3. Combine tomatoes with all other ingredients in a food processor until well blended.

---

**Tips & Tricks**—*You can make this salsa a day or two ahead from when you plan on serving/eating it, though I'm going to bet you'll want to eat it sooner rather than later. The flavors really do meld together after a day or two of being in the refrigerator.*

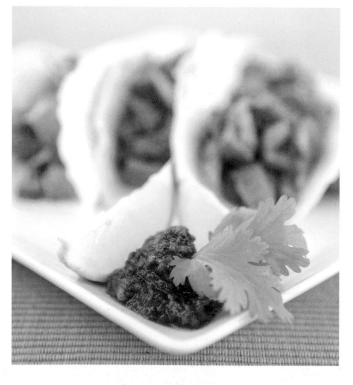

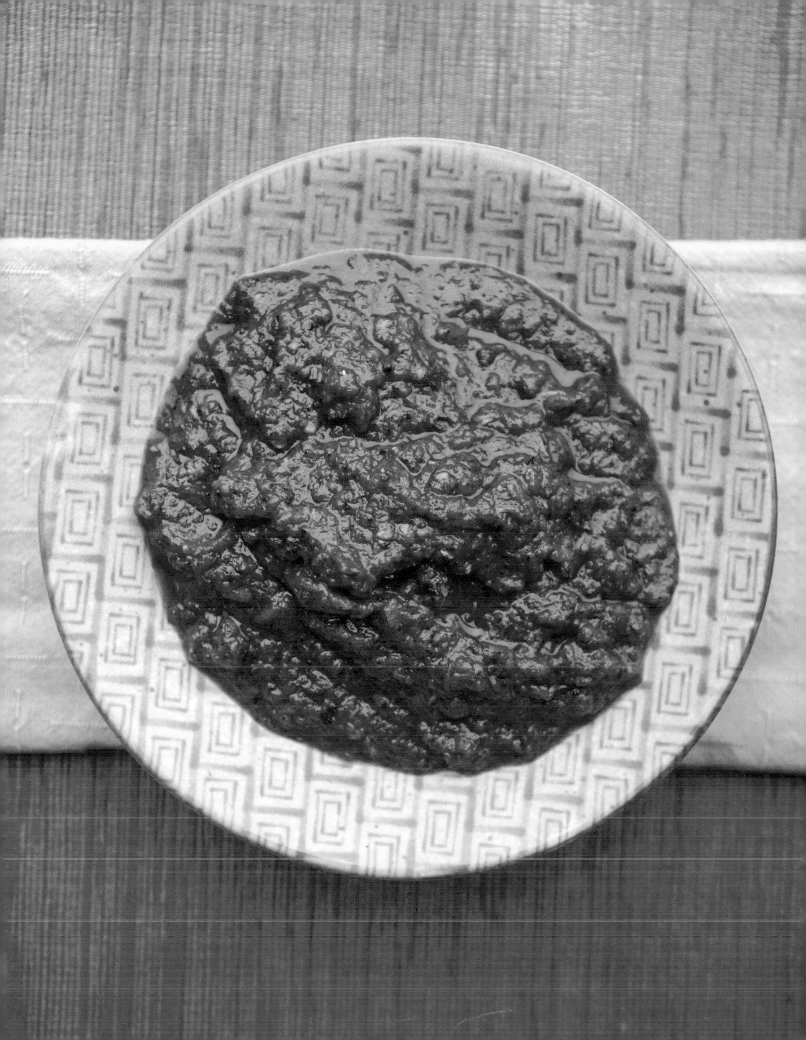

# paleo hummus, baba ghanoush, or "really tasty dip"

*Hummus (and all the various spellings) in Arabic means chickpeas, so technically you should call this recipe "baba ghanoush" (which is just really fun to say) or "really tasty dip." The point is that it will taste so much like hummus that you'll think it is hummus! Make it your own and call it "my super-secret world-famous dip." Bottom line: this is a great alternative to hummus, it gives those non-guacamole eaters some other kind of dip to enjoy, and it just plain tastes good.*

*A few notes on this one: if you are struggling with some autoimmune issues, ditch the eggplant (a nightshade) and use the zucchini or raw cashews instead.*

*Don't be afraid to play with flavorings. Hungarian smoked paprika and sumac are widely used in many Middle Eastern recipes, and go beautifully with this. Love garlic? Then add some more! Feel like using roasted garlic instead, or basil or some parsley or some other interesting mixture? Go for it!*

---

| | |
|---|---|
| 1 | large eggplant or 2–3 small Chinese eggplants |
| 2 | tablespoons tahini |
| 2 | tablespoons lemon juice |
| 1–2 | cloves garlic |
| ~ | pinch of cumin |
| 2 | tablespoons olive oil |
| ~ | salt to taste |

1. Preheat oven to 400°F (205°C).

2. Slice eggplant in half lengthwise and brush with some olive oil. Place on foil lined sheet pan and bake for 45 minutes or until soft.

3. Allow eggplant to cool, then scoop out insides of eggplant and combine in food processor with tahini, lemon juice, garlic and cumin, discarding the skins. Mix all until smooth.

4. Slowly drizzle in olive oil through feed tube until well combined.

5. If you have some smoked paprika or sumac at home, sprinkle a little bit of that over the mixture. Add salt to taste. Serve with some sliced veggies to dip in.

---

**Ingredient Notes**—*Tahini is sesame seed paste, and can be found in the ethnic aisle of most grocery stores (just check the label to make sure there aren't any added ingredients!). Sumac, should you choose to use, can be found in some Middle Eastern markets, cooking stores, and online stores (Penzey's and Surfas are two of my favorites). It has a slightly sour flavor and a reddish color. Great to use in spiced nut mixtures too!*

**Variations**—*If eggplant is not your thing, use 2 zucchinis (no cooking needed, but I find it preferred to peel). Spice things up and use some chili powder and lime juice for more of a "tropical" flair, or add in some sun-dried tomatoes or roasted red peppers to change up the flavor. To make things even creamier with a little more fat, replace the eggplant with ¾ cup of cashews that have been soaked in water for a few hours. Drain, place in processor, then add in remaining ingredients and enough water to reach your preferred consistency.*

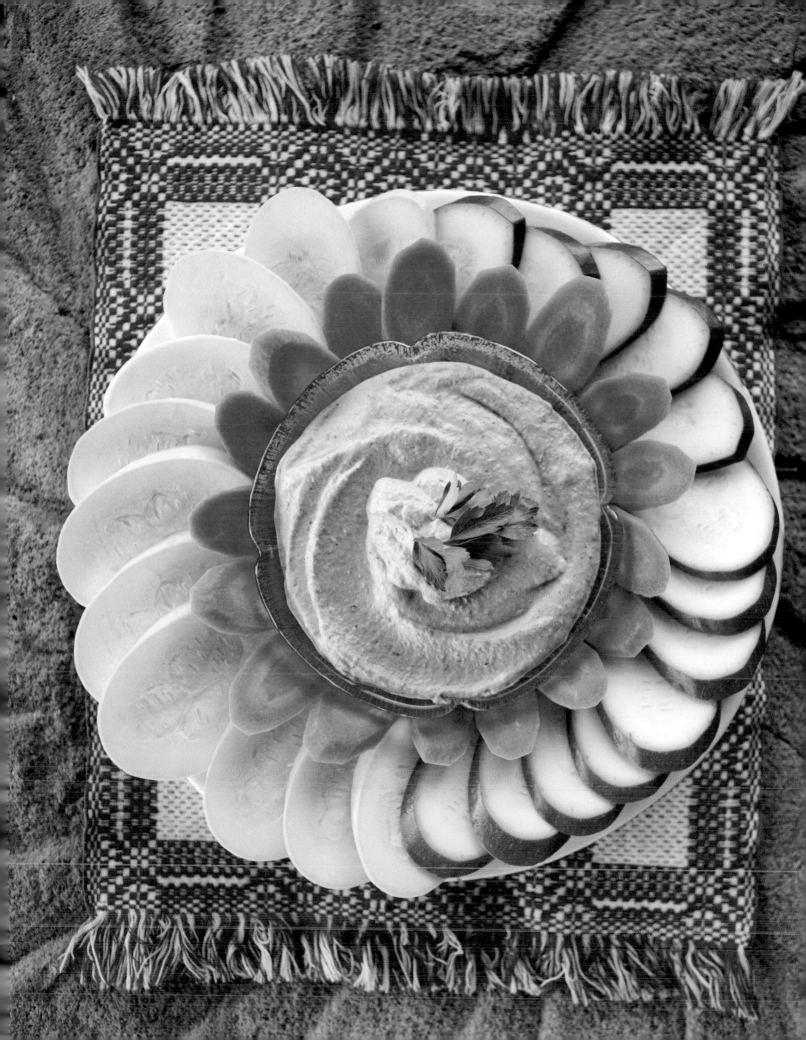

# salsa verde

*This is a super-easy salsa recipe—great for those who are tomato overloaded, as the taste is distinctively different. A member of the nightshade family, tomatillos have much more of a tart flavor as compared to their other nightshade relatives (tomatoes in particular).*

> There are a few ways you can cook the tomatillos for this recipe:
> - Broiling to char the onions and tomatillos (my preferred method)
> - Oven roasting to provide some of the roasting flavor
> - Charring on the grill or stovetop
> - Boiling in a saucepan
>
> The recipe below is written with the broiler method, as I find it's the quickest and easiest.

| | |
|---|---|
| 1 | pound (450 g) tomatillos, husked and rinsed |
| 1 | white onion, cut into large chunks |
| 1 | jalapeño, roughly chopped |
| ~ | juice of 1 lime |
| ½ | cup (12 g) cilantro |
| ~ | salt to taste |

1. Preheat oven broiler and line a sheet pan (cookie sheet) with aluminum foil.

2. Cut tomatillos in half, and place tomatillos and onions on sheet pan in oven. Broil for 5–7 minutes or until slightly charred.

3. Place tomatillos and onions in food processor along with the jalapeño, lime juice, cilantro, and salt.

4. Pulse until salsa is desired consistency (you can add water if you like a slightly runnier salsa and yours is too thick).

**Variation**—*This salsa is also really good with a little chipotle added, or some garlic. Get creative and make the recipe your own unique salsa! Try this salsa verde on your scrambled eggs next time.*

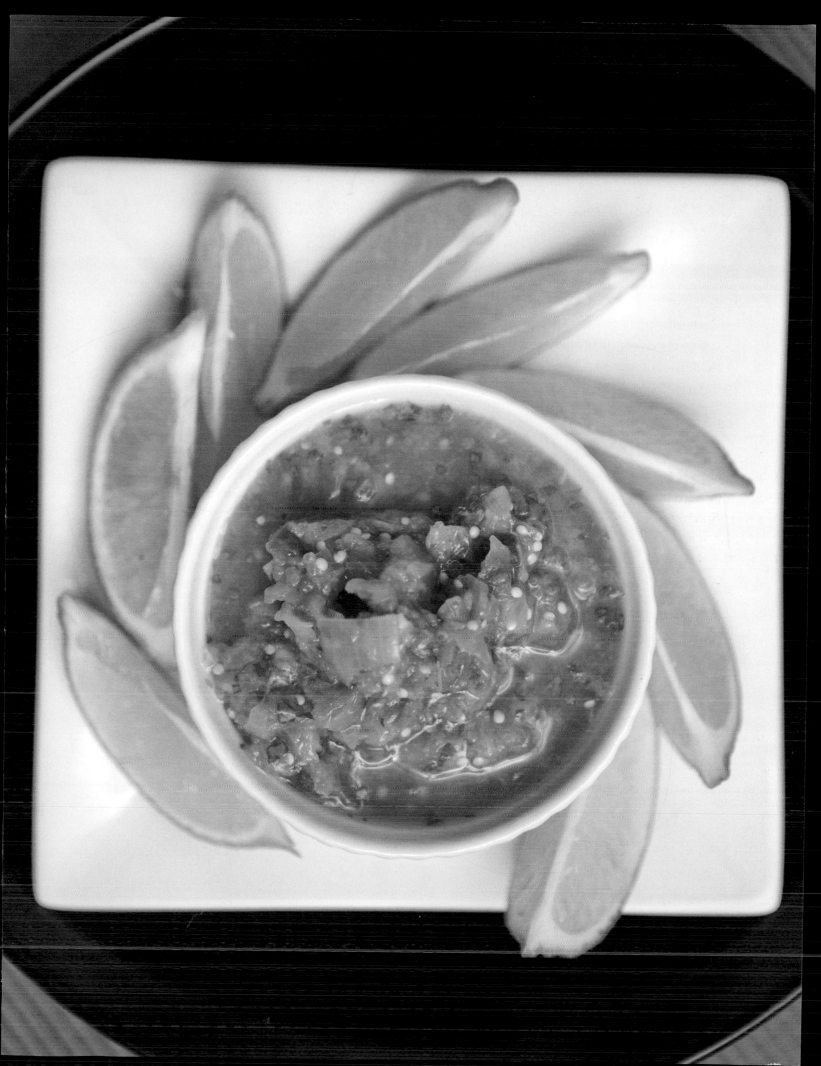

# pineapple salsa

*Fresh pineapple is one of those fruits that just makes you feel you are on a tropical island, even if you're thousands of miles away. We don't typically have pineapple too much throughout the year because of the sugar content, but when we do, this salsa is one that I love to create. It goes great over a piece of grilled fish (like a wild salmon or even some of the milder white fishes) or it can take ordinary grilled chicken or grilled shrimp to a more tropical place. If you don't have some fresh pineapple, this salsa is also delicious with some mangos.*

| | |
|---|---|
| 1 | medium pineapple |
| 1 | red pepper, diced |
| ¼ | cup (6 g) cilantro, chopped |
| 1 | tablespoon fresh mint, chopped |
| 1 | jalapeño, minced |
| 1 | lime, juiced |
| ¼ | teaspoon paprika |
| ¼ | teaspoon cayenne pepper (optional) |

1. Cut off top and base of pineapple, and peel, cutting out all the pineapple "sockets."

2. Cut pineapple in quarters lengthwise, removing core. Cut pineapple into small dice.

3. Combine pineapple dice with remaining ingredients in a medium-sized bowl.

**Ingredient Notes**—*When looking for a ripe pineapple, first check and smell the stem end of the fruit. It should smell sweetly of pineapple, and should have a yellow-gold color to it. Look for that color to be throughout the fruit, as that usually indicates ripeness throughout. We don't suggest using canned pineapple for this recipe, as most brands have a lot of added sugar, and fresh pineapple just plain tastes better. If you are adverse to salsas with a kick, keep the jalapeño out of the salsa!*

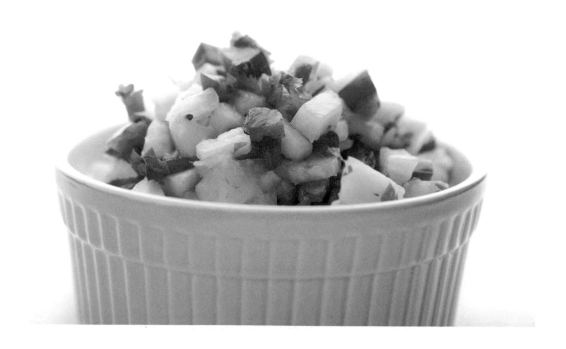

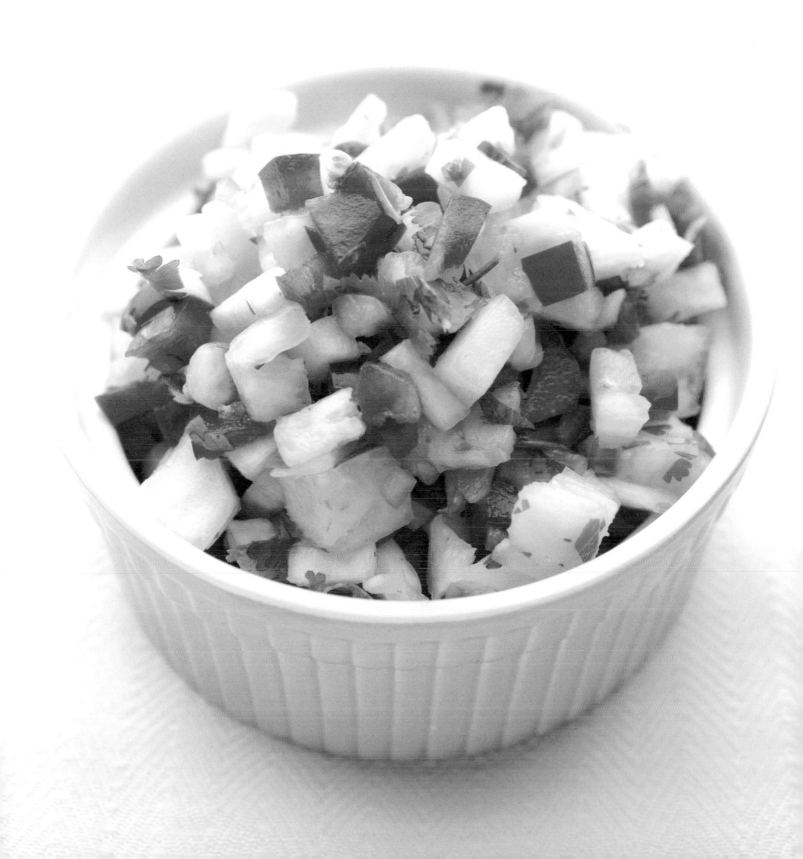

# homemade breakfast sausage

*I don't know about you, but finding a good breakfast sausage in our everyday grocery store is near to impossible. Most have added nitrites or nitrates in the ingredients, or MSG, or a whopping dose of sugar. Here's our take on making your own. It's really quite simple, and well worth the effort. My suggestion is to double or triple this recipe, vacuum seal the sausage you won't immediately use, and freeze until you need it.*

| | |
|---|---|
| 1 | pound (450 g) ground pork |
| 1 | teaspoon kosher salt |
| ¾ | teaspoon pepper |
| 2 | teaspoons fresh sage leaves, finely chopped |
| 1 | teaspoon fresh thyme, finely chopped |
| ¼ | teaspoon fresh rosemary, finely chopped |
| ¼ | teaspoon ground nutmeg |
| ¼ | teaspoon cayenne pepper |
| ¼ | teaspoon crushed red pepper flakes |

1. Take ground pork and mix with all the ingredients. Form into 2-inch-wide patties.

2. Heat a skillet over medium heat. Place sausage patties in skillet, and cook until browned, then flip over and continue cooking until sausage is fully cooked through.

**Variations**—*If you have a meat grinder, buy a pound (450 g) of pork butt along with ¼ pound (110 g) of fatback, dice those into chunks and combine with all the spices, and pass through the meat grinder. If you have a sausage stuffer, you can also buy your own casings and make sausage links. This recipe also works well with making turkey or chicken sausage.*

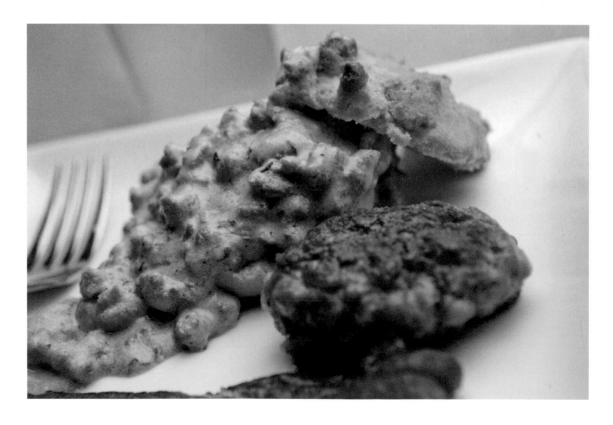

paleo comfort foods

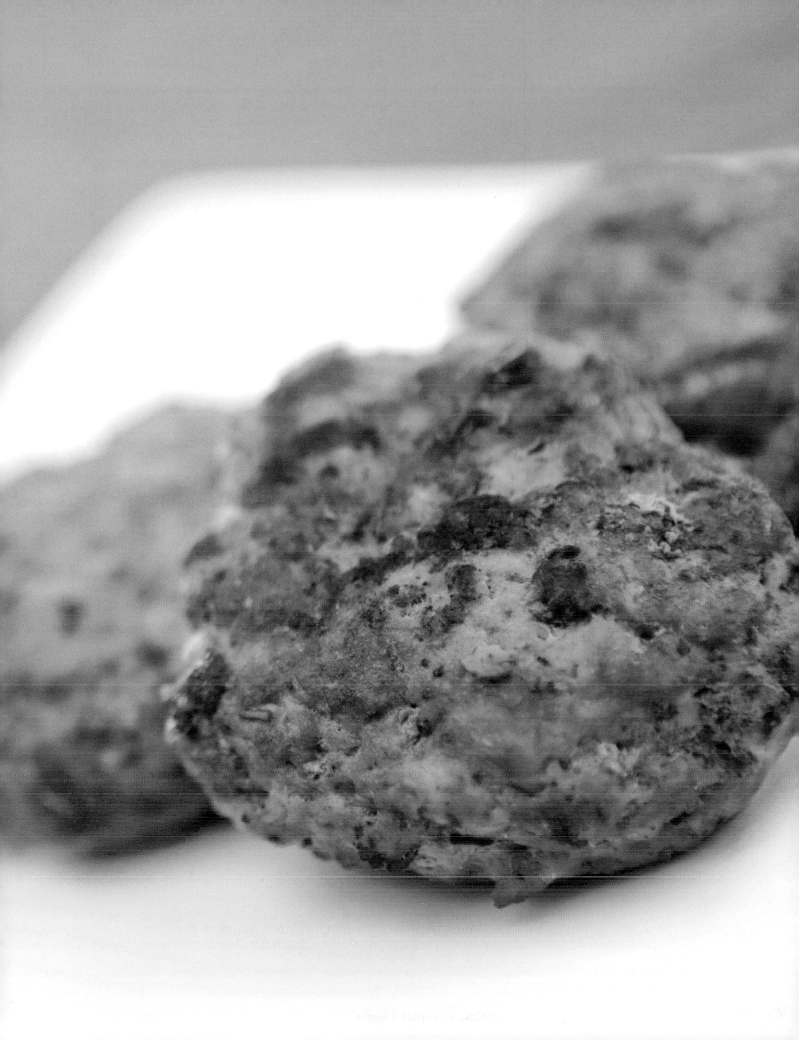

# prosciutto and asparagus bundles

*I love making these little bundles as appetizers for parties. Hard not to love vegetables wrapped in prosciutto . . . or really anything wrapped in prosciutto.*

*Some people avoid asparagus because they absolutely cannot stand the "smell" it causes when metabolized (most of you know the smell I'm talking about). Interestingly enough, some studies have shown that everyone gets "the smell," however, it has been stated that only about 22 percent of the population has the autosomal gene that enables them to smell the compounds.*

*Asparagus season is usually in the spring; however, you can very often find it available year-round. Look for asparagus to be firm to the touch, bright green stalks with tips that are tightly closed. Diameter is up to you, but I very much prefer the thinner stalks.*

| | |
|---|---|
| 3 | ounces (84 g) prosciutto |
| 1 | bunch thin asparagus, trimmed |
| 2 | teaspoons olive oil |
| ~ | pepper |
| ½ | cup balsamic vinegar |
| 1 | clove garlic, peeled and smashed |

1. Preheat oven to 425°F (220°C).
2. Working carefully, cut prosciutto pieces in half lengthwise, so each piece is about 1–2 inches (2–4 cm) wide and 3–4 inches (8–10 cm) long.
3. Cut asparagus spears to an even length (I like to make mine about 4 inches (10 cm) long, reserving the ends for use in other recipes).
4. Wrap 3 spears together in 1 piece of prosciutto, and place on large sheet pan.
5. Drizzle with olive oil and sprinkle with black pepper. Place in oven and cook for about 10 minutes or until asparagus is somewhat softened.
6. Meanwhile, in a small sauce pan, heat balsamic and garlic over medium heat until simmering.
7. Reduce heat and let simmer, reducing vinegar until syrupy, being careful not to burn.
8. Discard the garlic, and drizzle syrup over asparagus spears. Serve immediately.

**Variations**—*If dairy is part of your life or something you add in once in a while, these are really tasty with some goat cheese wrapped inside the prosciutto. You can also grill these to get more of a smoky flavor. If you prefer not to use the balsamic, these are extremely tasty as is!*

paleo comfort foods

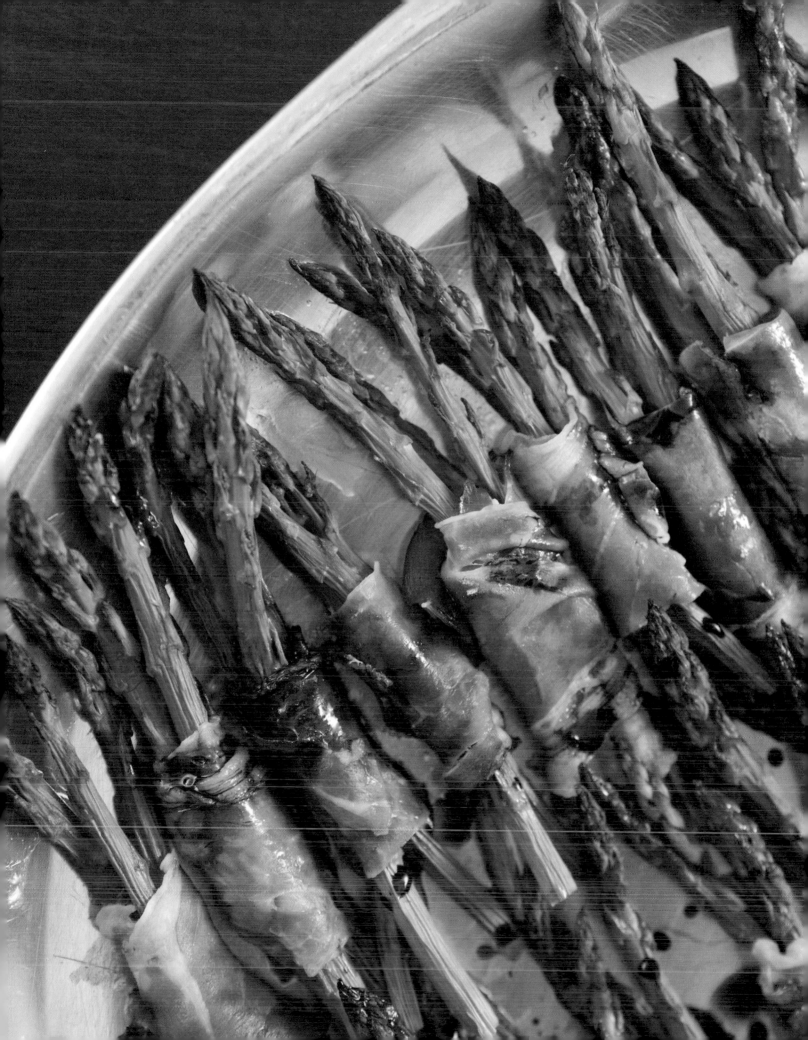

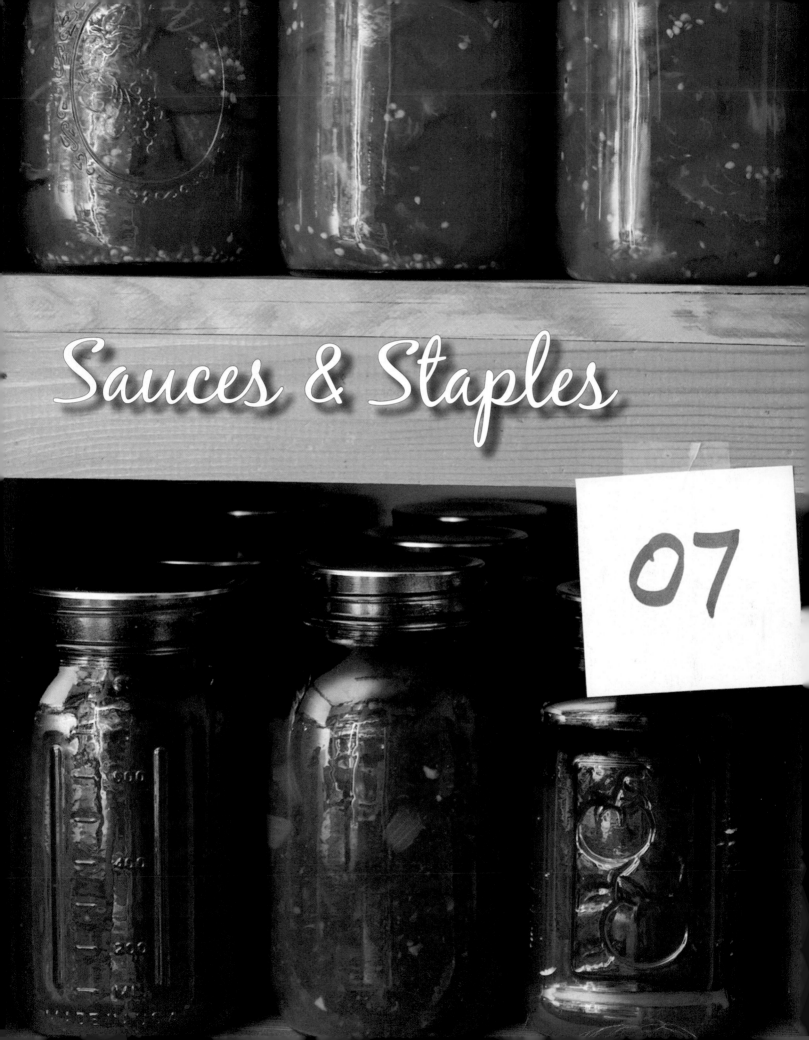

# Sauces & Staples

07

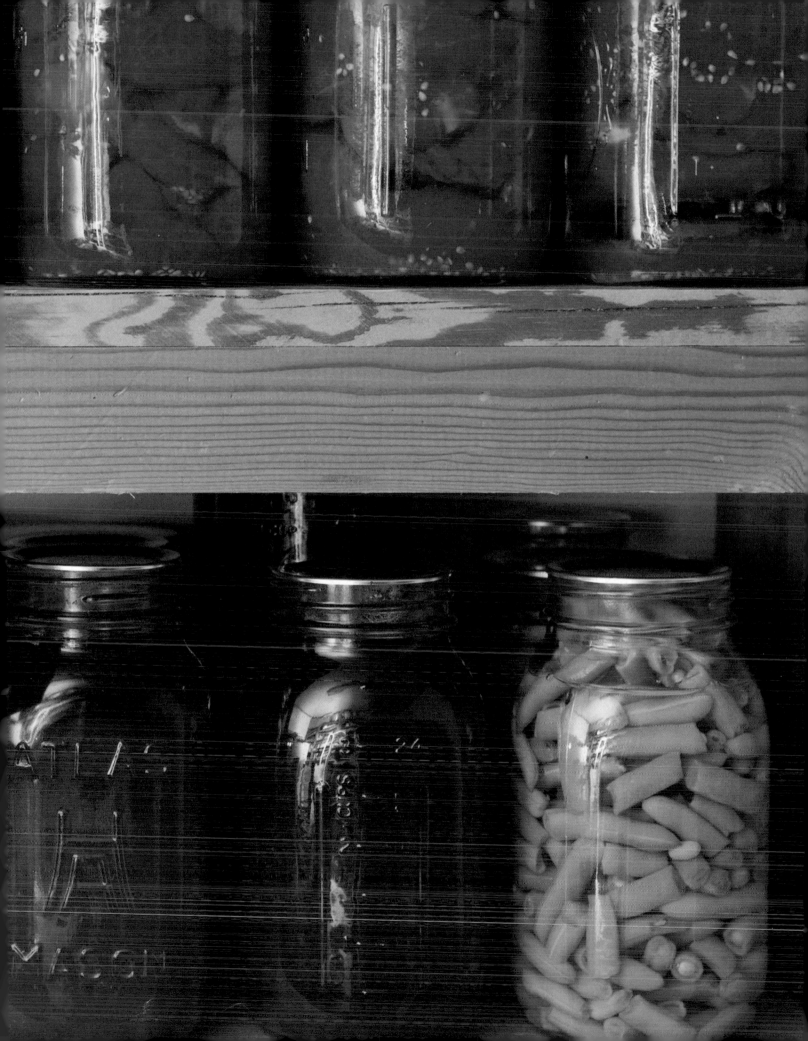

# nut butter

*There is a kind of guilt to publishing recipes like these. They are so incredibly simple. I do remember the very first time Julie told me how to make nut butter. I think I checked on it about 17 times to make sure it was OK. Really folks . . . just walk away for 5–10 minutes and come back to wonderful butter. If you're making a list of reasons to go get a nice Cuisinart food processor, put these recipes in the top 5.*

The sky is the limit on how many different combinations of nuts you can use. Below are our three favorites.

## Almond Butter

| 4–5 | cups (600–750 g) almonds |
|---|---|

## Pecash Butter

| 3 | cups (450 g) raw cashews |
|---|---|
| 2 | cups (200 g) pecan halves |

## Walecan Butter

| 2 | cups (200 g) walnuts |
|---|---|
| 3 | cups (300 g) pecans |

**1.** Make sure you have the chopping blade in your food processor (as opposed to the dough blade). Pour all the nuts in the bowl of the processor and turn on.

**2.** Allow the processor to run for 8 or 10 minutes or until you have nice creamy butter.

**3.** If you simply can't stand it, about 5 minutes in stop the motor and scrape all the nut fragments off the walls of the processor bowl. From there, just let it keep working.

**Variations**—*Consider adding ½ teaspoon of your favorite spice or taste. Examples include instant espresso, cinnamon, chipotle powder, nutmeg, vanilla, or citrus zest. You can also use roasted nuts to bring a different flavor to the butter. If you prefer a chunky nut butter, add in some whole nuts for the last minute or two until the desired texture is reached.*

paleo comfort foods

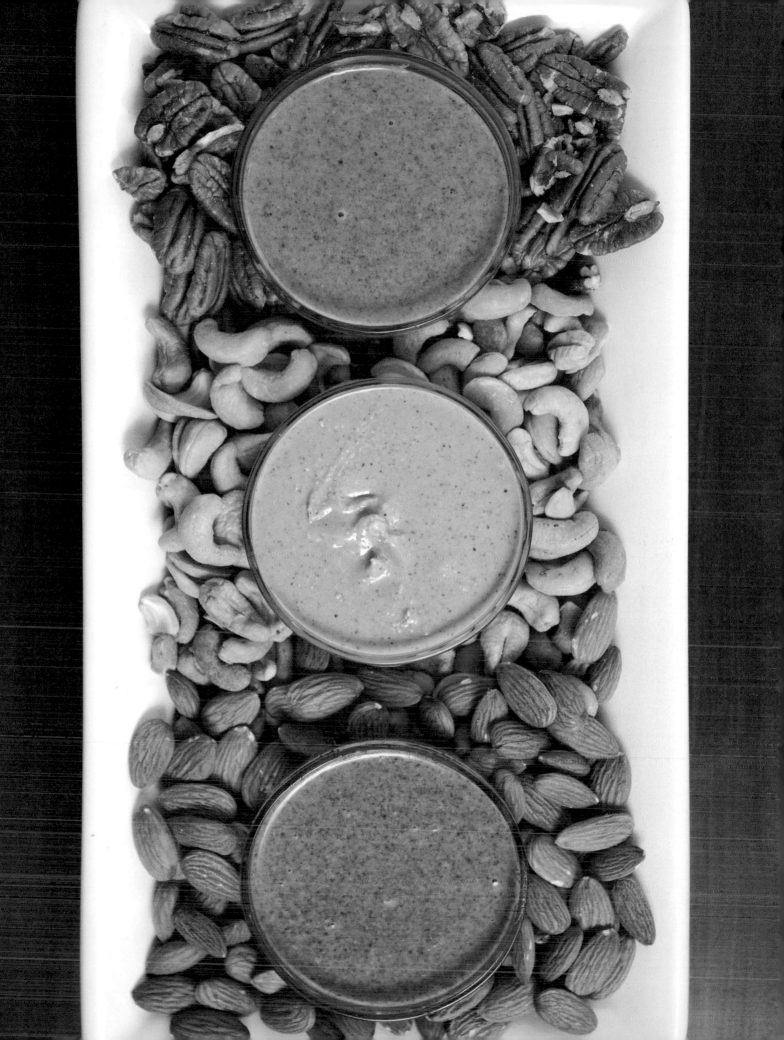

# chimichurri

*It all started on a girls' night in Los Angeles, where we were intentionally going to "bars and restaurants beginning with the letter L." Lola's, Luna Park, Lala's. It was the latter establishment—an Argentinean restaurant on Melrose Ave.—where I first tasted chimichurri, and my life was then and forever changed. What does the word mean? Lots of rumors abound regarding its origins, but the one I particularly like had to do with some British prisoners in Argentina saying "che-mi-curry" (give me curry)—asking for a condiment to go with their food. This was then corrupted to chimichurri. No matter its origins, the condiment is simply amazing and full of fresh flavors. A favorite appetizer of mine is grilled steak skewers with the chimichurri, and it's absolutely lovely served over some fresh grilled vegetables. It also makes a great marinade!*

| | |
|---|---|
| 1½ | cups (40 g) fresh flat-leaf parsley, trimmed of thick stems |
| 3–4 | garlic cloves |
| 2 | tablespoons fresh oregano leaves |
| 1 | teaspoon fresh thyme leaves |
| 1 | teaspoon smoked paprika |
| ½ | cup (125 mL) olive oil |
| 2 | tablespoons red or white wine vinegar |
| 1 | teaspoon sea salt |
| ¼ | teaspoon freshly ground black pepper |
| ¼ | teaspoon Tabasco or other hot sauce |

1. Place first five ingredients into a food processor and pulse until all herbs are finely chopped.

2. Remove to a mixing bowl and stir in the oil, vinegar, salt, pepper and hot sauce.

3. Serve immediately or refrigerate. If chilled, return to room temperature before serving.

**Tips & Tricks**—*If you want to get really authentic and feel like spending a lot of time with your knife, go ahead and do all the chopping of the garlic and herbs by hand and combine with the other ingredients by hand.*

**Variations**—*Feel free to add in some cilantro, or mix in some peppers of your choice (hot or sweet), some tomatoes, etc., though most of the so-called "authentic" Argentinean recipes will be much like the one stated above.*

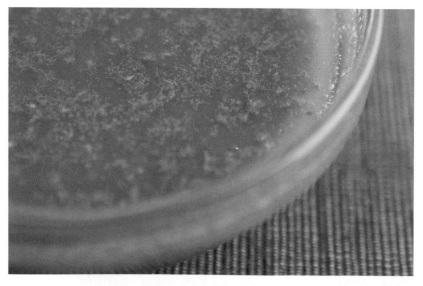

paleo comfort foods

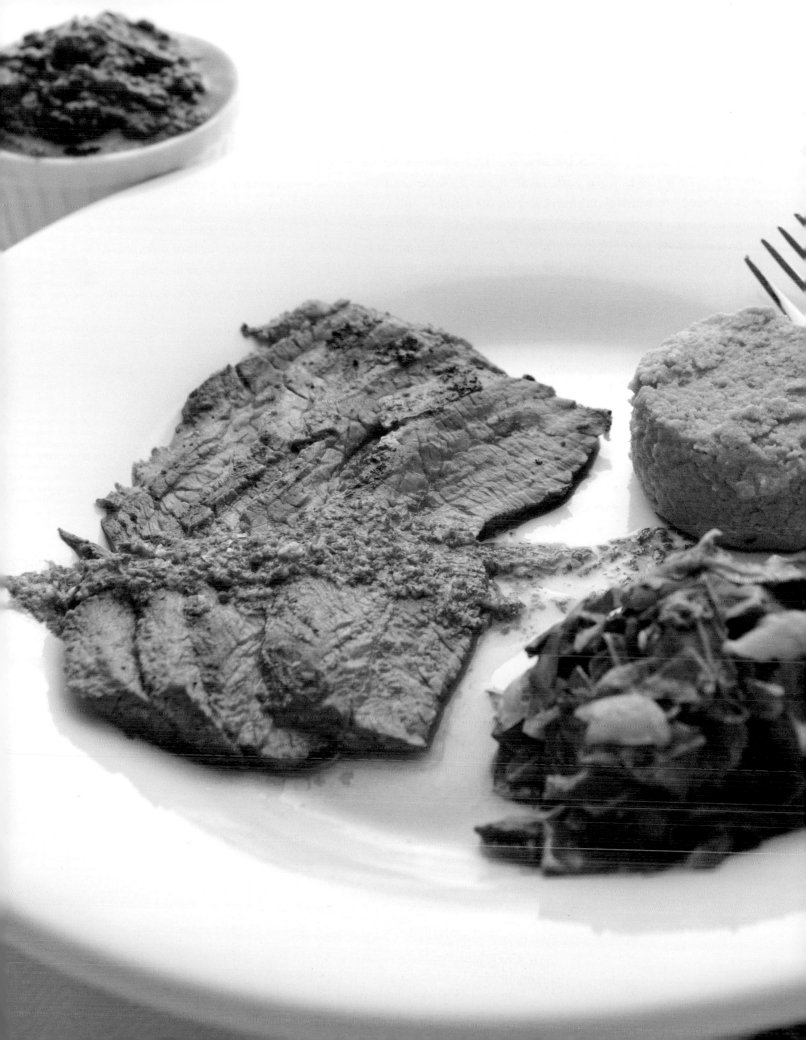

# chipotle dipping sauce
# (aka adobo sauce)

*This one is a dip/sauce/dressing/marinade all rolled in one. This recipe is a variation on one that my dear friends at Simple Gourmet used to make. The original recipe—if I recall correctly—called for mayo and sour cream. In adapting this to a more paleo palate, I first made this with no mayo—just the olive oil. It was good, but it wasn't the creamy sauce I wanted. Once I figured out a decent paleo mayo, I didn't even miss the sour cream. You can omit the mayo if you'd like too—it's still really tasty without! This sauce keeps in the refrigerator for at least a week and is incredibly tasty served on top of a fresh grilled burger or some fish tacos!*

| | |
|---|---|
| ½ | cup (125 mL) Paleo Mayonnaise (see recipe page 100) |
| ½ | cup (12 g) cilantro |
| 1 | clove garlic |
| 2 | tablespoons olive oil |
| 2 | chipotle peppers in adobo sauce |
| ~ | juice of 1 lime |

1. Combine all ingredients in a mini-blender or food processor until mixed well.
2. Keep refrigerated until ready to serve.

**Ingredient Notes**—*Chipotles (smoked jalapeños) in adobo (sauce) are found in the Mexican section of most grocery stores and at any Mexican mercados I've been to. Just check the ingredients, as some use less-than-ideal oils and others actually contain wheat flour. La Morena is one brand we like.*

**Variations**—*Tinker around with this one to get it as spicy as you'd like it (note well: even with the low amount of chipotles called for in this, for some palates this recipe will be like fire!). My BFF Melissa enjoys her sauce with some fresh squeezed orange juice and lots of cilantro. There are so many ways for you to make this sauce your own! If using the sauce as a dressing, you'll want to up the olive oil content some to get it more liquefied.*

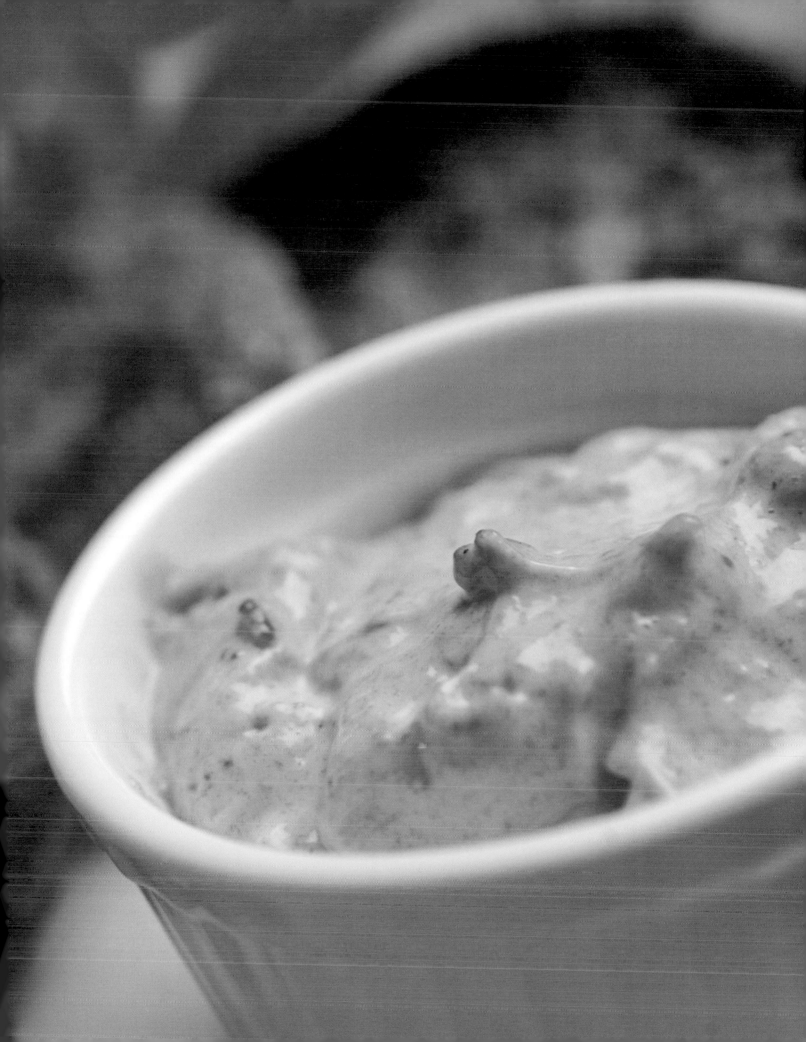

# not peanut sauce

*I can remember the first time I had a Thai chicken satay, and how the chicken itself was merely the vehicle to get more of that tasty Thai peanut sauce into my mouth. So delicious. Taking what my friend chef Jet had taught me about a good peanut satay, this recipe became my attempt at removing the peanut portion, replacing with an actual nut (since you all know peanuts are legumes), and giving it a shot that way. I was not in the slightest bit disappointed. This sauce was pure yum, and perfect with some leftover grilled chicken, steak, etc. My latest favorite? Sautéing up some red cabbage in a large wok with some of this sauce. This is one of those sauces that may in fact be life changing for you.*

| | |
|---|---|
| 1 | tablespoon coconut oil |
| ½–1 | tablespoon red curry paste |
| 2 | cups (500 mL) coconut milk |
| ½ | cup (125 mL) almond butter |
| 2 | teaspoons fish sauce |
| 1 | tablespoon apple cider or white vinegar |
| 1 | tablespoon honey (optional) |

1. In a medium saucepan, heat the coconut oil over medium heat, and stir in the curry paste until fragrant and slightly dried out.

2. Stir in the coconut milk, almond butter, fish sauce, vinegar (and honey if using), whisking constantly as sauce comes up to a boil.

3. Reduce heat to low and let simmer for 3–5 minutes, making sure it doesn't burn.

**Ingredient Notes**—*While yes, you could go and make your own red curry paste, there really is no need (unless you wish to experience that yourself for fun). The Mae Ploy and Maesri brands (found at many Asian supermarkets, or online at thaigrocer.com) are great with no added preservatives. According to my "expert" source chef Jet Tila (chefjet. com), most commercial kitchens use a paste, as these pastes have all the same ingredients that a homemade version would, and are without preservatives.*

**Variation**—*You could make this with cashew or hazelnut butter for a different nutty taste.*

**Plan Ahead**—*This sauce keeps in the refrigerator extremely well for about a week. You can make it ahead of time, then serve with chicken satay when you are ready to. You may need to add in some water to thin the sauce out some.*

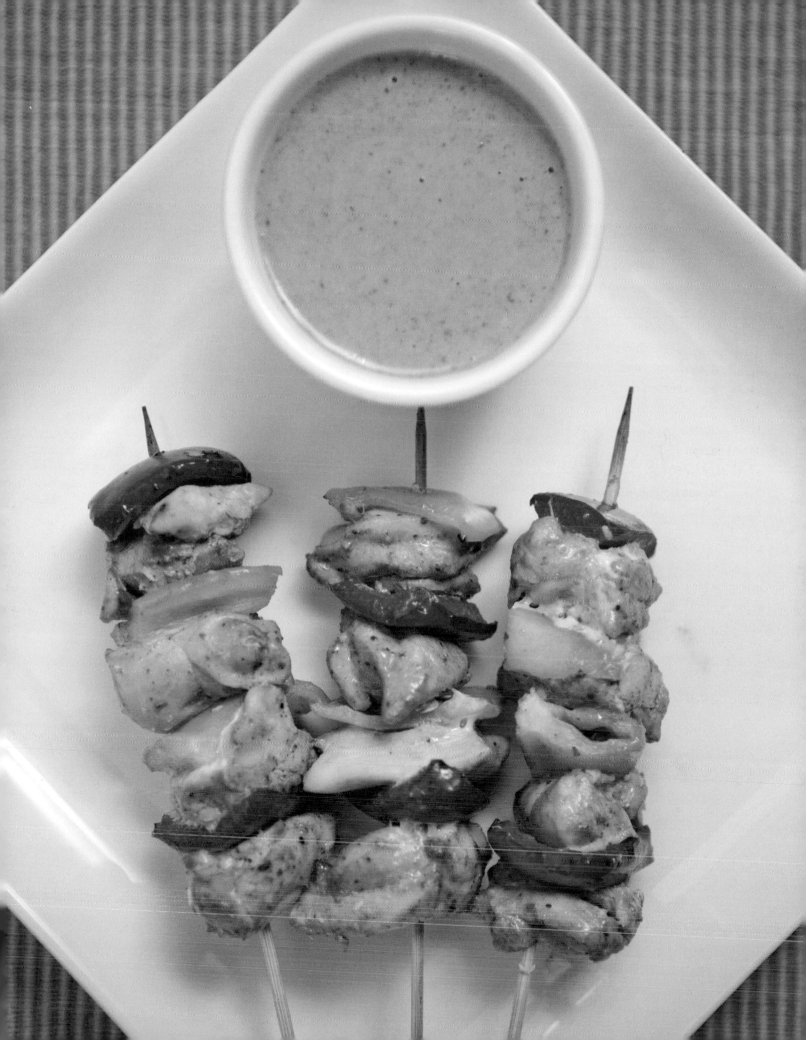

# remoulade sauce

*I like to think of remoulade sauce as the cousin of tartar sauce, only with even more of a flavor zing. Originally created in France as more of a white sauce with capers, anchovies, mayo, and more, the version you will most commonly find in the South takes more of its influence from Louisiana, where many restaurants will incorporate Creole mustard, ketchup, hot sauce, and a bunch of piquant ingredients.*

*Don't let the number of ingredients intimidate you. The great thing about this sauce is that you can get pretty creative with it, and if you find you are missing one of the ingredients, it will still taste pretty awesome.*

*Remoulade sauce goes great with peel-and-eat shrimp, fish sticks, crab cakes, and a host of seafood options. You can also toss this sauce over some grilled veggies, and you'll be amazed at how this sauce transforms even the most basic veggies into something incredible!*

---

| | |
|---|---|
| ¼ | cup (60 mL) fresh lemon juice |
| ½ | cup (125 mL) olive oil |
| ½ | cup (75 g) yellow onions |
| ½ | cup (35 g) green onions |
| ¼ | cup (25 g) celery |
| 2 | tablespoons fresh garlic |
| 2 | tablespoons prepared horseradish |
| 3 | tablespoons whole grain mustard |
| 3 | tablespoons prepared yellow mustard |
| 3 | tablespoons Paleo Ketchup (see recipe page 102) or substitute tomato paste |
| 3 | tablespoons chopped fresh flat-leaf parsley |
| 2 | tablespoons Paleo Mayonnaise (see recipe page 100) |
| 1 | teaspoon salt |
| ¼ | teaspoon cayenne |
| ⅛ | teaspoon freshly ground black pepper |

1. Place all ingredients in a food processor or blender.
2. Combine until well mixed.

---

**Variation**—*Give this sauce even more of a kick by adding in some hot sauce.*

**Plan Ahead**—*You can make this sauce ahead of time, as it will keep for up to a week refrigerated in an air-tight container.*

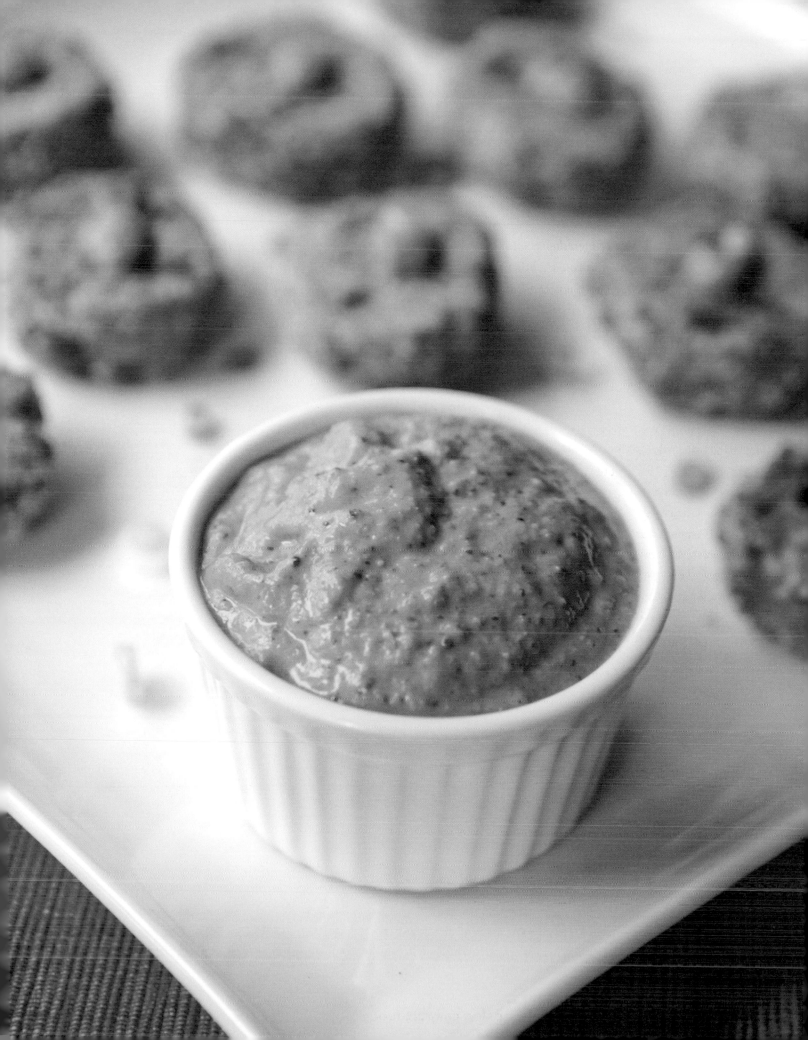

# paleo mayonnaise

*Truthfully, it is not hard to make your own mayo. I swear to you, it's not. Okay, if you don't have a food processor and you have to whisk the oil in by hand, yes that is more of a workout (which is reason 254 that you should go and get that food processor—now). Homemade mayo is great to have on hand for so many sauces, salads, aiolis, etc. Make some, store it in an air-tight container, and keep it for about a week. It's less expensive than the stuff with all kinds of nastiness in the ingredient list, and so much better for you!*

| | |
|---|---|
| 1 | large egg, brought to room temperature |
| 1½ | tablespoons lemon juice |
| ½ | teaspoon mustard powder |
| ½ | cup (125 mL) light or very mild tasting olive oil |
| ½ | cup (125 mL) avocado oil |
| ¼ | teaspoon white pepper (optional) |

1. Combine egg, lemon juice, and mustard in food processor and blend until frothy.

2. Using the drip hole in the top of the processor, or pouring teaspoon by teaspoon to start, drizzle the oil in drop by drop. *Do not rush this process, or you will end up with scrambled eggs mixed with oil!*

3. Once you have quite a few drops in there, you can pour the oil into the feed tube part of the food processor to let that useful drip hole control the rate of flow for you.

4. Refrigerate in sealed container. This will keep for a week or so.

**Variation**—*You can make spicy mayo simply by adding in some chipotle powder or chipotles in adobo.*

**Tips & Tricks**—*You will probably be tempted to dump all the oil in at one time. I restate this for emphasis: Do NOT dump the oil in at one time, or you will not find yourself with that nicely emulsified mayo. You will find yourself with runny, oily, slimy stuff that looks nothing like mayonnaise. Heed my warning! Start the oil drip by drip, and you'll end up with a great mayonnaise! If you find that you only have olive oil, you can use just that (without avocado oil), just be forewarned that the mayo may have a distinct olive taste.*

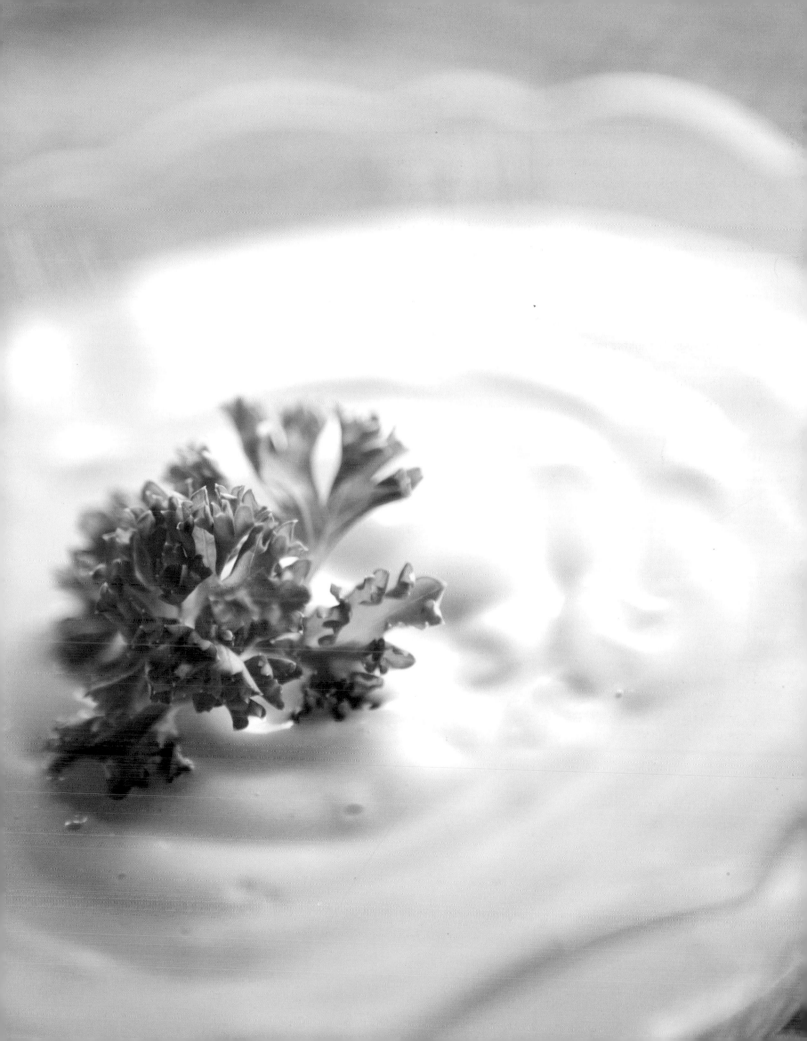

# cave ketchup

*Let's be honest, ketchup is king of all condiments. Most brands you buy off the shelf are loaded with sugar and preservatives. This version will keep in the refrigerator for at least a week—but if you're inspired, we recommend canning some big batches of this so you always have some ready to go. Consider doubling the batch and making more for down the road.*

| | |
|---|---|
| 6 | ounces (150 g) tomato paste |
| 2 | tablespoons apple cider vinegar |
| ¼ | teaspoon mustard powder |
| ½ | cup (125 mL) water |
| ¼ | teaspoon cinnamon |
| 1 | pinch allspice |
| 1 | pinch salt |
| ⅛ | teaspoon paprika (optional) |
| 1 | clove garlic |
| 1 | bay leaf |

1. Combine all ingredients (except garlic clove and bay leaf) in a medium sized sauce pan.
2. Bring to a boil stirring frequently.
3. Add in garlic clove and bay leaf (whole). Reduce heat and allow the mixture to simmer for 20–30 minutes stirring occasionally.
4. Watch for desired consistency, as this stuff will thicken quickly toward the end. If you overdo it, just add a tablespoon of water back to the mix.
5. Remove the bay leaf and garlic clove and allow ketchup to cool.

**Ingredient Notes**—*Use a tomato paste with no salt added.*

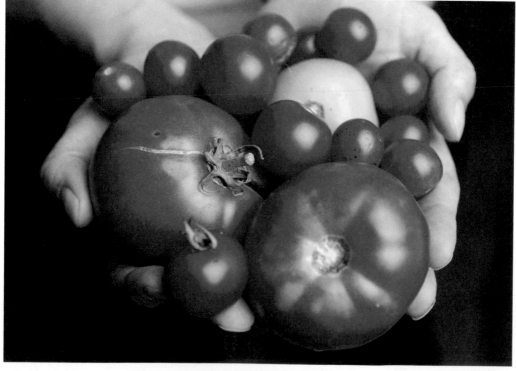

paleo comfort foods

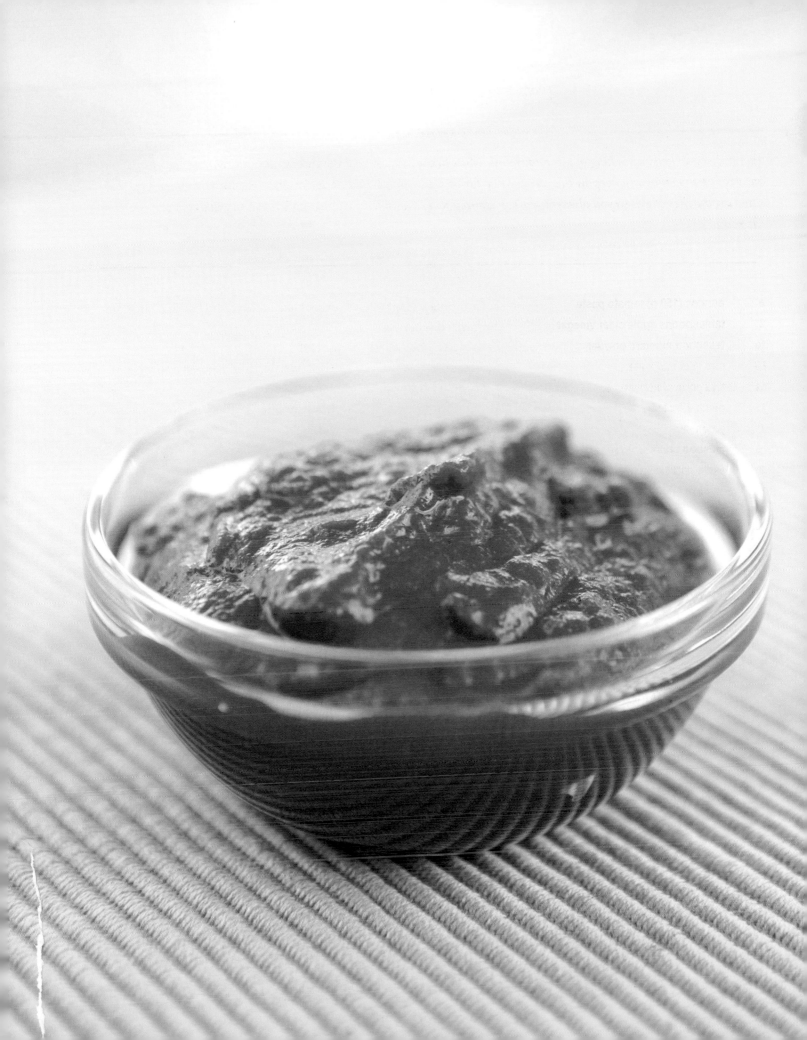

# barbecue sauce with some kick

*This recipe goes well with a variety of meats and what's not to love about barbequed chicken in the summertime? You can almost always count on us having at least a little container of this in the refrigerator. We put it on everything from eggs to salads. Don't be scared to throw this on top of a meatloaf or when sautéing vegetables.*

| | |
|---|---|
| 6 | ounces (150 g) tomato paste |
| 1 | cup (250 mL) beef stock |
| ¼ | cup (30 g) shallot, minced fine |
| 3 | cloves garlic, minced |
| 1 | tablespoon Dijon mustard |
| 1 | teaspoon prepared horseradish |
| 2 | tablespoons apple cider vinegar |
| 1 | tablespoon avocado oil |
| ½ | teaspoon salt |
| 1 | teaspoon red pepper |
| 1 | teaspoon cumin |
| 1 | teaspoon cayenne pepper |
| 1 | teaspoon black pepper |

1. Combine all ingredients into a sauce pan and bring to a quick simmer using medium heat.

2. Reduce to medium low and cover for 15–20 minutes. You'll want to stir frequently to keep it from sticking to the pan.

3. The longer you let this simmer, the more flavor you get in the sauce. If you aren't rushed and have at least 25–35 minutes, add an extra ½ cup (125 mL) of beef stock to the mixture at the beginning, then simmer 25-35 minutes or until the desired consistency is achieved.

**Tips & Tricks**—*No Garlic Press? Use a microplane grater for the garlic as you are certain to bring out more flavor in the sauce.*

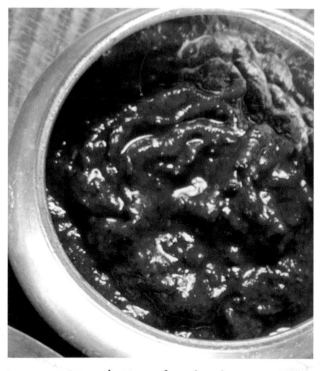

paleo comfort foods

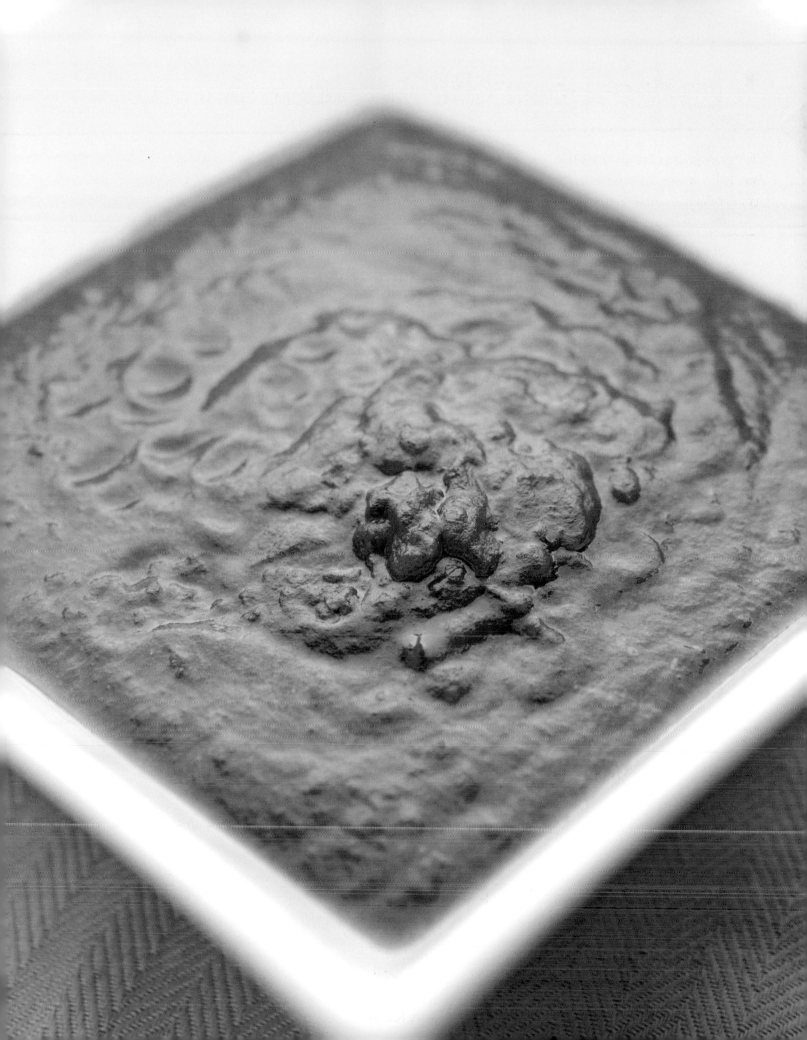

# red chile sauce

*My grandparents lived in New Mexico for many years, where the infamous chile reigns supreme. Of course, when they were still alive and living in New Mexico, my chile taste buds hadn't really come in yet.*

*This recipe pays tribute to those years they lived in Albuquerque, and the awesome New Mexico chiles you can find pretty widely available in the United States. I had the good fortune of spending some time in New Mexico for work a few years back and loved trying all the New Mexican chiles—so tasty! You can always make this sauce spicier, or get creative and add a host of other hot/dried peppers to see what you come up with. Use this sauce for our Chicken Enchiladas (recipe page 238).*

| | |
|---|---|
| 10–12 | dried red New Mexico chiles (found at most Latin markets) |
| 4 | cups (1 L) boiling water |
| 2 | tablespoons olive oil |
| 1 | medium onion, chopped |
| 2 | cloves garlic, chopped |
| 1 | teaspoon dried oregano, Mexican preferred |
| 2 | teaspoons apple cider vinegar |
| 1 | teaspoon ground cumin |
| ~ | salt to taste |

1. Rinse chiles and split to remove seeds. Place chiles on a sheet pan and bake for 10–15 minutes in a 275°F (135°C) oven (you should be able to smell the chiles—but do not burn them!).

2. Remove the stems from the chiles, place them in a heat-proof bowl and pour boiling water over. Allow them to sit for 5–10 minutes to soften them, then drain, reserving liquid.

3. In a medium-sized saucepan, heat the olive oil over medium heat, then add in the onion and garlic and sauté until soft. Add the chiles, about 3 cups (750 mL) of the water, oregano, vinegar, and cumin and simmer for 10–12 minutes.

4. Place the mixture in a food processor or blender and puree.

5. Strain the mixture through a coarse sieve. If the sauce is too thin, return contents back to sauce pan and reduce longer. If sauce is too thick, add more of the reserved soaking liquid.

6. Refrigerate until ready to use/serve.

**Variation**—*Definitely take a trip to your local Mexican grocer and get adventurous with some of the dried chiles! Guajillos, chile de Arbol, cascabel, California, ancho, mulato, pasilla . . . there are so many to choose from!*

**Tips & Tricks**—*Always use caution when combining hot ingredients in a food processor or blender. Oftentimes pressure will build up, causing the liquid to essentially explode. You do not want red chile sauce all over your kitchen . . . trust me!*

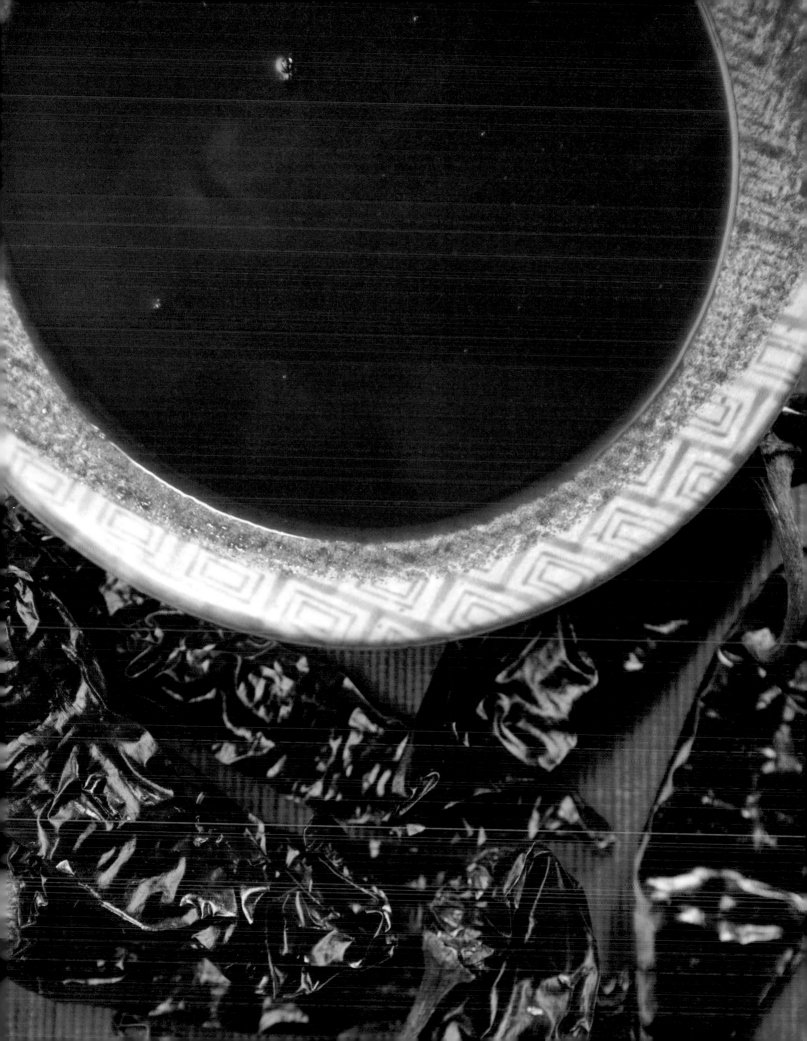

# tartar sauce

*Some of my fondest memories as a child were the week or so we would pack up the big blue van and head down to Mobile Bay to stay with my grandparents. If you don't know what a Mobile Bay Jubilee is, get out your computer and do a quick search. Papa (my grandfather) would come wake me up at 5 AM and out the door we would go. I held the lantern and the burlap sack. Papa and I would slide our feet along the shallows of the shoreline gigging flounder until the sun rose. Meanwhile, the rest of the family would be off catching shrimp and crab. When you bring back a bag of fifteen to twenty flounder, you had better have some tartar sauce handy for dinner that night. If you have your mayonnaise already prepared, this is a really simple concoction to whip up.*

---

⅔  cup (175 mL) Paleo Mayonnaise (recipe page 100)

2  tablespoons dill pickles, finely chopped

1  tablespoon fresh flat-leaf parsley, chopped

1  tablespoon onion, grated

1  teaspoon Dijon mustard

1  tablespoon lemon juice

1. Mix all ingredients in bowl (except lemon juice).
2. Once combined, slowly add the lemon juice, cover and store in refrigerator for at least an hour.

---

**Variations**—*Replace lemon juice with vinegar to sharpen flavor. Pickled jalapeños can add a nice kick. Consider using this sauce on chicken or grilled vegetables as a break from traditional flavors.*

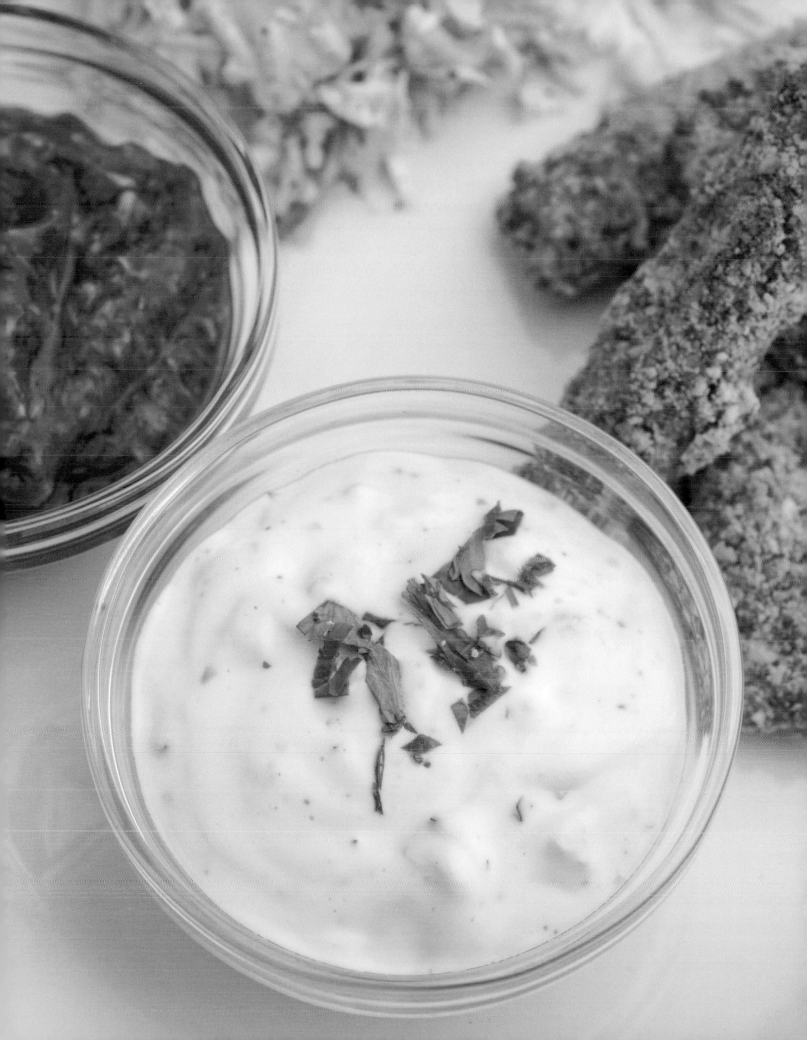

# turkey gravy

*You can make a really tasty gravy without demi-glace, flour, or a lot of tips and tricks professional chefs use, so don't be dismayed. The key to any good gravy is utilizing all those little browned bits (fond) in the bottom of your roasting pan and scraping them up and whisking with a roux and turkey stock. There are so many ways to make gravy, but this is our basic go-to that enables you to get a quick gravy on the table for Thanksgiving. The magic in this and really any gravy is the pan drippings, as that is where all the flavor can be found.*

| | |
|---|---|
| ~ | drippings in pan from Dry-Brined Turkey (page 240) |
| ½ | cup (125 mL) white wine |
| ¼ | cup (40 g) almond flour |
| ¼ | cup (40 g) arrowroot powder, mixed with ¼ cup water |
| 3–4 | cups (1 L) chicken or turkey stock |
| ~ | salt and pepper to taste |

1. Remove your roast turkey from the pan, and set the roasting pan over 2 burners. If you have a ton of excess fat in the pan, pour some of it off.

2. Turn the heat to medium-high, and deglaze the pan with the wine, whisking to break up all the browned bits off the bottom of the pan.

3. Meanwhile, in a small bowl, combine the almond flour, arrowroot powder and 1 cup (250 mL) of the stock, stirring until no lumps remain.

4. Slowly pour this "slurry" into the roasting pan, whisking to mix all.

5. Whisk in the remaining stock.

6. Once gravy starts to thicken, turn off heat and serve immediately. Season with salt and pepper.

**Variations**—*Add some fresh thyme, sage, or rosemary for extra flavor in the gravy. You can absolutely make this just using the stock to deglaze the pan (omitting the wine) if you so choose. If arrowroot powder is not something you have on hand, replace with additional almond flour mixed in with the stock as your thickening agent.*

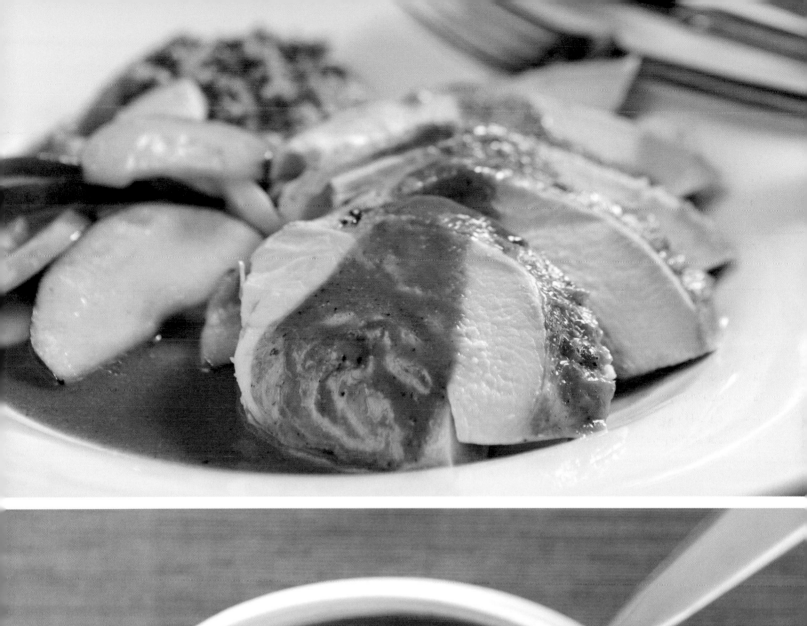
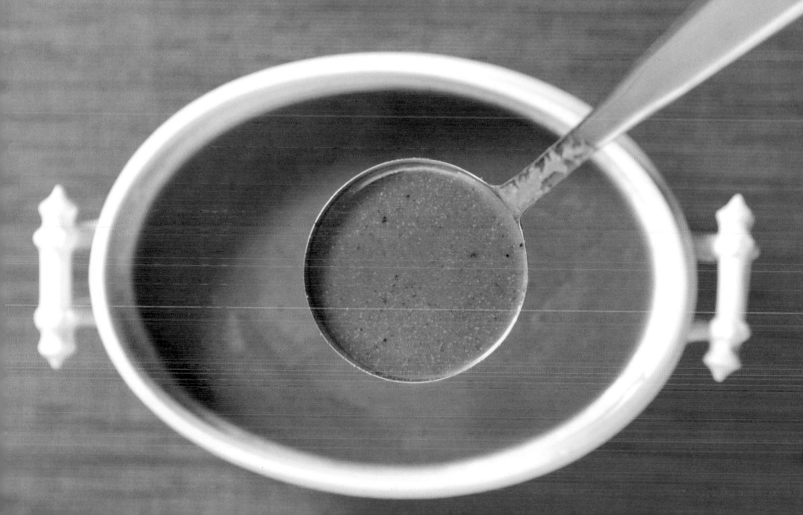

# crawfish stock

*Crawfish are available nearly year-round. Buy them fresh (alive) and keep them in a cool dry place until you are ready to cook. We prefer to purge our crawfish before we cook them. To do this, just before you turn on the stove top, place your crawfish in a sink full of cold water and about 1 cup (270 g) of salt. Don't purge them for too long (3–5 minutes). You want the crawfish alive when you toss them in the pot.*

*When cooking crawfish (to get the shells), bring the water to a boil and drop in a bag of Zatarain's Shrimp Boil. Add a few tablespoons of Cajun seasoning and boil for 3–5 minutes to allow the spices to mix well with the water. Drain and rinse your crawfish one last time before dropping them into the pot. You will boil them for about 4 minutes and then turn off the heat. Allow them to sit for another 5 minutes and then strain. Once the crawfish have cooled enough to handle with your bare hands, break the tails off and pull the meat out. Using a delicate touch, you can usually pull the tail fins off and the vein will come with it (think deveining shrimp). Place tail meat in a ziplock bag, reserve, and start to pull together your stock ingredients.*

| | |
|---|---|
| 1 | pound (500 g) crawfish shells |
| 1½ | quarts (1½ L) cold water |
| 3 | ribs celery |
| 1 | large onion |
| 1 | head garlic, halved |
| 2 | bay leaves |
| 1 | bunch thyme |
| 1 | lemon, halved |
| 1 | teaspoon black peppercorns |

1. Cover crawfish shells with cold water in stockpot. Bring to boil, then reduce to simmer for 10 minutes periodically skimming off any impurities that float to the top.

2. Add remaining ingredients and bring back to low boil. Reduce heat to low and simmer for 40–50 minutes.

3. You will want to cool the liquid quickly once done. Strain out any solids, and pour into a container or two and place in a cooler with plenty of ice. Allow to cool for an hour or two before storing. Do not place in your refrigerator until cooled.

**Tips & Tricks**—*Freeze filled water bottles (labels removed) ahead of time. You can then submerge these directly into the stock when ready to cool. This helps the stock to cool faster. We have Alton Brown to thank for this genius idea. Once cooled, you can freeze the stock in 2-cup (500 mL) measurements to have ready for your next étouffée or gumbo.*

paleo comfort foods

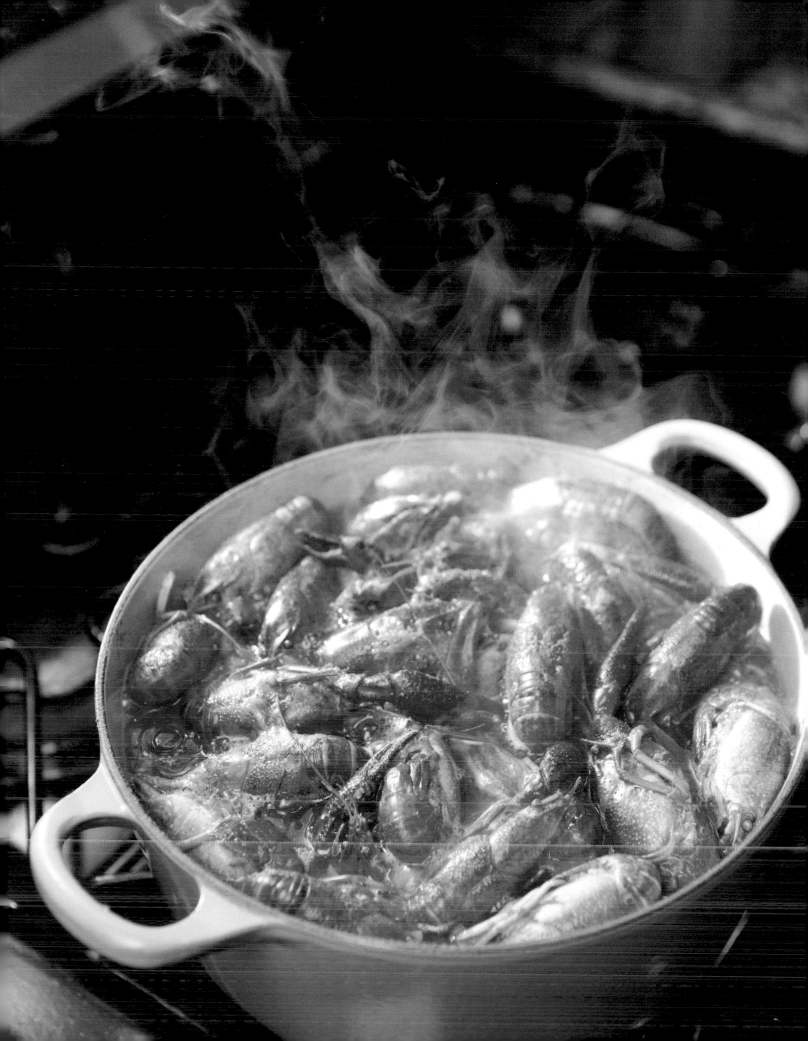

# chicken stock

*Yep, you can buy chicken stock off the grocery store shelf. You can buy lots of things off the shelf that don't taste nearly as good as what you can make at home. This recipe will net about 16 cups (nearly 4 liters) of delicious stock.*

*From the directions, you'll see we are pretty adamant about cooling the broth outside your refrigerator. There are several reasons for this. First, your refrigerator isn't nearly as good at cooling things down as it is in keeping them cool. Second, bacteria grow best in temperatures between 40-140°F (5-60°C). The quicker we can lower the temperature, the sooner we can avoid bacteria buildup. So be sure to have the cooler with an ice bath ready.*

*What's the difference between stock and broth? Typically broth is made with meat (often times along with some bones) whereas stock is usually just the bones. In the grocery store, you'll see both on the shelves, as the USDA does not differentiate between the two. In my humble opinion, stock has a richer flavor – especially when you make your own.*

---

| | |
|---|---|
| 3–4 | pounds (2 kg) chicken bones—necks, wings, whole carcass, etc. |
| 1 | onion, quartered |
| 3 | cloves garlic, peeled |
| 1 | celery heart, chopped |
| 3 | bay leaves |
| 3 | sprigs Italian parsley, chopped |

1. Place all ingredients into a large soup pot.
2. Add enough water to cover all the chicken and aromatics.
3. Invert a metal colander or steamer basket over the chicken and aromatics. This will make the skimming process much easier!
4. Bring water up to a fast simmer, and continue simmering for approximately 90–120 minutes, skimming scum off the top frequently.
5. Remove from heat and strain out all the solids.
6. Pour the stock into a container and place into a cooler with plenty of ice to surround the container.
7. Once the stock has cooled, the fat will congeal on the surface. Spoon off excess fat the following day and freeze whatever stock you don't need immediately.

---

**Variation**—*While this recipe is technically a stock, chicken broth is almost the same process—but you can reduce the simmer time to about 60 minutes in total. To make the chicken broth, use a whole chicken, and stuff the aromatics into the cavity of the bird. Then you have all that cooked chicken meat to use for some chicken salad, chicken soup, you name it!*

**Plan Ahead**—*Freeze a few bottles of water (please remove the labels). You can toss them in the container of your stock when you are ready to cool and they will help lower the temperature more quickly. Freeze your stock in smaller portions for future use with other recipes.*

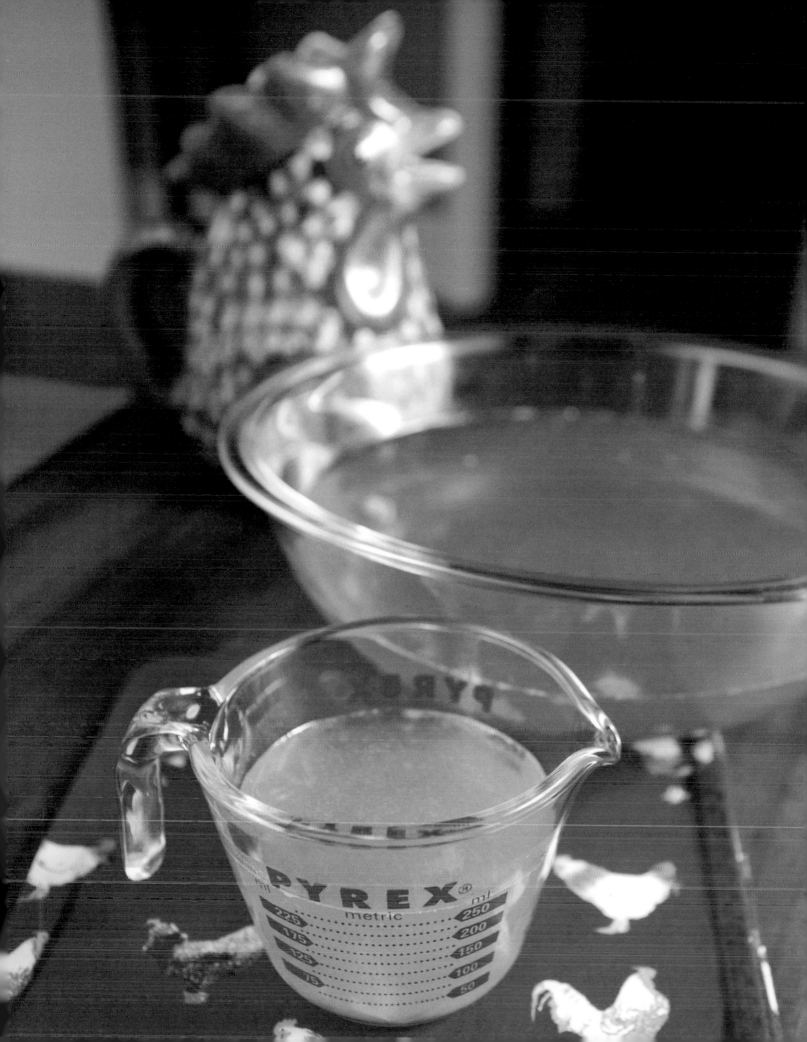

# basic biscuits

*We quoted this statement from Andrew Badenoch in the introduction, and we'll repeat it here: "Paleo is a logical framework applied to modern humans, not a historical reenactment."- I couldn't agree more with him. If it were to be a historical reenactment, I'd be without my Le Creuset and food processor . . . and that's where I draw the line.*

*Are most of the ingredients here ones that do not contain gluten, legumes, sugar, or dairy? If you use regular butter, there is a smidge of dairy from the milk solids, but other than that, yes, these are pretty much on the up and up. Eating them every day as a sausage-and-egg biscuit like that big chain with the golden arches isn't going to make you healthier. Once in a while, though, these are a great thing to bring to a brunch or serve on a lazy weekend for you and your family.*

| | |
|---|---|
| 6 | large egg whites |
| ¼ | cup (40 g) coconut flour |
| ¾ | cup (120 g) blanched almond flour |
| 1 | teaspoon baking powder |
| 1½ | tablespoons grass-fed butter or coconut oil |
| ~ | dash of salt (optional) |

1. In a bowl, whisk the egg whites until they are very frothy.
2. In a separate bowl, mix the two flours and baking powder, and then with a knife or fork, cut in the cold butter (or coconut oil) and add salt if using. You want to make a crumbly mixture. Let this sit in the refrigerator for 15–20 minutes.
3. Preheat oven to 400°F (205°C).
4. Remove flour/butter mixture from refrigerator, and gently fold in the egg whites, stirring to combine.
5. Spoon the biscuit batter onto a greased sheet pan or into muffin tins. Personally I like to form them into smooth biscuit shapes.
6. Bake for 12–15 minutes or until golden brown.

**Variations**—*If dairy is in your life, try these with some shredded cheddar cheese and chopped pickled jalapeños mixed in. Some crumbled-up crispy bacon in these is also awesome!*

**Tips & Tricks**—*If you ever have a need/hankering for "breadcrumbs," use these biscuits! Cut them in half and toast them in the oven to dry them out. Toss them in a food processor or blender to get them broken down into the crumbs, lay them out on a sheet pan, and toast until crispy.*

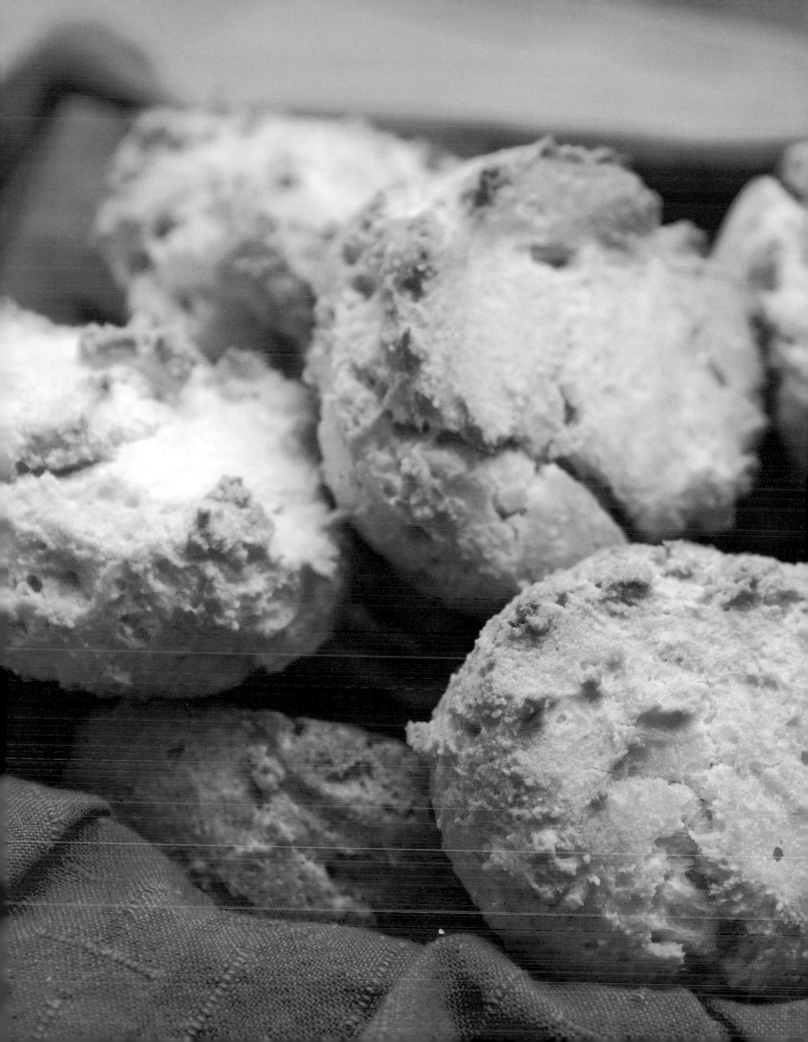

# coconut flour tortillas

*These tortillas opened a whole new door of possibilities for us. Given that they are a little bit labor intensive, they aren't something I suggest every day, but once in a while it's nice to have that tortilla to wrap some meaty goodness into.*

*I'm amazed at how well these tortillas hold up to heat (as in when baking enchiladas). Yes, they are much more fragile than typical corn or flour tortillas, but they still get the job done. We tested these out on some clients at our gym a while back and they indeed were a hit, especially when dipped in guacamole! It's really critical to have a good non-stick pan for these, as otherwise you'll have a heck of a time getting these tortillas to release from the skillet.*

| | |
|---|---|
| ¼ | cup (40 g) coconut flour |
| 8 | large egg whites |
| ¼ | teaspoon baking powder |
| ½ | cup (125 mL) water |
| ~ | coconut oil |

1. Whisk all ingredients together in a bowl, making sure no lumps remain. If you want thinner tortillas, add 1–2 teaspoons more water.

2. Preheat a small nonstick skillet over medium heat. Place about 1 teaspoon coconut oil in the pan. Swirl around to coat.

3. Pour about 3 tablespoons of the batter into the pan, tipping the pan from side to side while you pour in the batter (to get a very thin tortilla). Do not attempt to flip the tortilla unit you are sure the first side is golden brown. Otherwise, the tortilla will rip.

4. Once nice and golden brown, flip over and brown on opposite side. Remove to plate, and repeat process (adding in some coconut oil, the batter, etc.). You should get about 8–10 medium-sized tortillas (if you make yours very thick, you will get less).

**Variations**—*You could try doing cumin-spiced tortillas, chili-spiced, or for more of a treat, some cinnamon or nutmeg would be lovely.*

**Do Ahead**—*Make these a day or two in advance, store them in a ziplock bag, and then reheat when you need them.*

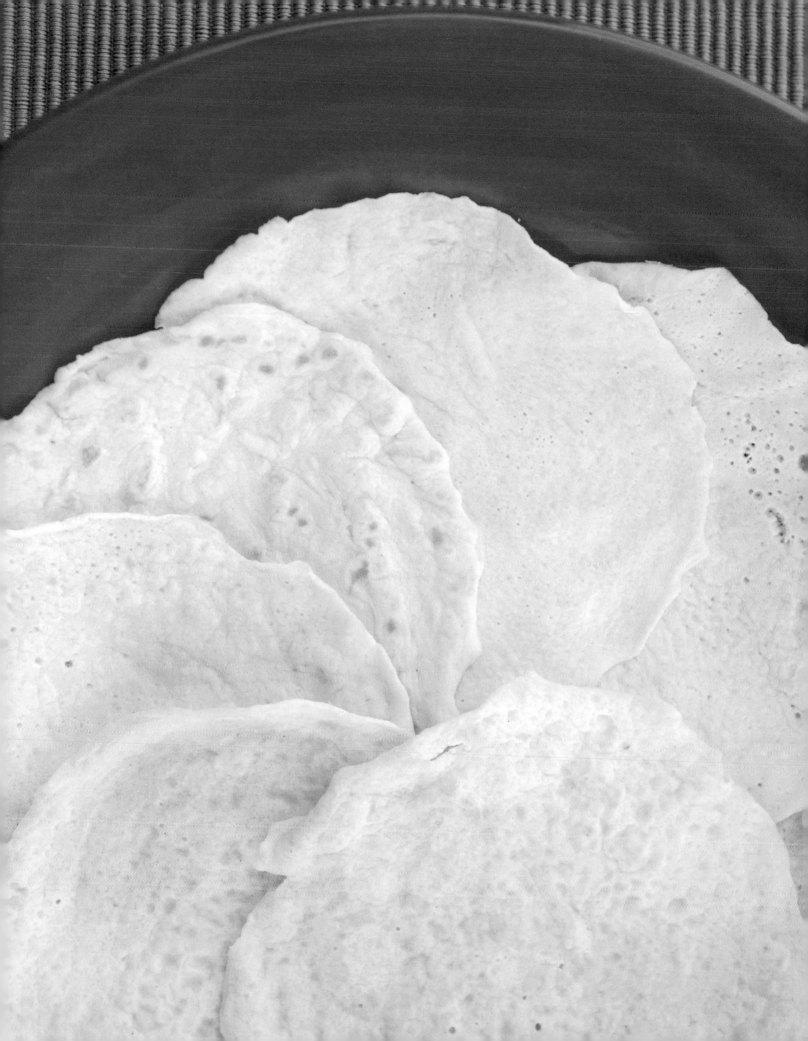

# pumpkin pancakes

*Sometimes, life calls for some pancakes. Yes, these are paleo friendly, but if leaning out is your objective, save these for special occasions and do not make them your everyday breakfast. That said, for those mornings that do call for a little dose of comfort, whip up a batch of these, and serve with a dense protein source. I like to serve these pancakes with turkey or chicken sausage.*

| | |
|---|---|
| 4 | large eggs |
| 4 | large egg whites |
| 1 | cup (250 mL) canned pumpkin |
| ½ | cup (75 g) almond flour |
| 1 | teaspoon baking powder |
| ¼ | cup (125 mL) coconut milk |
| 1 | teaspoon vanilla |
| ½ | teaspoon nutmeg |
| 1 | teaspoon cinnamon |
| ½ | cup (50 g) pecans, crushed (optional) |
| 1-2 | tablespoons butter or coconut oil |

1. Mix all ingredients in large bowl except optional pecans.

2. Heat a griddle or large skillet to medium heat and coat griddle/pan with butter or other fat source when hot.

3. From here, traditional pancake rules apply with a slight modification. These will not bubble like your traditional pancakes. The batter is a bit thicker. On medium heat the first side takes about 2-3 minutes to brown then another 1-3 minutes on the other side.

**Variations**—*We're fans of adding a few chopped nuts on top of a freshly poured pancake. You can also top a stack of these beauties with a few berries, or mix into the batter some finely chopped apples for a little sweetness.*

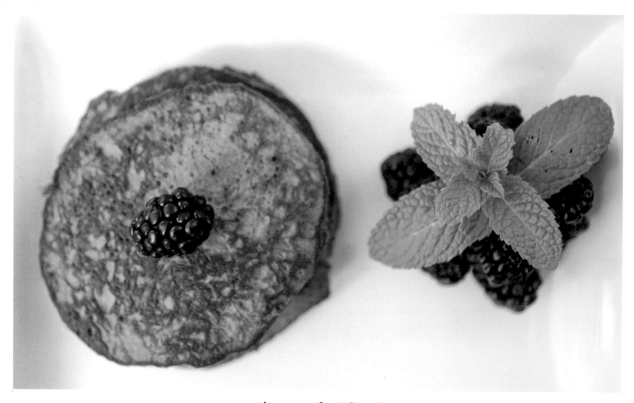

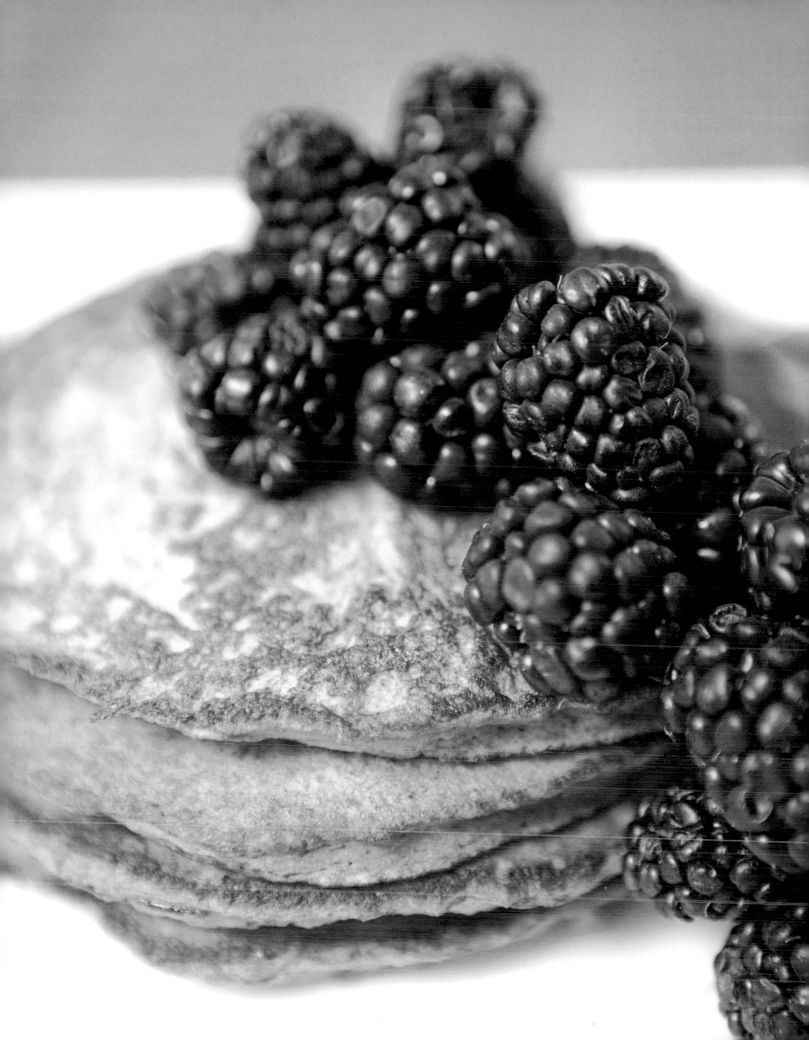

# nutty pie crust

*Whenever my mom would ask me to make "Sullivan's Apple Pie" for a holiday meal, my least favorite part was making the crust. Not because it wasn't easy, because it was (we had a super-easy recipe from the Women's Guild in my hometown). I was simply never a fan of crust However, this recipe changed all that for me. The crunch of the pecans and the slight bit of sweet make this crust delicious. The only drawback I've seen with some of these nut flour–based crusts is that they aren't as flakey as you'd get with a standard flour-based crust, and they are a little more fragile, but since they won't upset your tummy for days, I think it's a great compromise.*

| | |
|---|---|
| 1 | cup (150 g) almond flour |
| ½ | cup (60 g) pecans, roughly chopped |
| ~ | pinch sea salt |
| ¼ | cup (65 mL) coconut oil (melted) or butter (softened) |
| 2 | tablespoons honey (optional) |
| 1 | teaspoon vanilla extract |

1. Preheat oven to 350°F (175°C).

2. Combine the almond flour, pecans and pinch of salt in a large bowl.

3. In another bowl, combine the oil (or butter), honey, and vanilla extract.

4. Stir the wet ingredients into to the dry until completely combined. Using your fingers, press the dough into a 9½-inch (24 cm) pie pan.

5. Bake for 12–14 minutes or until the crust is golden brown.

6. Remove and set on baking rack to cool, making certain to let it cool completely before filling.

**Variations**—*You can use Steve's Paleo Krunch (www.stevesclub.org) in place of the pecans, which is super tasty. Just pulse the Krunch a few times in the food processor to eliminate any super-big chunks. Just about any nuts would be wonderful in this crust.*

**Do Ahead**—*You can always make this crust a day or two in advance before you make your pie.*

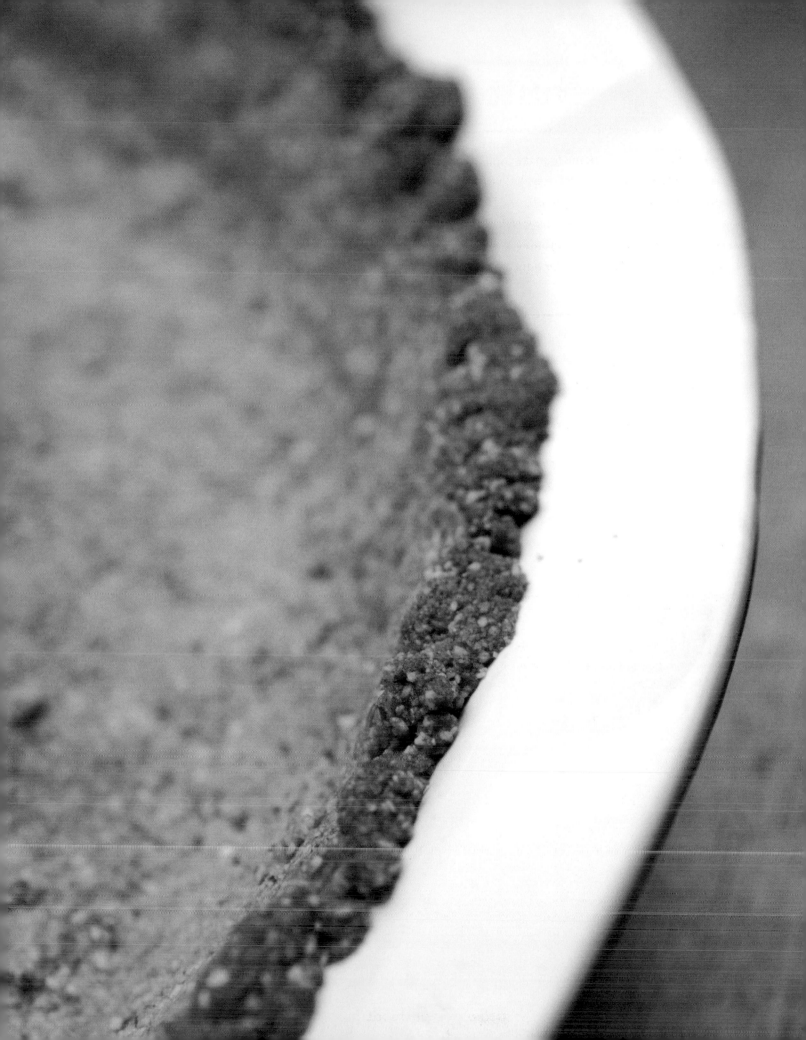

# basic bread loaf

*Bread and paleo don't really go together. But every once in a while—like the one time I've been sick since going paleo— toast just sounded good. Here's a recipe for those times that you're wanting a comforting slice of toast but without some of the irritation from a gluten-containing bread. It won't taste like the Wonder bread of your youth, but it still gets the job done. If I had kids, I might even be inclined to make a school snack of a slice of this with some almond butter and apple slices as a "sandwich."*

| | |
|---|---|
| 3½ | cups (500 g) almond flour |
| ¾ | teaspoon baking soda |
| ¼ | teaspoon salt |
| 4 | large eggs |
| 1 | tablespoon honey |
| ¾ | teaspoon apple cider vinegar |

1. Preheat oven to 300°F (150°C).
2. Combine all the dry ingredients.
3. In a separate bowl, whisk the eggs, then add in the honey and apple cider vinegar.
4. Pour the batter into a well-greased loaf pan.
5. Bake for 45 minutes or so, or until bread is golden brown and a wooden skewer comes out clean when inserted.

**Variation**—*This bread variation is great to use in making a paleo-friendly stuffing for Thanksgiving. Simply stir about 1–2 teaspoons each of sage, rosemary, and thyme into the bread mixture. When the loaf is done cooking, dice the bread into cubes, toast them in the oven (to dehydrate and make crispy) and use like you would other bread for stuffing (aka dressing).*

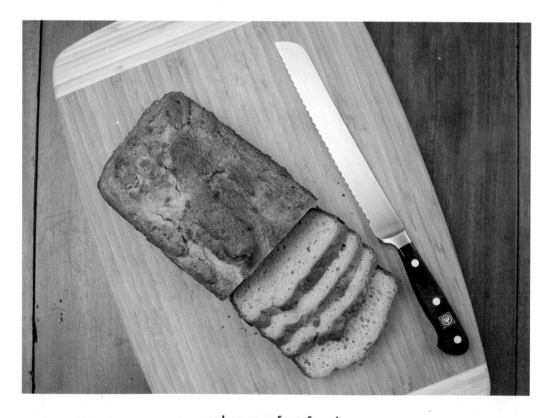

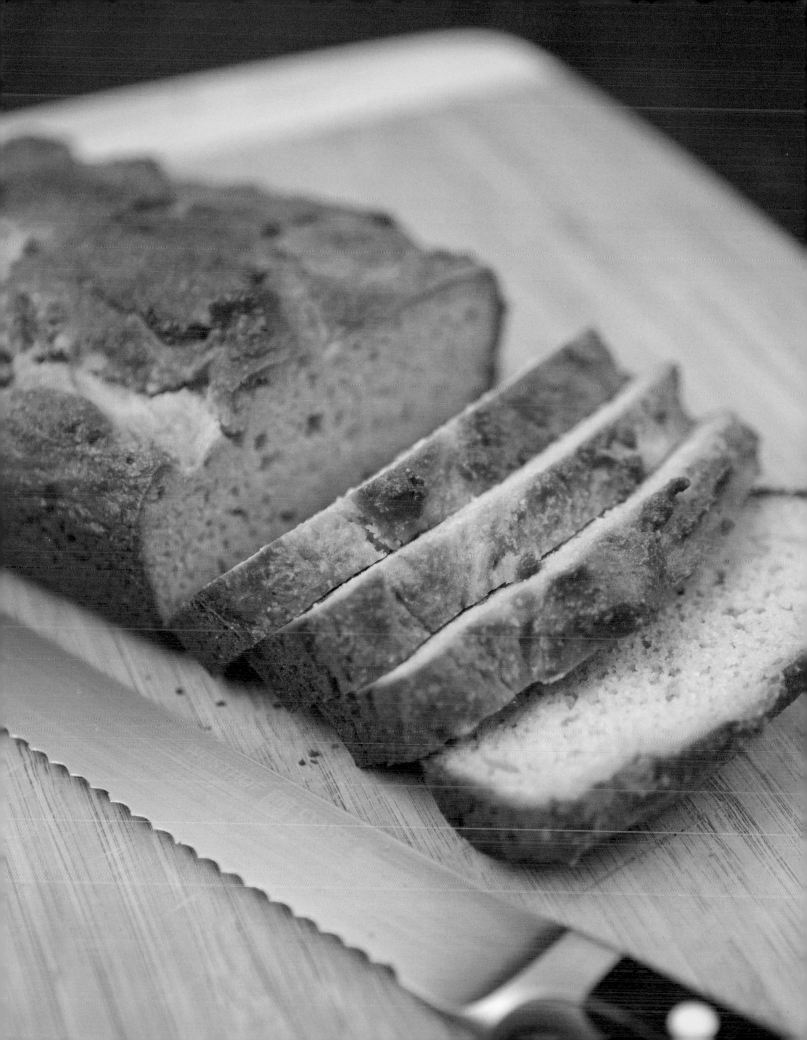

# dad's famous secret dry rub

*My dad, Scottie Mayfield, does a number of things extremely well. Smoking, barbecuing, and grilling meat are definitely things he does well. When dad is cooking, it usually involves a large quantity of meat. I will say that having this mixture in the kitchen can come in very handy in a pinch. When you are finished making this big batch of tastiness, seal some of it up in smaller containers and tuck them away for later.*

*Dad orders most of his spices from Penzey's (penzeys.com). If you haven't been to a store or their website, you don't know what you're missing. They have it all and at very reasonable prices. This recipe will set you back about $60 and can last your average griller well over a year.*

---

| | |
|---|---|
| ½ | cup (12 g) French thyme |
| ½ | cup (12 g) Four Peppercorn Blend, ground |
| ½ | pound (230 g) sea salt |
| 4 | ounces (113 g) onion powder |
| 4 | ounces (113 g) ground cumin |
| 4 | ounces (113 g) ancho chili powder |
| 4 | ounces (113 g) turmeric, powdered |
| 4 | ounces (113 g) minced garlic |
| 4 | ounces (113 g) sweet paprika |
| 4 | ounces (113 g) cracked rosemary |
| 8 | ounces (226 g) mustard powder |
| 8 | ounces (226 g) California seasoned pepper, Penzey Special |
| 4 | ounces (113 g) cayenne pepper, ground |

1. Combine all ingredients into large container.
2. Shake it on your favorite meat anytime to remember why you made it in the first place.

---

**Variations**—*For those Paleo perfectionists, cut the salt out of this rub. Feel free to cut this recipe in half or fourths if you like.*

**Tips & Tricks**—*If you have a vacuum sealer, bag up smaller portions of this and seal them to retain freshness.*

# easy dry rub

*If my dad's famous recipe seems a bit daunting, try this one on for size. All of these ingredients can be found in your local grocery store. There is really no wrong way to do a dry rub. You'll always want to pay attention to how much salt you add and you always have the option of omitting. Other than that, let your creativity flow far past this recipe. This keeps great in an airtight container for several weeks. It's also a great gift to a host or hostess for those summertime barbeques.*

| | |
|---|---|
| 3 | tablespoons black peppercorns |
| 1 | tablespoon rosemary leaves |
| 1 | tablespoon chipotle powder |
| 2 | teaspoons garlic powder |
| 1 | teaspoon paprika |
| 1 | tablespoon mustard powder |
| 1 | teaspoon sea salt |

**1.** Blend peppercorns and rosemary in coffee grinder, Magic Bullet or Mortar & Pestle.

**2.** Combine all ingredients in small bowl and store in an airtight container until ready to use.

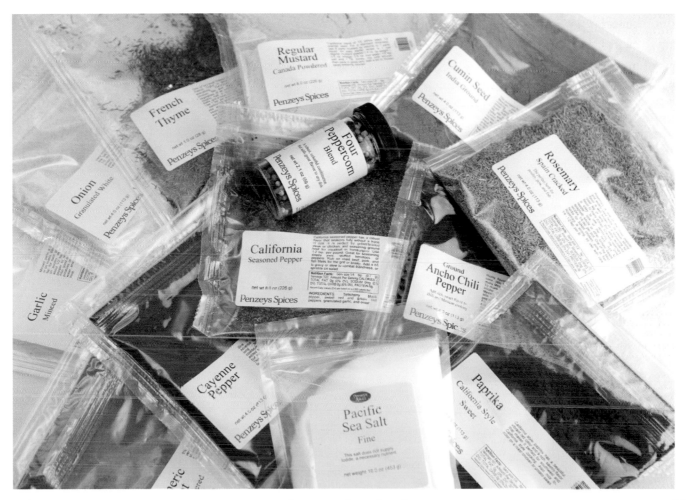

# dill pickles

*Our canning endeavors always include pickles. My (Charles') brother Michael grew the most amazing cucumbers a few years ago. We were in Tennessee buying up some of his produce and picked up a batch of the ones labeled "Canning Cukes." They are great to garnish any summertime meal with and a perfect snack on the go. Be careful. The canning bug can get a hold of you and not let go.*

| | |
|---|---|
| 5 | pounds (2.25 kg) cucumbers, sliced into spears, ends removed |
| ½ | cup (100 g) salt |
| 3 | cups (300 g) ice cubes |
| 2 | cups (500 mL) water |
| 4 | cups (1 L) distilled vinegar |
| 10 | cloves garlic, peeled |
| 2 | tablespoons dill seed |
| 1 | teaspoon celery seed |
| 2 | teaspoons peppercorns |
| 6 | 1 pint (473 mL) jars, along with 6 new jar caps and canning jar bands |

1. Once the ends are removed from the cucumbers, cut them to fit into pint-size jars. In a large bowl, layer cucumbers, salt, and ice cubes. You'll want to drain and rinse them in about 2 hours.

2. Boil enough water in large pot to cover standing jars.

3. Once water is boiling, use canning tongs to lift jars in and out of the water. On your first jar, pour the boiling water into a bowl containing your jar caps to soften the rubber seals.

4. Place the hot, sterilized jars on a towel-covered kitchen surface.

5. Combine water, vinegar, garlic, dill seed, celery seed, and peppercorns in medium saucepan. Be sure you have a nonreactive pan.

6. Bring the brine to a boil. Meanwhile, drain/rinse your cucumbers and stuff them snuggly into each jar. Once brine is boiling, pour mixture over cucumbers in jars. You'll want to leave some space toward the top of the jar (about ½ inch).

7. Using a chopstick or skewer, poke and prod around the jars to release any bubbles that may still be lingering.

8. Once you have the jars filled, use a magnetic tool to place the caps on each jar. Be careful to put them on straight. Screw on bands to just fingertip tight. If you don't have a canning rack to lay in the bottom of your pot, just lay some extra jar rings in the bottom so the water can boil around your jars.

9. Gently place jars into pot of hot water (from before) You'll want there to be 1–2 inches of water covering the tops of the jars when they are all in there. Bring water to boil and leave boiling for 10 minutes. Turn heat off, remove lid to pot and let sit for 5 minutes.

10. Using canning tongs, remove jars individually onto towel and let sit for 24 hours. Check seals and store in cool place for up to a year.

**Variation**—*Throw a hot pepper in a jar or two to add some kick.*

**Tips & Tricks**—*Bite the bullet and get a canning kit. You can find them online for around $20. You'll also need the jars and tops. You can reuse the jars and bands each year, but you will need new caps.*

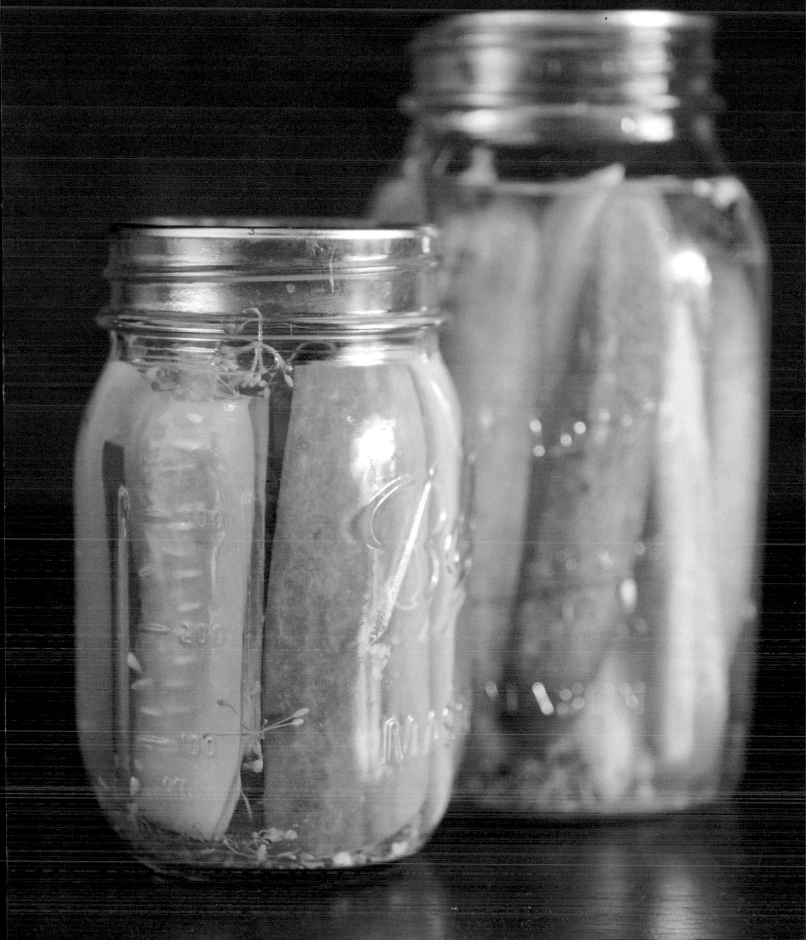

# tomato sauce

*We have two approaches to this wonderful sauce and it all depends on whether or not we are eating it that day. If you can't wait, serve this simple sauce over spaghetti squash and enjoy.*

*Our other approach with this is to double or triple the batch and can the sauce for the colder months when fresh tomatoes aren't available. Chances are you can find a local market or farm to buy a box of Roma tomatoes to turn into something you'll enjoy all winter long. Any tomatoes will do. We grow quite a few heirloom tomatoes in the yard. They can add color and sweetness (depending on the type) if you throw in a few different kinds.*

| | |
|---|---|
| 20 | tomatoes, peeled and chopped |
| ¼ | cup (65 mL) olive oil |
| 3 | cloves garlic, minced |
| 1 | large onion, chopped |
| 1 | green pepper, chopped |
| 1 | tablespoon fresh basil |
| 1 | teaspoon dried oregano |
| ½ | teaspoon salt (optional) |
| 1 | teaspoon pepper |

**1.** To peel tomatoes, submerge in hot water for 1-2 minutes, then remove immediately to a bath of ice water. Skins should peel off very easily.

**2.** Chop tomatoes and place in a large bowl.

**3.** Heat olive oil in large pot and sauté garlic, onions, and peppers until onions become translucent. Throw in your basil and allow it to darken.

**4.** Add in your tomatoes, oregano, salt, and pepper. Bring entire mixture to a boil, reduce heat and simmer for about 2 hours.

**5.** Stir occasionally to keep things from sticking to the bottom.

**Variations**—*Add chopped jalapeños for hot, habaneros for super hot. Be sure to sauté them a bit. If you are looking for some protein, throw in two pounds (1 kg) of your favorite cooked ground meat for the last 20 or 30 minutes of simmering.*

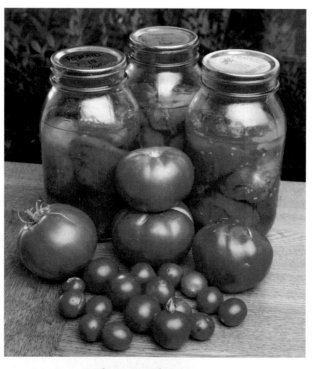

paleo comfort foods

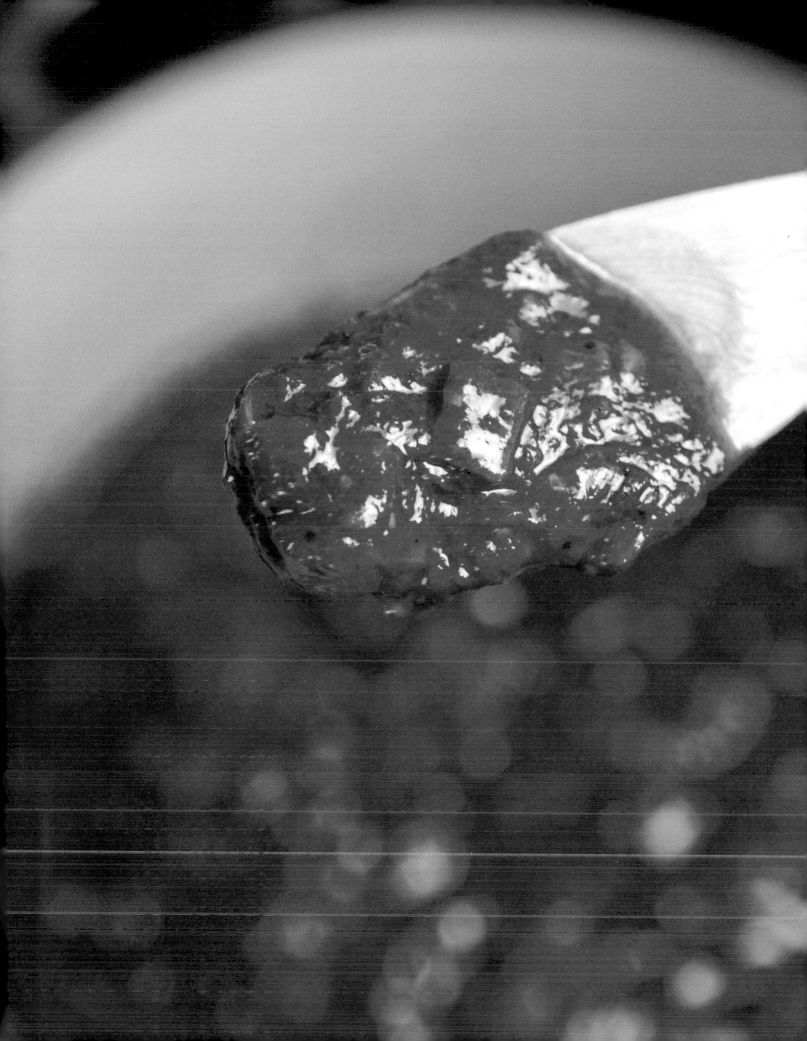

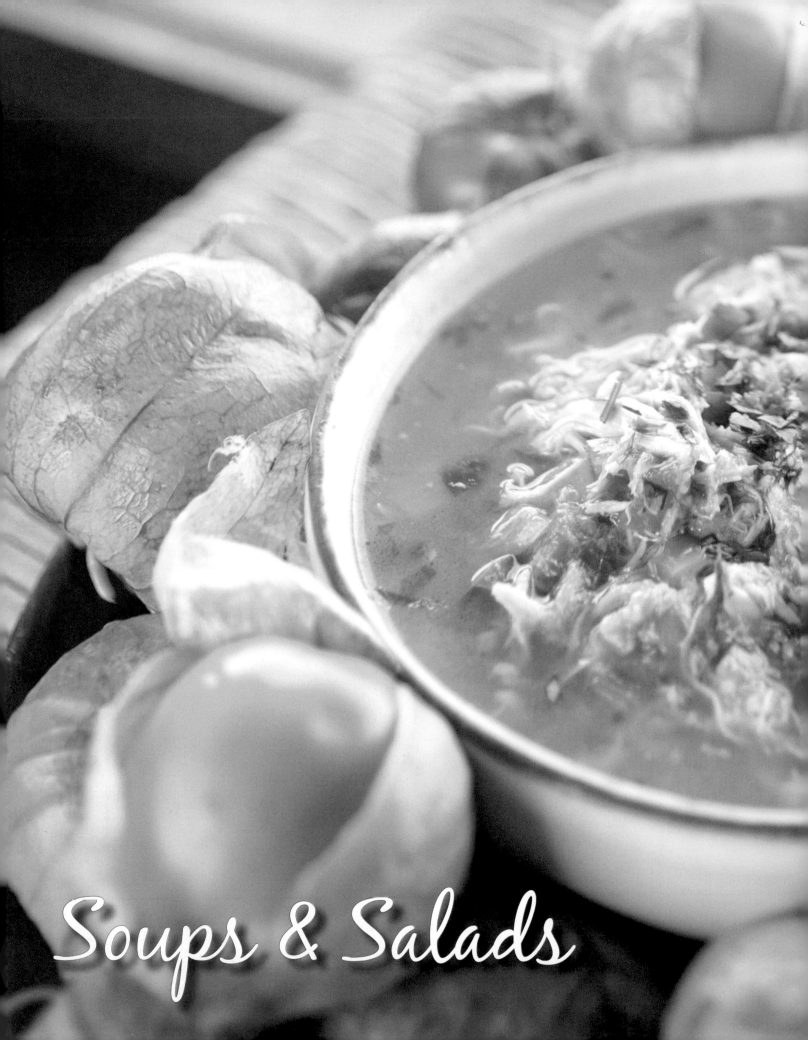

Soups & Salads

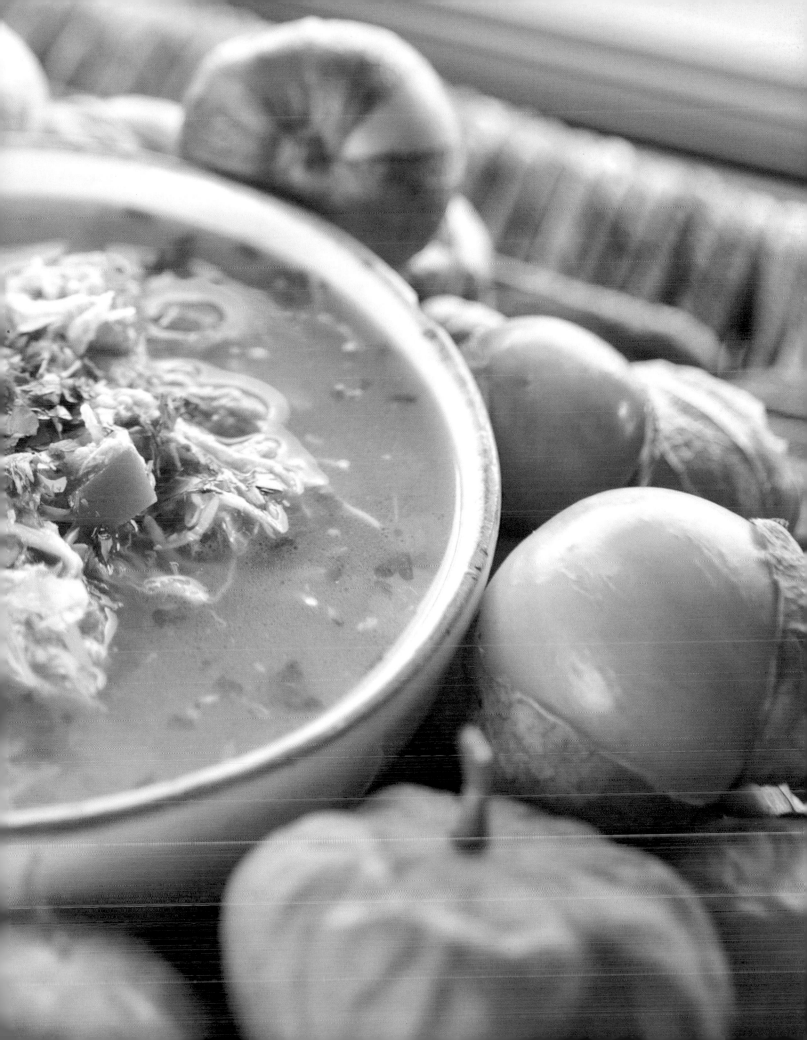

# chicken & grape salad

*Great for picnics and tailgating, chicken salad is a Southern staple. There are a thousand different ways to make this stuff. This recipe is a bit chunkier than most folks are used to. Serve on sliced cucumber or zucchini as an appetizer or spoon into romaine lettuce leaves and serve as a meal.*

| | |
|---|---|
| 1½–2 | pounds (1 kg) chicken breasts |
| 1 | cup (100 g) celery, finely chopped |
| 1 | small onion, minced |
| 1 | cup (175 g) seedless grapes, sliced |
| 1 | tablespoon Dijon mustard |
| ⅛ | teaspoon salt (optional) |
| 1 | teaspoon ground mustard |
| ½ | teaspoon black pepper |
| 1½ | cups (375 mL) Paleo Mayonnaise (recipe page 100) |
| ½ | cup (60 g) walnuts, chopped |

1. Preheat oven to 350°F (175°C). Coat casserole dish with butter or olive oil.
2. Place chicken breasts in dish, sprinkle a pinch of black pepper/salt over the top and cook uncovered for 45 minutes or until chicken is cooked through.
3. Remove chicken from oven and let cool.
4. Mix all other in ingredients in large bowl.
5. Once chicken has cooled, roughly chop and combine with all other ingredients.

**Ingredients**—*Skinless chicken breasts are ideal for this recipe.*

**Variations**—*Boiling chicken also works but removes some flavor. You can also use leftover chicken in this recipe, which will spare you the cooking of the chicken step! Pressed for time and don't have access to pastured chicken? Use some store-bought precooked chicken (rotisserie, baked, etc.)*

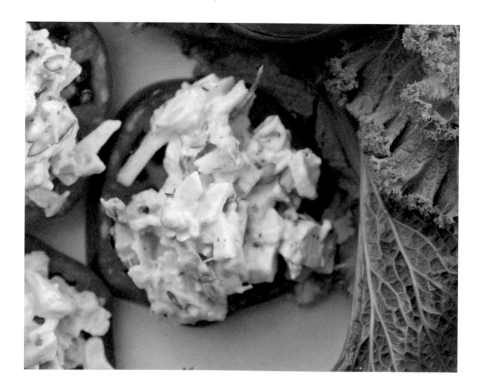

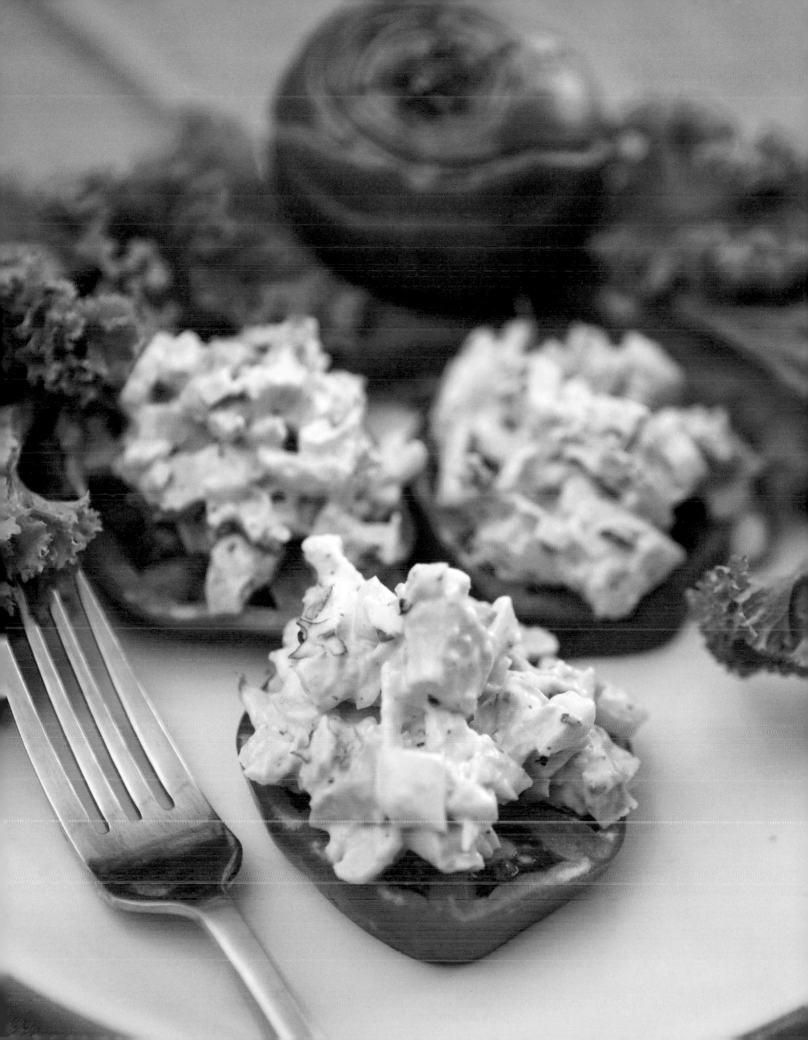

# shada's kale salad

*My (Julie's) sister-in-law, Shada, has a kitchen and cookbook collection I covet. Not to mention that she's also the one who first introduced me to Donna Hay and the Australian cooking magazine,* Delicious. *Shada is Australian, but perhaps more like a sibling to me than her husband—my brother—when it comes to our love of cooking and food.*

*Shada made this recipe when I was in town one autumn weekend. Kale has always evaded me as far as recipes were concerned, in that I was rather bored of braising it with some smoked paprika, garlic, etc. This recipe made use of fresh kale, and the resulting salad is so fresh, light, and delicious. Kale—a cooler weather green—is pretty prevalent in Georgia in the fall/winter, and I love serving this salad during that time of year, as it's almost like a taste of summer.*

| | |
|---|---|
| 1 | bunch kale washed and tough stems removed |
| 4 | radishes, chopped |
| ¾ | cup (75 g) sun-dried tomatoes, minced |
| 2 | Granny Smith apples, chopped |
| ¾ | cup (20 g) flat-leaf (Italian) parsley, chopped |
| ¾ | cup (12 g) mint, chopped |
| 1 | cup (100 g) toasted pecans |
| ~ | salt and pepper to taste |
| ½ | cup (125 mL) fresh lemon juice |
| ½ | cup (125 mL) olive oil |

1. Chop the kale into very small pieces.
2. Mix the rest of the ingredients except for the lemon juice and oil in a large bowl.
3. Whisk together lemon juice and olive oil, then pour over salad and toss (I like to massage it all with my very clean hands).
4. Refrigerate until ready to serve.

**Variations**—*There is no limit to what you can add or subtract from this salad. My sister-in-law served it with some of her homegrown and dried tomatoes, feta cheese, and a few other items. I've been meaning to try some chopped up jicama in this, some fresh avocado, or some toasted pine nuts. The other night I used some pears and cucumber, and it was—as expected—really tasty!*

**Tips & Tricks**—*If you plan on doing this ahead and having some leftovers, make sure the apple gets doused well in some lemon juice, or else it will brown. Or, you can just leave it out and add at the last minute.*

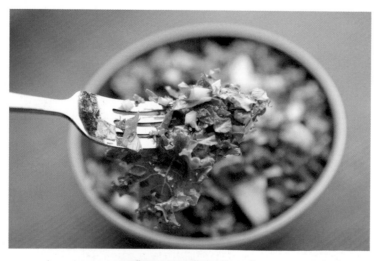

paleo comfort foods

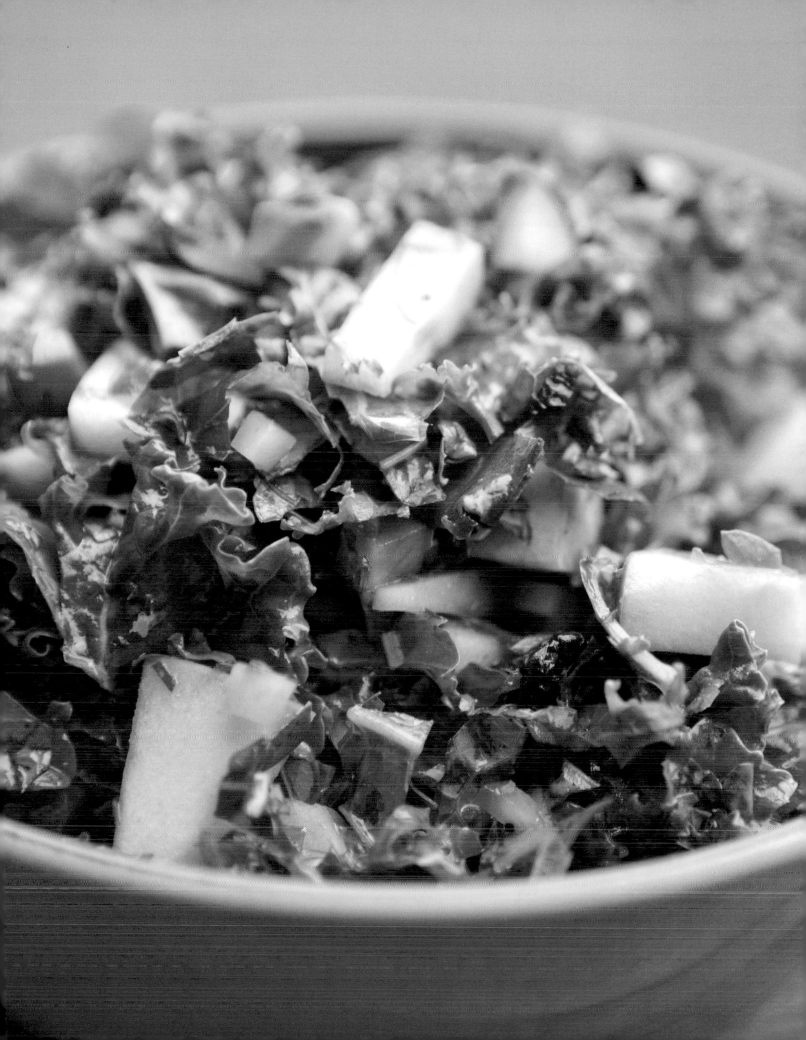

# creamy caesar salad

Yes, it is very random that the Caesar salad was reportedly first made in Tijuana, Mexico. Almost as random as the fact that I spent one New Year's Eve eating really good Chinese food in Tijuana followed by seeing a Beatles cover band.

I digress. As the story goes, Caesar Cardini ran a restaurant in Tijuana back in the early 1920s that catered to Southern California clientele, who would go to Mexico to be free of Prohibition and get their drink on. As some of the lore has it, on a busy July 4th in the 1920s, Cardini's ran out of most restaurant staples, so the folks in for dinner just asked him to make whatever he could. Cardini evidently concocted his namesake salad, prepared tableside, and thus the salad was born. Rumor has it that Cardini was very much opposed to anchovies in his dressing, and the original recipe did not call for such. However, anchovies—which are very rich in that lovely "umami" taste—are a natural source of glutamate, and they add a complex, salty flavor that is hard to replicate without a bunch of unnatural stuff.

I do call for some Worcestershire sauce in this. You can make your own version of the sauce, or look for a brand that does not have any gluten contained. I found one brand that has no wheat/gluten, but had a smidge of evaporated cane juice. I was okay with that. If you aren't, just keep it out!

Many recipes call for coddling the egg before adding it to the dressing. Essentially, this is almost like poaching the egg (you can coddle the egg either in its shell or in a special egg coddler). I usually just use the freshest eggs I can and skip the coddling!

---

| | |
|---|---|
| ~ | juice of ½ lemon |
| 1 | teaspoon Worcestershire sauce |
| 4 | anchovies |
| 3 | garlic cloves minced |
| 1 | large egg |
| 1 | teaspoon Dijon mustard |
| 1 | tablespoon Paleo Mayonnaise (page 100) |
| ½ | cup (125 mL) olive oil |
| 1 | head romaine lettuce, leaves torn into bite-sized pieces |

1. Take all dressing ingredients except olive oil and blend in food processor.

2. When mixed well, slowly add the olive oil while the processor is running.

3. Place some of the dressing in the bottom of a wooden bowl, and toss in lettuce leaves to combine. Add more dressing as desired. Serve immediately.

---

**Variations**—If I was going to be cheating with some dairy, or following a lacto-paleo diet, I'd for certain add in some fresh shaved Parmigiano-reggiano to my Caesar salad! To make this salad into a meal, top your salad with some grilled chicken, grilled salmon, or grilled shrimp.

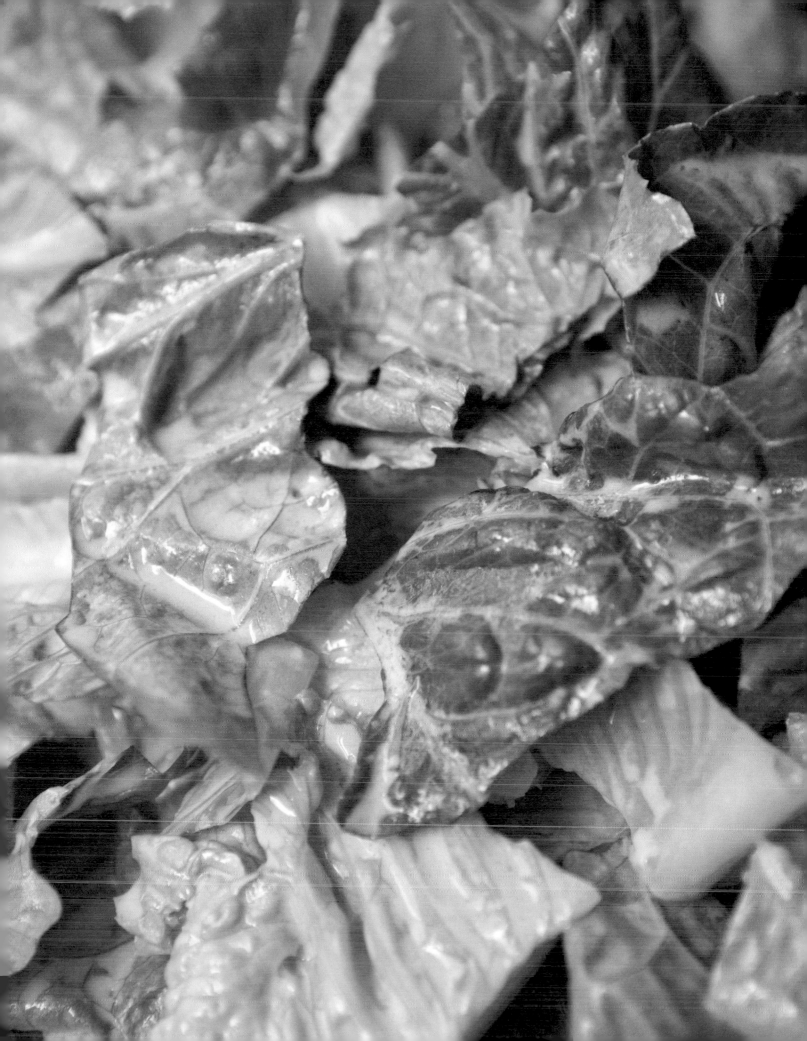

# summertime tomato salad

*I love tomatoes, and love that Charles and I both take great pride in our tomato crops. So much so that in the summer it became our ritual on Friday nights after work to go and pick fresh tomatoes out of our garden, and we would then go and make a fresh salad with the bounty. On one such Friday night, we were out picking tomatoes and Charles told me that he thought there was a ripe Cherokee purple tomato around the corner . . . and there were several, along with a beautiful engagement ring. Whether it's an engagement ring, or some of the ripe tomatoes from our 15+ varieties in the garden, I love going out to our garden and seeing what treasures await! Tomatoes prepared in their most natural state—like in this recipe, sliced up with some fresh basil from the garden—is indeed our definition of summertime on a plate and is what this recipe is all about!*

| | |
|---|---|
| 1–2 | pounds (.5–1 kg) assorted fresh tomatoes, sliced into wedges |
| ½ | cup (12 g) fresh basil, chopped |

### For the vinaigrette

| | |
|---|---|
| 1 | tablespoon balsamic vinegar |
| 1 | clove garlic |
| 3 | tablespoons olive oil |
| ~ | fresh cracked pepper to taste |

1. Place sliced tomatoes and basil onto a platter or in a large bowl.
2. In a Magic Bullet or other mini-chopper, combine the balsamic and garlic, and then add in the olive oil. You can also just whisk by hand, and chop the garlic by hand.
3. Pour the dressing over the tomato/basil mixture, and season with some fresh cracked pepper. Eat immediately and enjoy!

**Variations—***If you are allowing some dairy into your life, fresh mozzarella is absolutely sublime with this dish. If you want more "zing" with this recipe, add in some sliced-up red onions.*

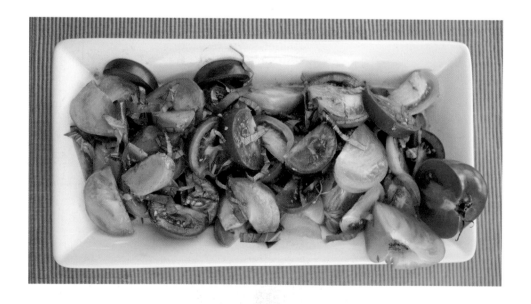

paleo comfort foods

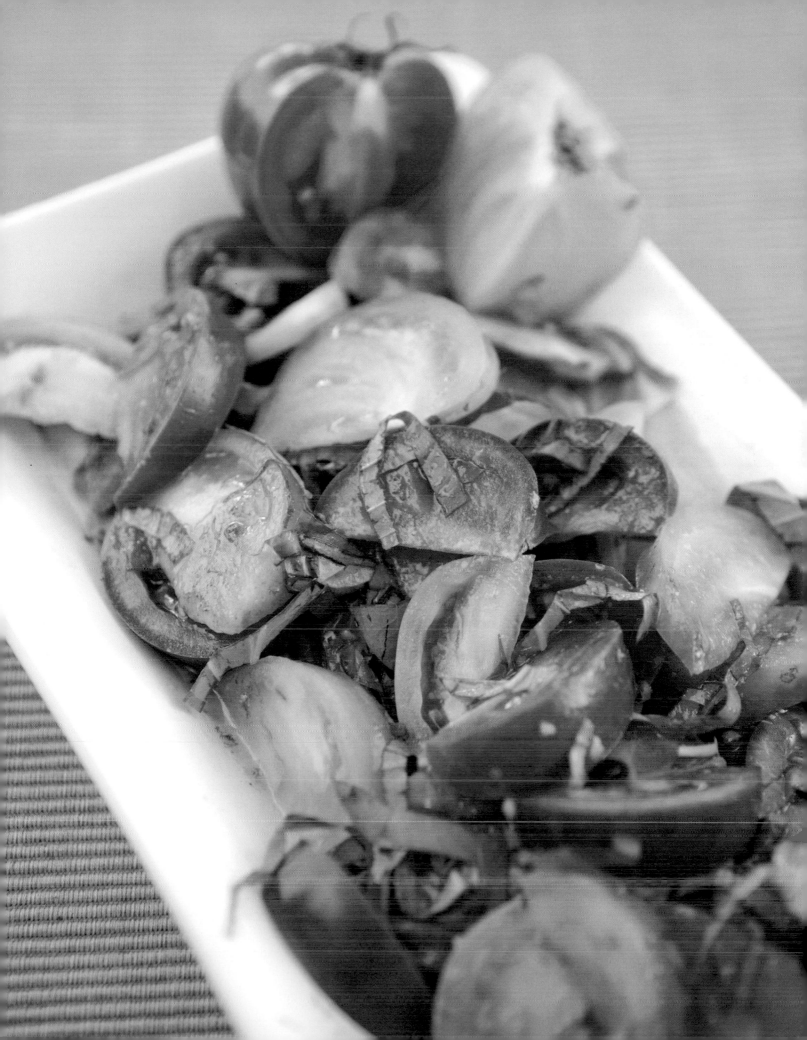

# cucumber & watermelon salad

*Watermelon combined with the crunch of cucumber makes for a light, almost spa-like side salad, one that's almost sweet enough to be classified as dessert. This salad is great for your summertime picnics and potluck brunches.*

*It's a little known fact that Cordele, Georgia, is the watermelon capital of the world. This might explain why there are always so many watermelons available in this neck of the woods come summertime. Some tips for picking a ripe watermelon: look for symmetry (whether round or oval), firmness, and no bruises, as well as for the end that was touching the ground during growing to have a slight yellow color (as opposed to white). As watermelons are composed mostly of water, a ripe watermelon will feel heavy for its size.*

*Watermelon is pretty much nature's candy, so depending on your insulin issues, you might want to go easy on this one and save as a special treat.*

---

| | |
|---|---|
| 4 | **cups (600 g) watermelon, deseeded and either cubed or shaped into balls using a melon baller** |
| 2 | **cups (300 g) English cucumber, sliced** |
| 3 | **tablespoons fresh mint, chopped** |
| ¼ | **cup (60 mL) fresh squeezed lime juice** |
| 1–2 | **teaspoons balsamic vinegar (optional)** |

**1.** This truly is as easy as it sounds. Take the watermelon, cucumber, mint, and lime juice, and mix in a bowl.

**2.** Season with salt and pepper to taste.

---

**Variations**—*If you are personally okay with dairy, try this one with some feta cheese. This recipe is also tasty with about a tablespoon of balsamic vinegar added in.*

**Do Ahead**—*You can prep the watermelon, cucumber and mint ahead of time, but don't add the lime juice or any salt until it is close to time to serve.*

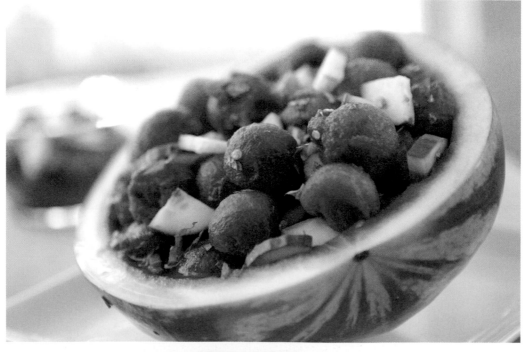

paleo comfort foods

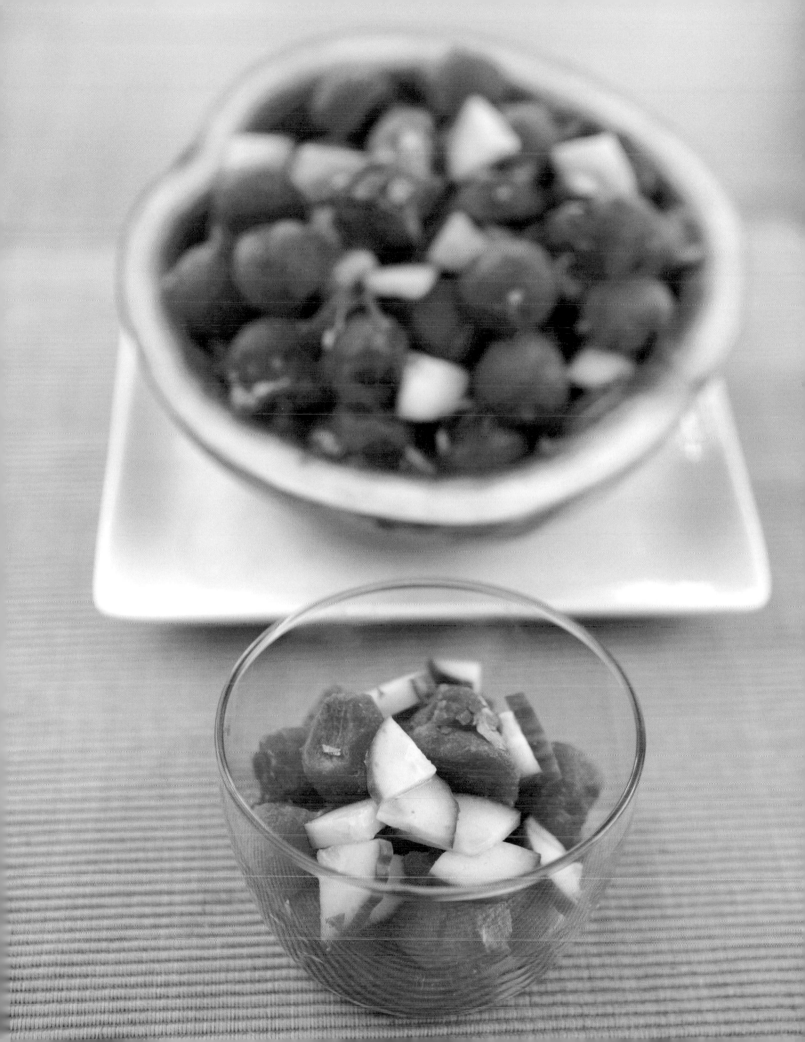

# simple shrimp salad

*Eating a hearty beef stew when it's 90 degrees in the shade isn't really my cup of tea. Summer is typically chock full of salads and things that have little to no heat required—save for grilled items. Shrimp salad, chicken salad, tuna salad, these are all great variations on a theme to add to your recipe repertoire. Having different ways to prepare these will enable you to stave off boredom by eating similar—but very different—salads in the summer.*

| | |
|---|---|
| 1 | pound (450 g) shrimp, boiled, peeled and deveined |
| ½ | cup (125 mL) Paleo Mayonnaise (recipe page 100) |
| 1 | teaspoon Dijon mustard |
| ½ | teaspoon white wine vinegar or white wine |
| 2 | teaspoons fresh parsley or dill, minced |
| 2 | tablespoons minced green onions |
| 1 | stalk celery, minced |

1. Chop the cooked shrimp into small chunks and place in a bowl along with the mayonnaise, mustard, vinegar, dill, green onion, and celery.

2. Stir until well combined, then refrigerate until ready to serve.

**Variation**—*Grilled shrimp or pickled shrimp in this recipe add an entirely new flavor dimension that is super tasty as well.*

**Hint**—*This goes great served over mixed greens, or as an appetizer on top of cucumber rounds.*

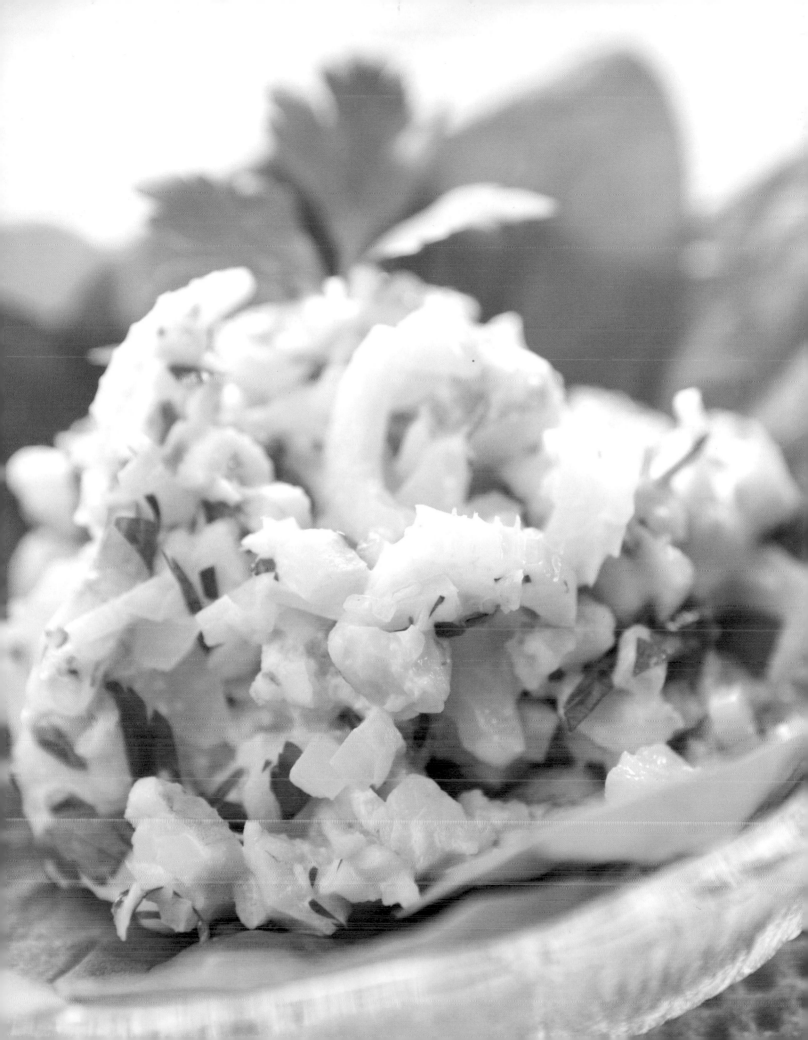

# tomato and orange salad

*This recipe stems from my days working with Melanie and Taji of Simple Gourmet—way before I had ever heard of paleo. I think one summer we must have had close to fifty groups make a variation of this recipe for their culinary team-building events. Regardless of how many times I've made it, I have never tired of it.*

*This salad pairs exceptionally well with some simple grilled chicken or salmon. And nothing beats tomatoes from your own garden for this creation!*

| | |
|---|---|
| 2 | pints (1 L) grape, cherry or sungold tomatoes, halved crosswise |
| 1 | small shallot, minced |
| ~ | zest of 1 orange |
| 2 | teaspoons fresh-squeezed orange juice (from the orange you just zested) |
| ⅓ | cup (80 mL) olive oil |
| 1 | tablespoon red wine vinegar |
| 2 | tablespoons fresh basil, chopped |
| ~ | salt and pepper to taste |
| 1 | bag arugula, washed |

1. Place all tomatoes in large mixing bowl.
2. Add shallots and orange zest.
3. Using a potato masher, mash tomatoes so they release their juices.
4. Stir in orange juice, olive oil, red wine vinegar, basil, salt, and pepper.
5. Serve on top of arugula.

**Variation**—*You can either serve the tomato orange mixture on top of arugula without any real mixing, or you can toss the arugula with some of the juices from the tomato/olive oil/vinegar mixture, then top with the tomatoes.*

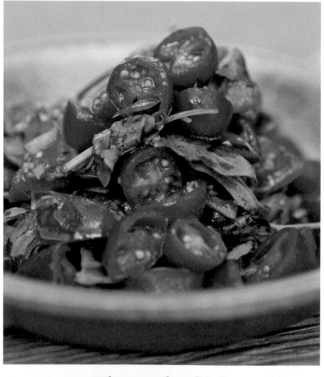

paleo comfort foods

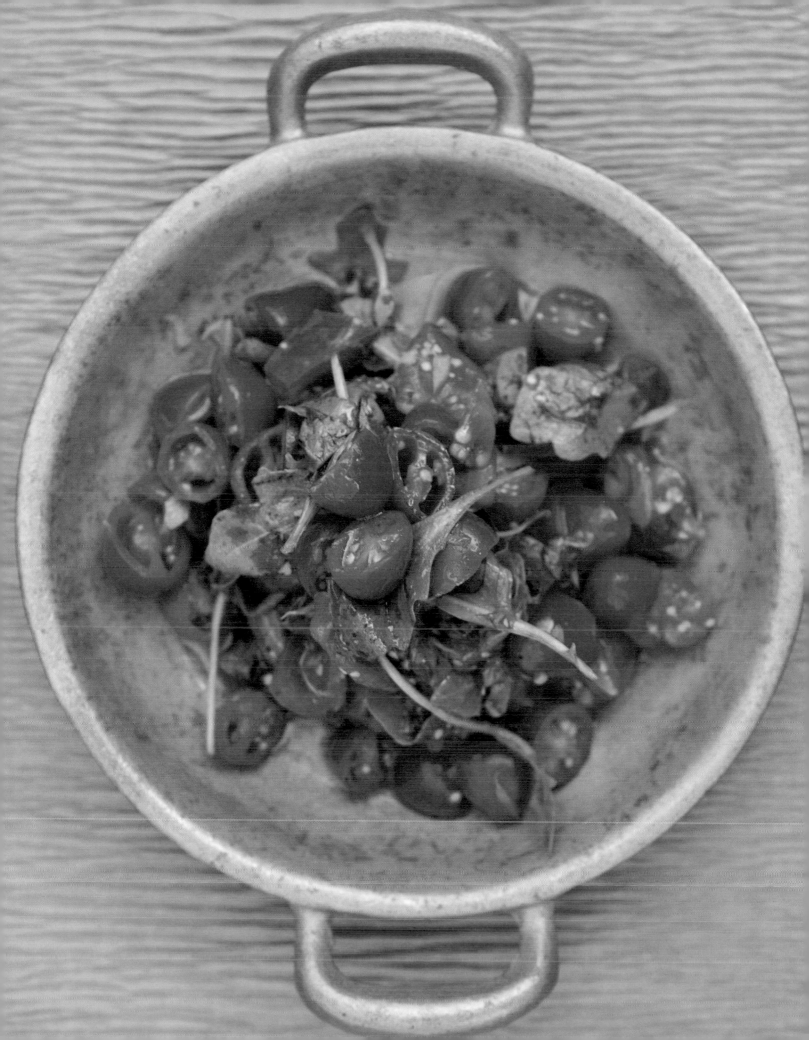

# gingered butternut squash soup

*Ah, butternut squash . . . fall comfort food, or baby food made acceptable for adults? Your choice. However, in the fall when squashes are abundant, this soup is a perfect start off to a dinner party.*

*What I love about this soup is that it's super easy to tweak the flavors. Add in some coconut milk to give it more of that delicious coconut-y flavor. Or add in some Granny Smith apples to the mixture and cook those with the squash, pureeing into the mix. Mix in some of your favorite curry to give this more zip. Whatever your choice, know that the butternut squash is chock full of good vitamins. It is a little high on the carb side, so best not to overdo it with this stuff. If your objective is leaning out, save this one for when you reach that optimal leanness!*

| | |
|---|---|
| 1 | butternut squash peeled and seeded |
| 1 | tablespoon olive oil |
| 1 | medium onion, diced |
| ½ | cup (50 g) chopped leeks (white and green parts) |
| 1 | tablespoon ginger, peeled |
| 5 | cups (1.25 L) chicken stock |
| 2 | teaspoons nutmeg |

1. Cut butternut squash into about 1 inch (2 cm) even sized cubes.
2. Heat a large pot or Dutch oven over medium heat. When hot add olive oil and once oil is hot add in onions and leeks.
3. Add in squash, ginger and chicken stock and bring to a simmer, cooking until the squash is tender (about 15 minutes or so).
4. Pour off most of the stock and reserve.
5. Carefully add squash, onions, ginger, and leek mixture to blender or food processor and puree (using caution as the heat of the ingredients will very often cause the blender top to want to pop off and make a mess all over your kitchen).
6. Once pureed, add contents back to pot, and add in the chicken stock until the desired consistency is attained.
7. Stir well and add in nutmeg, salt, and pepper to taste.

**Hint**—*This soup freezes exceptionally well. Just make sure to refrigerate it for a day first to allow it to fully cool before freezing.*

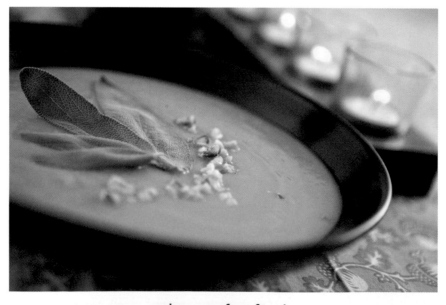

paleo comfort foods

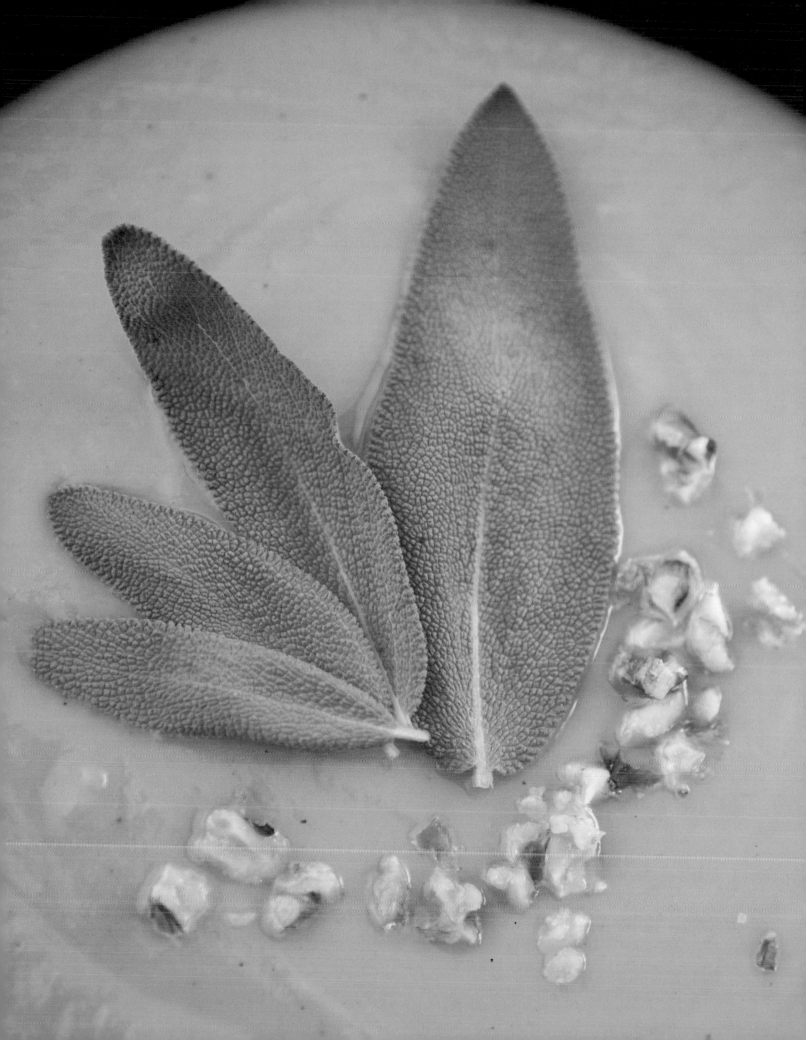

# tom kha gai
## (aka chicken coconut soup deliciousness)

*As I mentioned in the beginning of this book, I was fortunate enough while living in Los Angeles to befriend some chefs who are way more talented/knowledgeable than me. Chef Jet Tila is one such person. Jet is the executive chef at the Wynn Encore's Wazuzu restaurant, has been featured on the Food Network's "Best Thing I Ever Ate" and "Iron Chef America." He is of Thai/Chinese descent, and his family owns and runs the first Thai market ever opened in Los Angeles. He knows his stuff and is just an awesome dude. I had a blast getting to cater events with him and explore the hole-in-the-wall Thai joints around LA under his supervision. I am fairly certain that the knowledge he imparted to me regarding making really good curry scored me a husband.*

*Jet taught me what I know about Thai cooking and ingredients, and this is one recipe that reflects such. Much of Thai food is about balance, and getting the correct balance of spice, coconut (sweet), and "umami" (mostly from the fish sauce) is quite a feat. While you could theoretically make this soup without the fish sauce, you'll be missing that subtle umami flavoring.*

*I could go on and on about Jet and his food, what he taught me, but I will spare you that and suggest that you check out Jet's website (www.chefjet.com) and where he might be appearing next!*

| | |
|---|---|
| 3 | cups (250 mL) chicken stock |
| 3 | Kaffir lime leaves, torn |
| 3 | 2-inch (5 cm) pieces of lemongrass, bruised to help release the flavor |
| 2–3 | 1-inch (2 cm) pieces of fresh ginger, peeled |
| 2 | tablespoons fish sauce |
| 2 | tablespoons fresh squeezed lime juice |
| 1–2 | Thai chili peppers, thinly chopped (optional) |
| 1 | cup (75 g) sliced mushrooms |
| 2 | cans coconut milk |
| 2 | pounds (1 kg) chicken breasts, thinly sliced |
| 2–3 | tablespoons cilantro, chopped (optional) |

1. Bring all the ingredients up to and including the chili peppers (if using) to a boil.

2. Reduce to a simmer and let it cook for about an hour or so to really get those flavors melding.

3. Add in the mushrooms and coconut milk. Bring to a simmer.

4. Add in the chicken and simmer until the chicken is cooked through.

5. Finish off with some cilantro and extra chili peppers (if you want) and enjoy!

**Ingredient Notes**—*If you cannot find Kaffir lime leaves (Charles bought us two Kaffir lime trees for Christmas one year—yay!) you can use some lime zest and it will get close to a similar flavor—but not exactly the same. My suggestion is this: when you can find some Kaffir lime leaves in the store, buy a bunch and put them in a plastic bag, freezing them until you need them. Many Asian markets carry Kaffir lime leaves in the produce section (where you might find other fresh herbs). Galangal is more commonly used in such recipes as opposed to ginger, but is a little harder to find.*

**Variation**—*By all means use shrimp instead of the chicken and it would be mighty tasty too!*

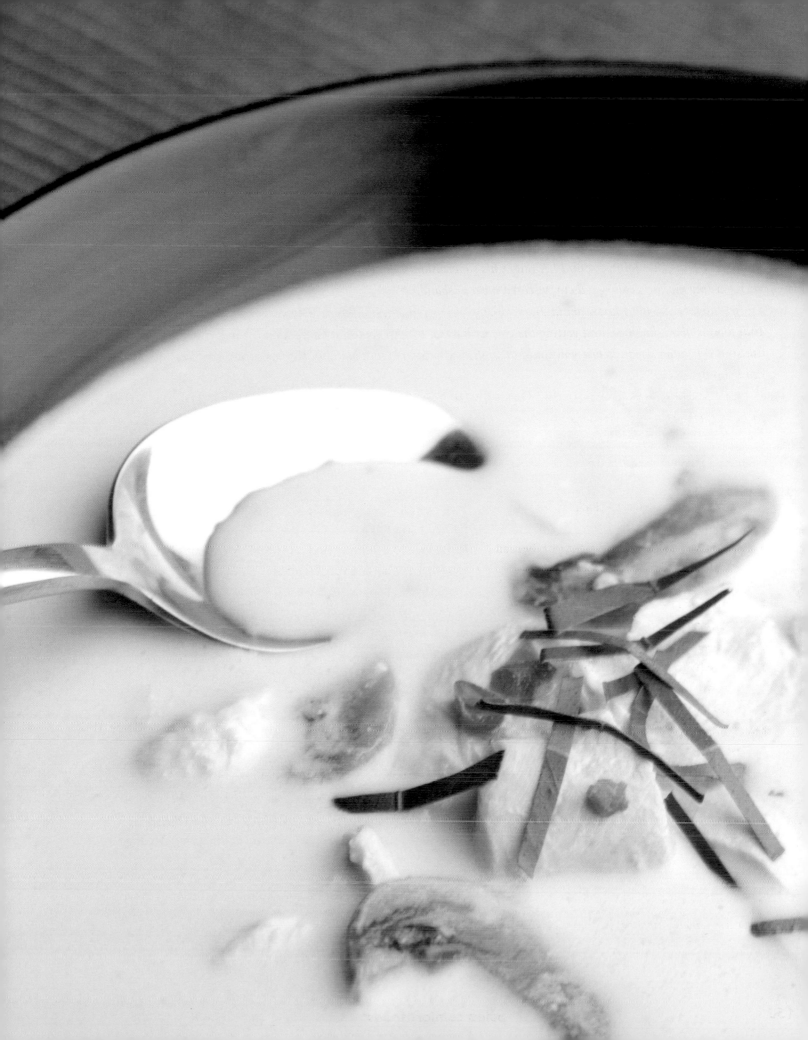

# chili—as it should be!

*You can start a pretty heated argument with certain people about whether chili should or shouldn't have beans in it. Our vote is pretty obvious. Sitting down to a bowl of this on a cold winter day just seems right. Double or triple the batch for big parties. Perhaps having a diced red onion or chives for garnishing would be appropriate.*

| | |
|---|---|
| 1 | ancho chili, dried |
| 2 | red chile peppers, dried |
| ½ | cup (125 mL) olive oil |
| 1 | pound (450 g) beef (chuck, tenderloin), cubed |
| 1 | tablespoon cumin seed |
| 1 | teaspoon garlic powder |
| 1 | teaspoon cayenne pepper |
| 2 | chipotle peppers in adobo sauce |
| 1 | pound (450 g) ground beef |
| 2 | cups (300 g) onion, chopped |
| ½ | cup (125 mL) beef stock |
| 28 | ounces (825 mL) canned crushed tomatoes |
| 28 | ounces (825 mL) canned whole tomatoes |
| 3–4 | tablespoons tomato paste |
| 4 | cups (700 g) bell pepper, chopped |

1. Place the dried ancho and dried red peppers in a bowl of hot water to soak for at least 30 minutes. Drain.

2. Add ¼ cup (60 mL) of oil into large pot and get it good and hot. Take cubed meat and brown in pot on all sides. Remove browned cubes from pot and set aside.

3. Combine remaining olive oil, cumin seeds, garlic powder, cayenne pepper, reconstituted peppers and chipotle peppers in food processor and process for 30 seconds to 1 minute.

4. Return your large pot to medium heat, and brown ground beef. Once browned, add spice/seasoned paste from processor and onions. Cook until onions are slightly translucent, then add the beef stock. Bring to a simmer and cook until stock is reduced slightly.

5. Add in both cans of tomatoes (crushed and whole), tomato paste, chopped peppers and the browned cubed meat.

6. Stir to mix all ingredients and simmer for 1½–2 hours. The longer you cook the more flavor you get.

**Variations**—*Ground turkey or sausage can be substituted for the ground beef.*

**Tips & Tricks**—*If you don't want to stand over the stove for a few hours, dump everything in a slow cooker after step 4. Set the cooker to high. You can freeze chili in individual servings and enjoy it for weeks to come.*

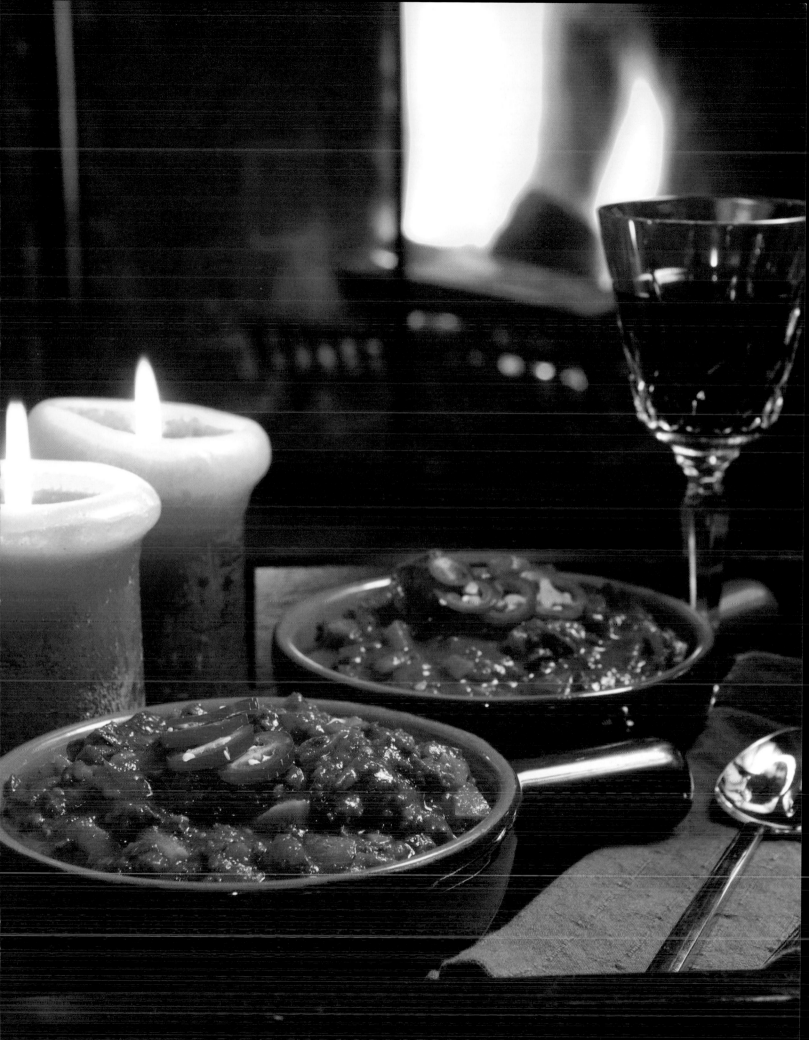

# shrimp (or crab) bisque

*Yes, there are a lot of ingredients here. I promise you . . . they are worth it! This is a rich, velvety soup that people will swear is thickened with flour and must have heavy cream in it.*

*The thing that really stands out to me in this recipe: tomato paste. Tomato paste is one of those fantastic foods that has a naturally high level of free glutamate acids—providing that richness in flavor to the dish that might not otherwise be there (anchovies, fish sauce, and nori are other high sources of free glutamate).*

| | |
|---|---|
| 1 | pound (450 g) raw large shrimp |
| 3 | cups (750 mL) seafood or chicken stock |
| 1 | cup (250 mL) water |
| 2 | tablespoons olive or coconut oil |
| ½ | cup (50 g) chopped leeks (white and light green parts) |
| 1 | small onion, diced |
| 4 | cloves garlic, chopped |
| 2 | teaspoons Old Bay seasoning |
| ½ | teaspoon cayenne pepper |
| ¼ | cup (60 mL) brandy |
| ¼ | cup (60 mL) dry sherry |
| 2 | tablespoons grass-fed butter or coconut butter |
| 2 | tablespoons bacon fat |
| ¼ | cup (40 g) almond flour |
| 1 | tablespoon arrowroot powder |
| 1 | can coconut milk (full fat) |
| ½ | cup (110 g) tomato paste |

1. Peel and devein the shrimp, reserving shells. In a large pot, heat the stock and water along with the shells from the shrimp. Simmer for approximately 20 minutes. Strain the shells out, reserving all the liquid.

2. Meanwhile, in a separate pot, heat the oil over medium/medium-low heat. Add the leeks and onions, stirring frequently, and cook for about 10 minutes or until the leeks and onions are soft and translucent and somewhat caramelized (being careful not to brown).

3. Add the garlic and cook for about 2 more minutes.

4. Add the Old Bay, cayenne pepper and shrimp and stir. Cook for about 3 more minutes or until shrimp are pink.

5. Add brandy to mixture and stir. Stir for a minute or two then add the sherry. Stir for about 2 minutes more.

6. Add all contents of pan to food processor or blender, and blend until smooth.

7. In the pan you just had the shrimp/leeks/onions in, add the butter/bacon fat and melt over medium heat.

8. Add in almond flour and arrowroot powder, stirring for a few minutes until it starts to brown.

9. Add the mixture from the food processor, the coconut milk, and the strained stock liquid into the pan with the flour/fat mixture.

10. Stir in the tomato paste, and let simmer until heated through. Taste and season as you'd like.

**Tips & Tricks**—*If you are using a gas stove, use extreme caution when pouring in the brandy as brandy can ignite and set your eyebrows on fire. I suggest turning the flame off, adding the brandy, stirring, and then turning heat back on. No one wants to be sporting a face with no eyebrows.*

**Variations**—*If you're feeling adventurous, use some crab meat and crab roe along with or instead of the shrimp, and you've for the most part just transformed this soup into the Southern favorite of She Crab soup. You can always skip the brandy and sherry, but the flavor won't quite be the same.*

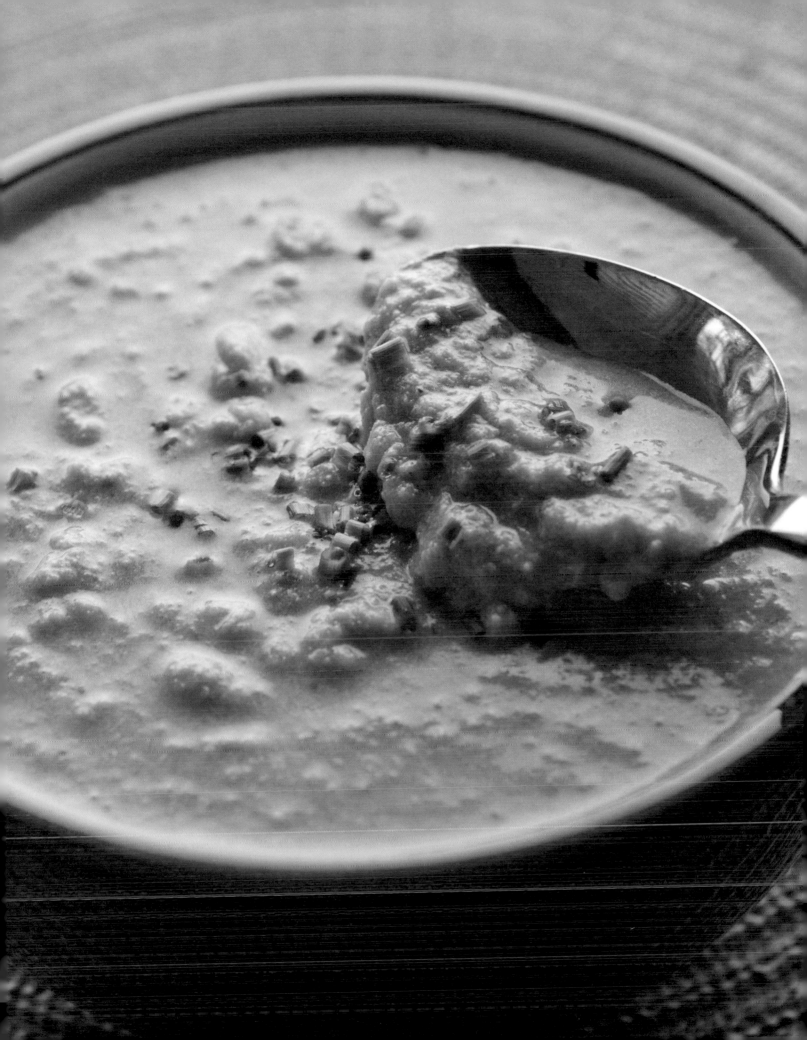

# melon gazpacho

*For me, being the non-tomato kid growing up, I pretty much thought V-8 was a punishment much like soap in your mouth. Which is why sweet, fruity dishes like a melon gazpacho hit a homerun with me. This is absolutely delightful on those dog days of summer when it is simply too hot to make any kind of dessert. Light, refreshing, cooling, this one has it all.*

| | |
|---|---|
| 6 | cups (1 kg) watermelon, seeded and cubed |
| 2 | medium cucumbers, peeled, seeded and cubed |
| 1 | honeydew melon, cubed |
| ¼ | cup (6 g) chopped fresh basil |
| ¼ | cup (6 g) chopped fresh mint |
| 2 | tablespoons minced shallot |
| ¼ | cup (6 g) chopped flat-leaf parsley |
| 3 | tablespoons red wine vinegar |
| 2 | tablespoons extra-virgin olive oil |
| ¾ | teaspoon salt (optional) |

1. Working in batches, combine some of the melons, cucumber, basil, mint, shallot, and parsley in a blender or food processor. Be careful not to fill too high or you will have a mess!

2. Puree until smooth.

3. Remove the first batch and pour into a large bowl.

4. Repeat process for 2 or 3 more times until all melon has been pureed.

5. Stir all together, and mix in the vinegar, olive oil and salt to taste.

**Variations**—*Add some tomatoes, other varieties of melons, some pears, whatever works for you to change this up.*

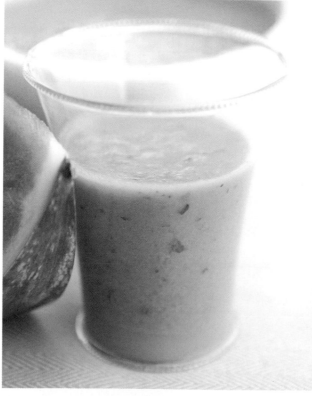

paleo comfort foods

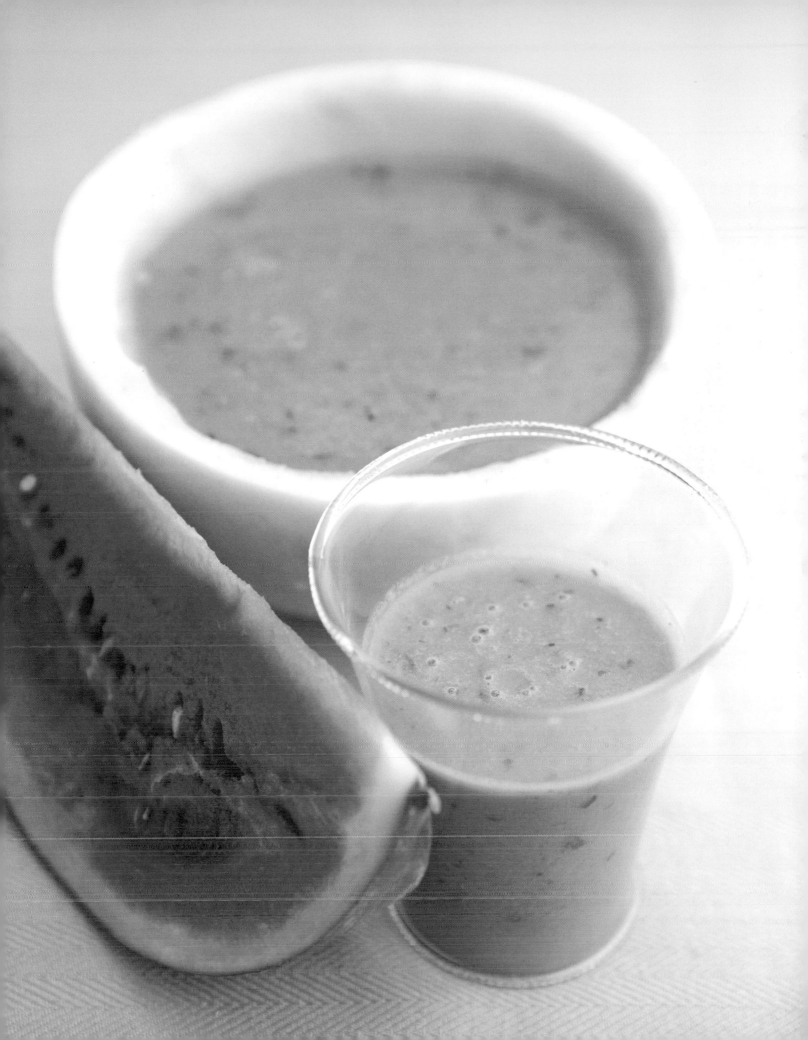

# vidalia onion soup

*I know what you're likely thinking: the only purpose for French onion soup is to have something to drown a piece of baguette with melted Gruyere into. Reinvent your tastes just a bit here, and enjoy the soup for the taste it delivers sans bread and cheese.*

*There are thirteen counties in Georgia—and parts of seven other counties in Georgia—that are the only ones in the country authorized to grow the ever-popular and sweet Vidalia onions. What makes Vidalias so sweet? Evidently it's due to the low amount of sulfur in the soil in the areas where these sweeties are grown.*

*This recipe is loosely adapted from Cook's Illustrated. By caramelizing the onions in the oven, you avoid having to stir all the time, and you enable the onions to keep even more of their delicious flavor.*

---

| | |
|---|---|
| 3 | tablespoons grass-fed butter, clarified is preferred |
| 4 | Vidalia onions |
| 2 | cups (500 mL) red wine |
| 2 | cups (500 mL) water, + more for deglazing pan |
| ½ | cup (125 mL) sherry |
| 3 | cups (750 mL) beef broth |
| 4 | sprigs fresh thyme |
| 1 | bay leaf |

1. Preheat oven to 400°F (205°C).

2. Use some of the butter to grease the bottom of a large Dutch oven, and place remainder of butter and all onions into the Dutch oven. Cover and cook in oven for 1 hour.

3. Remove the pot from the oven, stir the onions and butter scraping the sides and bottom, and place back into the oven with lid slightly ajar for another 60–90 minutes.

4. Meanwhile, in a small saucepan, heat wine over medium heat, and reduce down until it's about ¼ cup in total volume. Remove from heat.

5. Remove the pot of onions from the oven, and place uncovered on stove on medium-high heat. Scrape the sides and bottom of pan frequently, until the liquid mostly evaporates and the onions are browned.

6. Continue to cook until the bottom of the pan has a brown crust, about 6–8 minutes.

7. Stir in about ¼ cup (60 mL) of the water, being sure to scrape up the crust on the bottom of the pan.

8. Cook until the water has evaporated and you have another dark crust. Repeat this addition of water until the onions are dark brown.

9. Mix in the wine and sherry and cook, stirring frequently, until the liquids evaporate.

10. Mix in the beef broth, 2 cups (500 mL) water, thyme, and bay leaf, scraping up any bits of fond that may be on the bottom and sides of pan.

11. Bring the liquid up to a boil, then reduce heat to a low simmer, cover, and allow to simmer for about 30 minutes. Remove thyme and bay leaf, and season as you prefer with salt and pepper.

---

**Ingredient Notes**—*If you don't have access to Vidalias (usually only available in the spring and summer months), you can use any other sweet onions.*

**Variation**—*This recipe is a little more labor-intensive process than some. You can absolutely tweak this to make it a little easier. To do so, skip the oven cooking of the onions and simply sauté the onions in a pot on the stove, following along from step 4 above.*

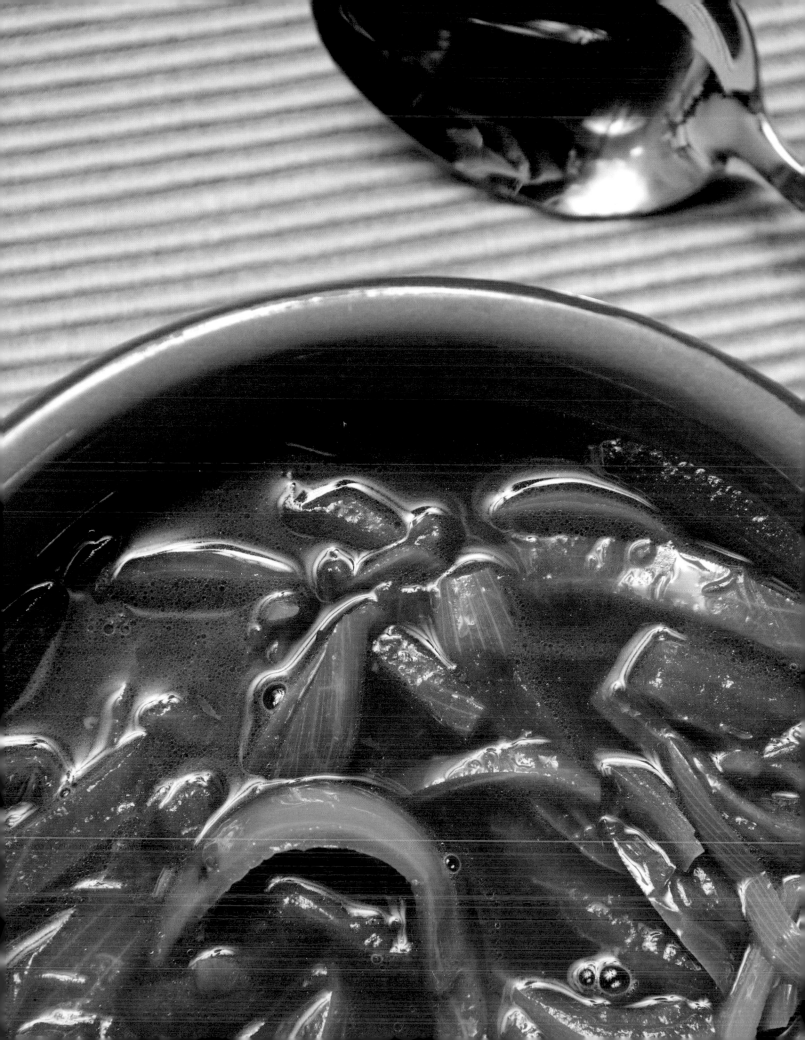

# chicken tomatillo stew

*The first time I made this recipe, I was still Zone-ing my paleo portions (at least in respect to the protein content), and I was amazed at how big a portion turned out to be. This soup is awesome on those cold winter days, and is one that does well simmering in the crock pot too.*

*If you have access to fresh tomatillos, use about 1½ pounds (¾ kg). Just be certain to remove the husks!*

| | |
|---|---|
| 1–2 | tablespoons coconut oil |
| 2–3 | poblano peppers, chopped |
| 2 | yellow onions, chopped |
| 1–2 | jalapeños (or more to taste) chopped |
| 2 | cloves garlic, minced |
| 2–3 | green or red peppers (optional) |
| 1 | cubanelle pepper (optional) |
| 2 | teaspoons chipotle powder |
| 2 | teaspoons chili powder |
| 1 | tablespoon cumin |
| 2 | teaspoons smoked paprika |
| 1 | 28-ounce (794 g) can tomatillos, drained and coarsely chopped |
| 2 | pounds (1 kg) cooked chicken, shredded |
| 4 | cups (1 L) chicken broth |

1. Heat coconut oil over medium heat in large Dutch oven or pot.
2. Add ingredients up to and including the cubanelle peppers and sauté until onions are translucent.
3. Add next ingredients up to tomatillos. Mix spices in until well-incorporated.
4. Add tomatillos, chicken and broth.
5. Bring to a simmer and let cook for an hour or two. Taste and adjust seasonings to your liking.

**Ingredient Notes**—*More jalapeños = more heat! If you don't like your food with any kind of kick, avoid the jalapeños, go easy on the poblanos, and maybe just use extra bell peppers. Tomatillos are part of the nightshade family, so if you are struggling with some autoimmune issues, your best bet is to steer clear of this particular dish.*

**Variations**—*You can use pork (this recipe is especially tasty with smoked pulled pork!) instead of chicken, and add or detract as many vegetables as you like.*

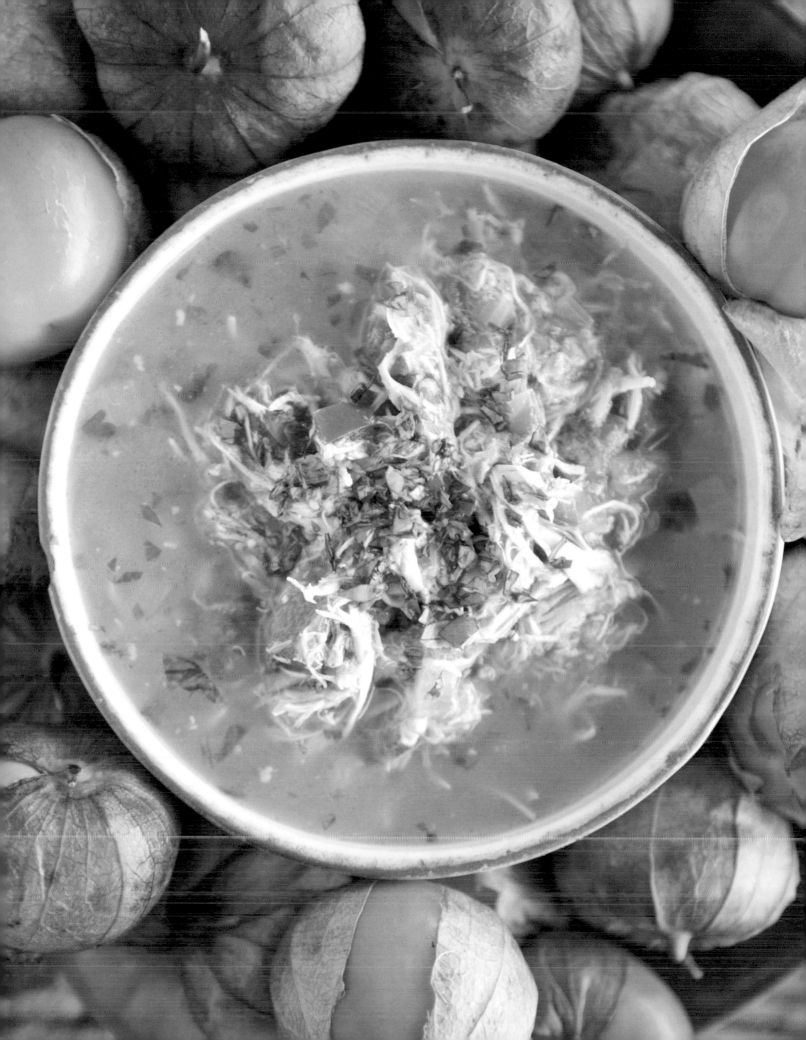

# chicken soup

*Nothing says comfort quite as well as that first cup of chicken soup as the weather begins to turn chilly. Sometimes the simplest things bring the most pleasure in life. This is a great recipe to get cooking in the slow cooker and let go for a few hours!*

*For tackling this recipe in the tastiest way possible, go find the recipe for chicken stock in this book (page 114) and follow the instructions for broth (cook the whole chicken to get your broth and cooked chicken meat all in one fell swoop). By doing this step the day before, you can also chill the broth some, and skim off any unwanted fat.*

| | |
|---|---|
| 2 | tablespoons bacon grease |
| 2 | cloves garlic, minced |
| 2 | medium onions, chopped |
| 1 | quart (1 L) chicken stock (or broth) |
| 4 | cups (400 g) celery, chopped |
| 4 | cups (300 g) carrots, chopped |
| ½ | cup (12 g) Italian parsley, chopped |
| 3–4 | pounds (1.5 kg) chicken meat, cooked and shredded |
| 1 | teaspoon salt |
| 1 | teaspoon black pepper |

1. Heat a large pot over medium heat, and add in bacon grease. When hot, stir in garlic and onions and sauté.

2. When onions are slightly translucent, add stock (broth), celery, carrots, parsley, and chicken.

3. Sprinkle salt and pepper and give one good stir.

4. Bring to a boil then reduce heat and let simmer for 1 hour stirring occasionally.

**Plan Ahead**—*Have carrots, celery, and parsley chopped and bagged a day ahead. Especially if you choose to make the broth a day ahead, you'll have time to chop while that is cooking.*

**Variations**—*Using turkey for the soup is really tasty too, and gives you something to do with all that leftover Thanksgiving turkey and the carcass.*

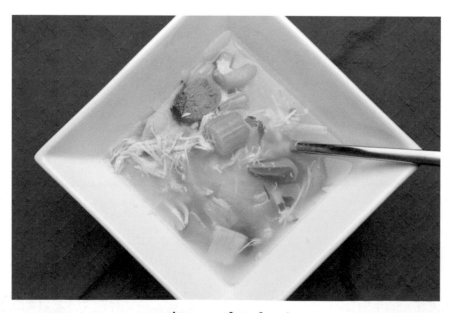

paleo comfort foods

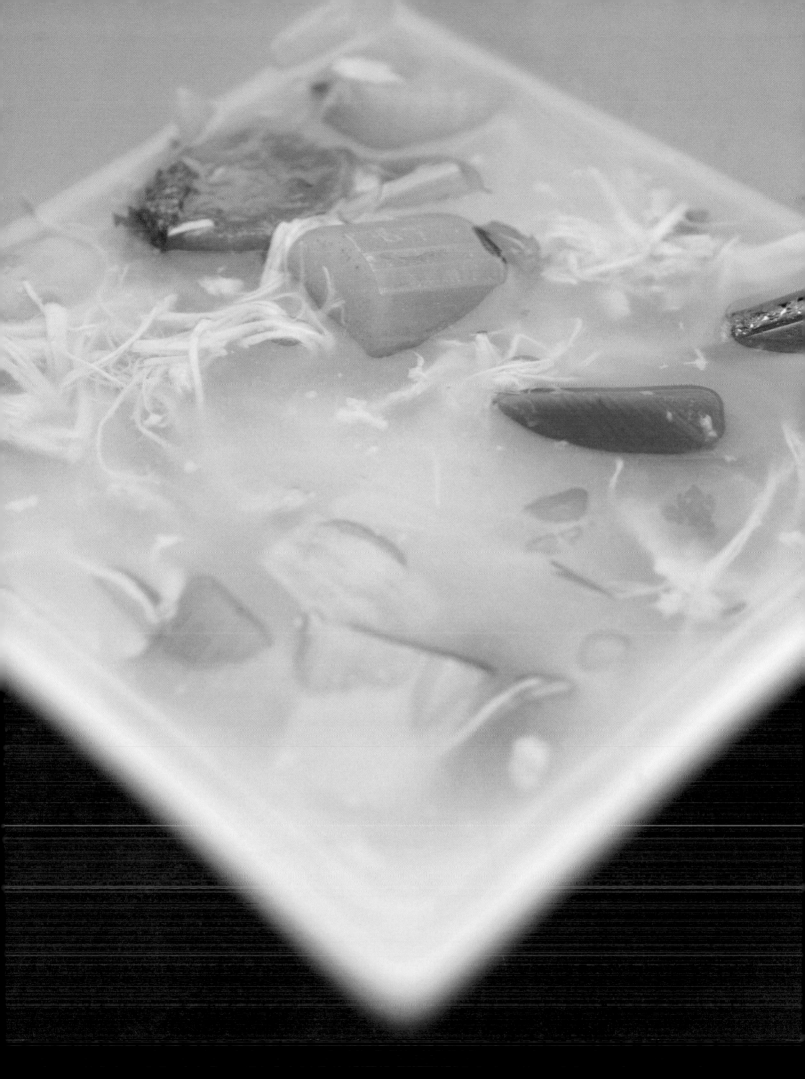

# jambalaya

*This bayou classic combines so many wonderful flavors and textures. We didn't have to tweak this classic too terribly much to make it paleo friendly. Traditionally, the rice for this meal will soak up a fair portion of your liquid. Cauliflower rice does some of that for you here, and is a lot less inflammatory and is far lower in carbohydrates.*

| | |
|---|---|
| 2 | tablespoons coconut or avocado oil, divided |
| 1 | tablespoon Cajun seasoning |
| ¾ | pound (340 g) andouille sausage, sliced into rounds |
| 1 | pound (450 g) boneless skinless chicken breasts, cut into 1-inch (2 cm) pieces |
| 1 | large onion, diced |
| 1 | green pepper, diced |
| 3 | stalks celery, diced |
| 1 | tablespoon garlic, minced |
| 16 | ounces (475 mL) crushed tomatoes |
| ½ | teaspoon red pepper flakes |
| ½ | teaspoon ground black pepper |
| 1 | teaspoon celery salt |
| ½ | teaspoon Tabasco |
| 2 | teaspoons Worcestershire sauce |
| 1 | teaspoon filé powder |
| 2 | cups (500 mL) chicken broth |
| 1½ | cups (225 g) riced cauliflower (see page 200) |

1. Heat 1 tablespoon of oil in a large heavy pot over medium heat.

2. Keeping the sausage and chicken separate from one another, toss both with Cajun seasoning to coat. Sauté sausage until browned. Remove with slotted spoon, and set aside.

3. Add 1 tablespoon oil, and sauté chicken pieces until lightly browned on all sides. Remove with a slotted spoon, and set aside.

4. In the same pot, sauté onion, bell pepper, celery, and garlic until tender.

5. Stir in crushed tomatoes, and season with red pepper, black pepper, celery salt, Tabasco, Worcestershire sauce and filé powder. Stir in chicken and sausage.

6. Cook for 10 minutes, stirring occasionally.

7. Stir in the chicken broth. Bring to a boil, reduce heat, and simmer for 25 to 30 minutes, or until liquid is slightly reduced.

8. Serve with riced cauliflower.

**Variations**—*Absolutely try this using turkey or duck in place of chicken.*

**Ingredient Notes**—*As mentioned elsewhere in this book, you'll want to keep an eye on the Worcestershire sauce you use, as some do contain gluten. We find the Lea & Perrins reduced-salt brand seems to be okay for our standards (no gluten/soy, minimal amounts of sugar).*

**Plan Ahead**—*Have the cauliflower rice already prepared, and you can sauté it a bit beforehand if you'd like your cauliflower cooked.*

**Hint**—*Individual servings of this dish freeze well.*

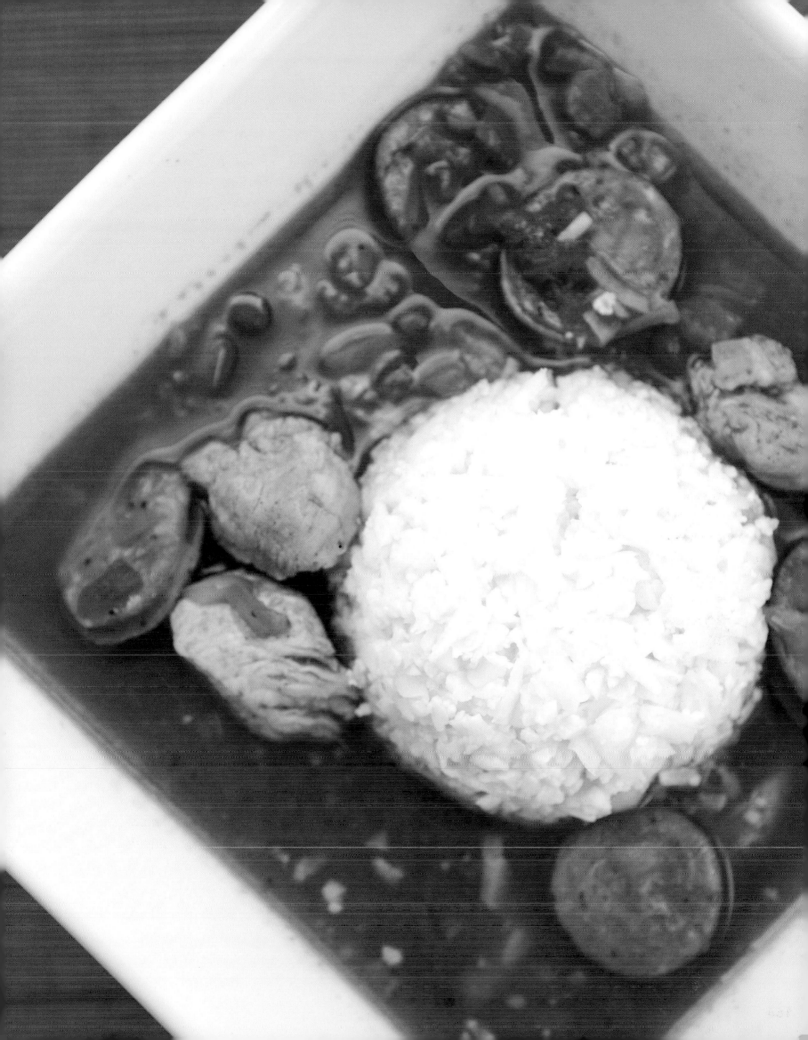

# beef stew

*Beef stew was a staple in our house growing up, with the primary ingredients being the meat, carrots, peas, and potatoes. I think if my mom had told me there were anchovies in her beef stew (there were not) I would have refused to eat it. However, now that I'm an enlightened, mature cook of my own, I have to say that anchovies are very often that secret ingredient that give certain dishes a taste that you can't quite figure out. It's that whole "umami" principle. Nigella Lawson and Cook's Illustrated both have varieties of this stew, and I have to say it's a keeper! Don't tell your guests about the anchovies, and they will never know they are there. They will just think it tastes amazing.*

| | |
|---|---|
| 3 | medium cloves garlic, minced |
| 4 | anchovies |
| 1 | tablespoon tomato paste |
| 2 | tablespoons avocado or coconut oil |
| 3–4 | pounds (2 kg) chuck roast, cubed and patted dry |
| 3–4 | pieces thick cut bacon, cut into small pieces |
| 2 | large onions, chopped |
| 4 | medium carrots, peeled and cut into 1–inch pieces |
| ¼ | cup (40 g) almond flour |
| 2 | cups (500 mL) red wine |
| 4 | cups (1 L) chicken broth |
| 2 | bay leaves |
| 4 | sprigs fresh thyme |
| 2 | cups (300 g) green beans (optional) |

1. Preheat oven to 300°F (150°C).

2. In a small bowl, mash together the garlic and anchovies. Stir in the tomato paste and set aside.

3. Heat the oil in a large Dutch oven over medium-high heat, and working in batches, add the chuck roast meat.

4. Brown for 5–6 minutes per side, then flip over with tongs. Remove from pot and add other meat and repeat process. Set meat aside on a plate.

5. Fry bacon pieces in the pan until crispy.

6. Add the onions and carrots to the pot, stirring to loosen any of the browned bits on the bottom of the pan. Add in the anchovy/garlic paste and stir until well combined.

7. Add in the almond flour and cook until it is rather dried out.

8. Stir in the wine, and simmer to let the wine reduce somewhat.

9. Add the broth, bay leaves and thyme, and bring to a boil. Add the meat back to the liquid mixture and cover.

10. Place in the oven for 1½–2 hours or until meat is super tender.

11. Stir in the green beans (if desired) and let cook another 5–10 minutes or until beans are cooked.

**Variations**—*You can add to or take away just about any ingredients you so choose here. Mushrooms would be lovely in this, as would some cauliflower. The beans don't really do much except add some color and additional carbs, so feel free to do away with those if you choose. You can also cook this stew in a slow cooker or crockpot. Follow the instructions through step 8, then in step 9 combine everything in your slow cooker and turn on high for 3-4 hours.*

**Tips & Tricks**—*As with most stews, this tastes even better after sitting for a day in the refrigerator!*

**Hint**—*This recipe reheats very well, so feel free to store some in the freezer.*

paleo comfort foods

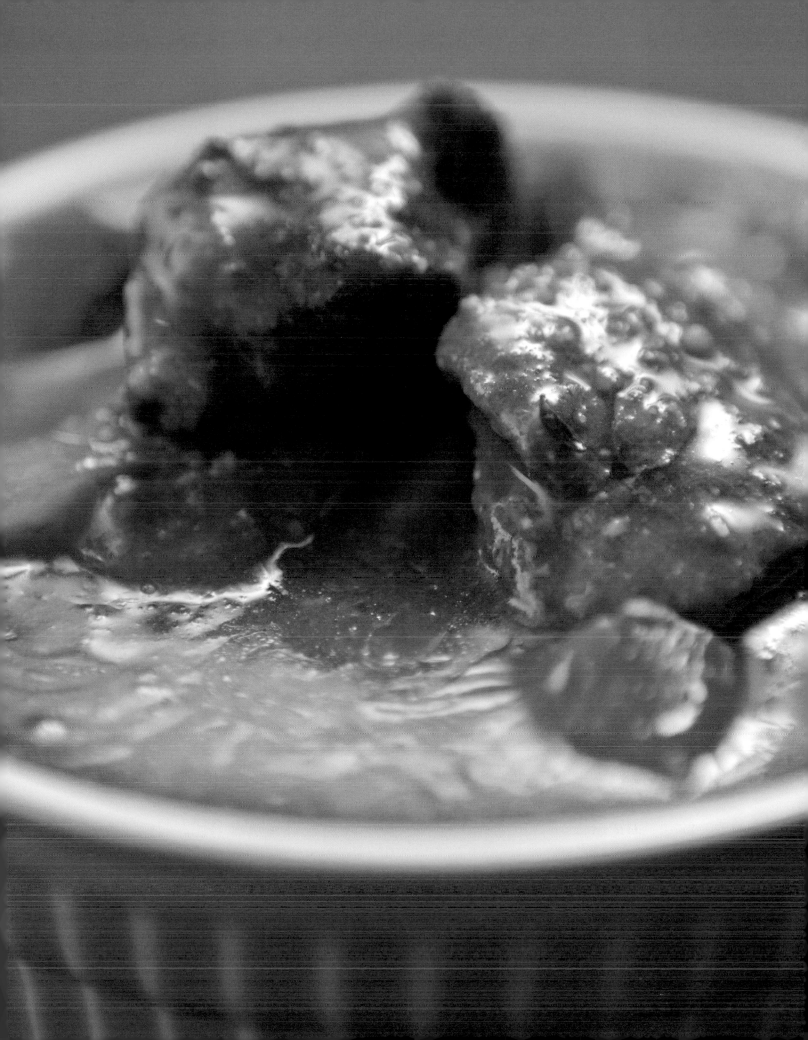

# paleo gumbo

*Shortly before Charles popped the big question, he brought me down to Mobile, Alabama for a few days with his family. There are two things about that trip that stood out to me: me catching a really big speck trout (and Charles saying that's why he asked me to marry him), and his mom's gumbo (which may have been why I said yes to Charles!). All kidding aside, his mom makes an amazing gumbo, with a roux that is pure perfection. This had me incredibly intimidated to even attempt roux without the usual flour. I was surprised with the outcome, and found this gumbo even met Charles' approval.*

| | |
|---|---|
| ¼ | cup (60 mL) bacon grease |
| 3 | tablespoons coconut flour |
| 3 | tablespoons almond flour |
| 2 | cups (300 g) onions, chopped |
| 2 | cups (200 g) celery, chopped |
| 2 | cups (350 g) green pepper, chopped |
| 3 | cloves garlic, minced |
| 1 | quart (1 L) can tomatoes |
| 2 | cups (500 mL) chicken or seafood stock |
| 2 | bay leaves |
| ½ | pound (225 g) lump crab meat, picked over for shells |
| 1 | pound (450 g) shrimp |
| ½ | pound (225 g) andouille sausage, sliced |
| 1 | tablespoon filé powder |

1. To make the roux, heat the bacon grease over medium heat and whisk in coconut flour and almond flour. Stir continuously until the roux has a dark brown color but is not burnt (think dark peanut butter color).

2. Add the onions, celery, peppers, and garlic and sauté until onions are translucent and celery somewhat soft.

3. Add in the tomatoes, stock, and bay leaves, and bring to a simmer.

4. Stir in the crab meat, shrimp, and andouille, cooking until shrimp are cooked through.

5. Remove from heat and add filé' powder.

6. Stir and serve with cauliflower rice.

**Variations**—*If you don't have any crabmeat, you can up the shrimp or sausage quantities. Chicken also works great in gumbo.*

**Hint**—*This freezes well as individual servings.*

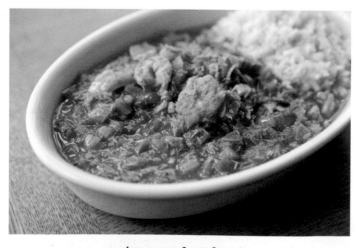

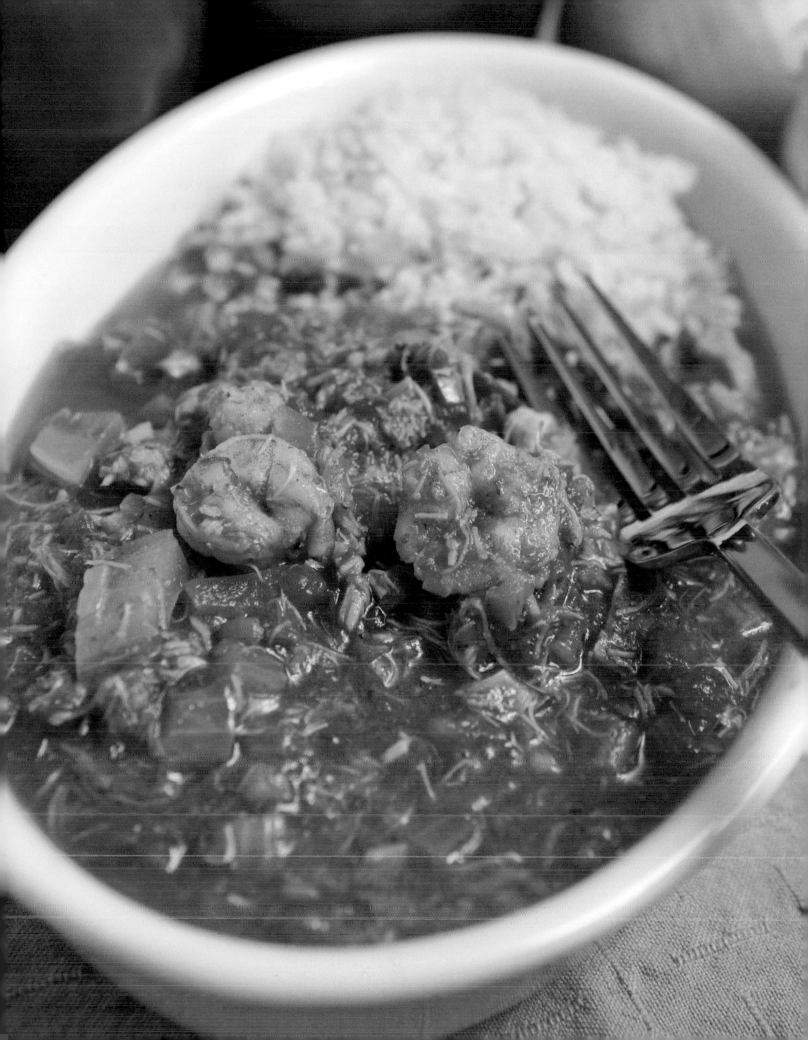

# crawfish étouffée

*Down on the Bayou, étouffée is pretty synonymous with comfort food. You'll have a hard time waiting to eat this one. Your kitchen will smell so very delicious. Two things to consider are how to get your crawfish tails and what stock you will use. The good news is that you can answer both questions with the same answer . . . boil your own crawfish. If you can stand not to eat all those tails up in the process, you'll be left with plenty of shells/heads to make your own stock. If you don't have time to do both steps, enjoy the tail meat and just use chicken broth. Going the extra step will give you enough crawfish stock to bless your kitchen with several attempts at mastering this Cajun delicacy.*

| | |
|---|---|
| 4 | tablespoons butter or oil |
| 1½ | cups (225 g) onions, finely chopped |
| ½ | cup (50 g) celery, finely chopped |
| ½ | cup (85 g) bell pepper, finely chopped |
| 2 | teaspoons Cajun seasoning |
| 2 | pounds (900 g) crawfish tail meat |
| ½ | cup (75 g) almond flour |
| 2 | cups (500 mL) crawfish stock, or chicken stock |
| ¼ | cup (35 g) garlic, minced |
| 2 | tablespoons fresh thyme, chopped |
| 2 | teaspoons Worcestershire sauce |
| ½ | teaspoon salt and freshly ground black pepper |
| 1 | teaspoon hot sauce |
| ½ | cup (12 g) green onion, thinly slices |
| 1 | tablespoon fresh lemon juice |
| 3 | cups (700 g) riced cauliflower |

**1.** Melt butter in large skillet or pot. Add onion, celery, bell pepper, and 1 teaspoon of the Cajun seasoning, sauté until onions are translucent.

**2.** Add the crawfish meat and other teaspoon of Cajun seasoning. Cook for 3 to 5 minutes or until meat starts to let off liquid.

**3.** Add the almond flour stirring constantly for another 3 to 5 minutes. Pour in a small amount of the stock and vigorously stir into a paste.

**4.** Add remaining stock slowly, whisking constantly. Bring to boil and then reduce heat to simmer. Have some extra stock on hand. You may need it to get the consistency just right. Think gravy.

**5.** Add the garlic, thyme, Worcestershire, salt, and black pepper.

**6.** Simmer for 20–30 minutes. Mix in the hot sauce and green onions and simmer for 5–10 more minutes.

**7.** Stir in the lemon juice and adjust seasonings to taste.

**8.** Serve over the riced cauliflower.

**Variation**—*Shrimp étouffée is also really tasty.*

**Ingredient Notes**—*Read the label of your Worcestershire sauce. We use low-sodium Lea & Perrins.*

**Hint**—*This is a great, freezer-friendly meal!*

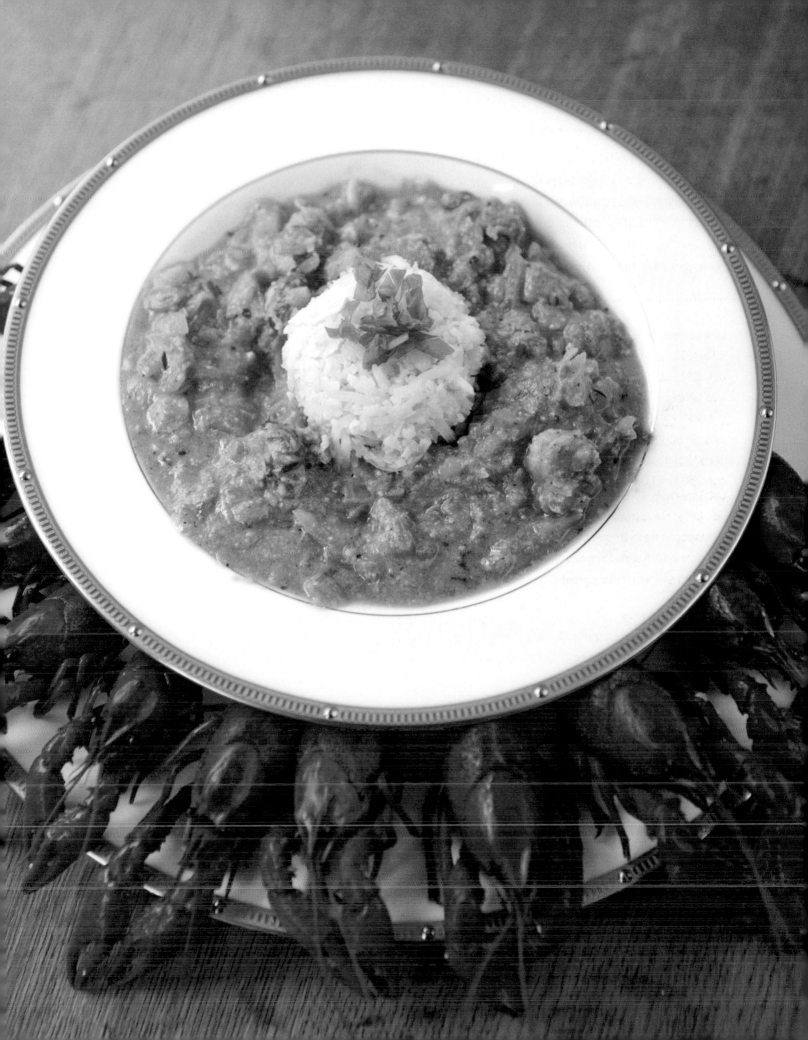

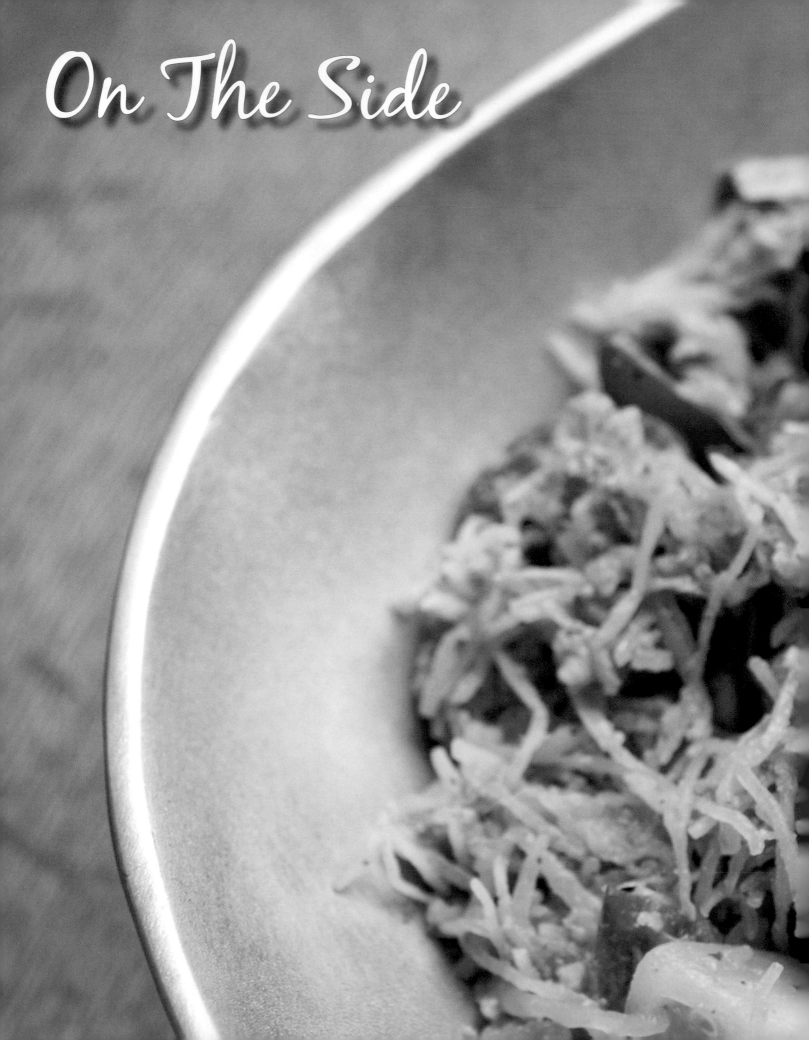

On The Side

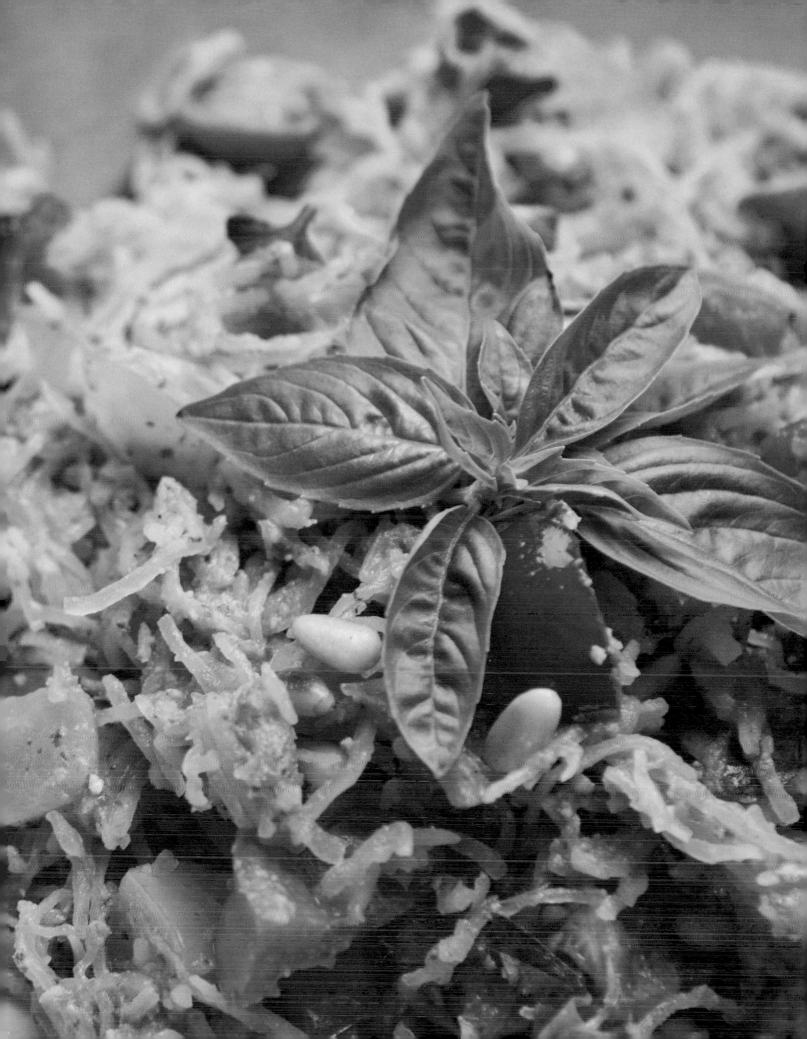

# brussels sprouts slaw

*As a child, and on into adulthood, I thought Brussels sprouts were vile food items that were only served soggy and overcooked with that nasty sulfuric smell. And then, a miracle happened: one Thanksgiving, my friend Peter made a Brussels sprouts dish that was simply divine and turned me into an instant fan. From there, I sought them out on menus, in recipes, everywhere I could. I'd say now, when in season, we eat them at least once a week. The following recipe is a take on a Brussels sprout slaw we had at Muss & Turners here in Atlanta a few years back.*

| | |
|---|---|
| 1 | cup (100 g) large pecan halves, toasted |
| ½ | pound (230 g) thick-cut bacon, cut into small pieces |
| ¼ | cup (60 mL) Dijon mustard |
| 2 | tablespoons apple cider vinegar |
| 3 | tablespoons fresh lemon juice |
| ¼ | cup (60 mL) olive oil |
| ¼ | teaspoon freshly ground black pepper |
| 1½ | pounds (700 g) Brussels sprouts, trimmed |
| 2 | green onions (scallions), cut on the bias |

1. Preheat oven to 325°F (165°C). Place pecans on small rimmed baking sheet. Bake nuts until toasted—about 5–10 minutes (be careful not to burn!).

2. Meanwhile, in a large sauté pan, cook bacon over medium-high heat until crispy. Drain on paper towels, and save the extra bacon fat for future use.

3. Whisk mustard, vinegar, and lemon juice in a small bowl; whisk in oil. Season with pepper.

4. Using processor fitted with ⅛- to ¼-inch slicing disk, slice Brussels sprouts (alternately, you can slice with knife). Transfer to large bowl.

5. Preheat large skillet over medium heat, and add in 1–2 tablespoons of the leftover bacon fat. Add in Brussels sprouts and sauté until softened and slightly brown.

6. Pour the mustard/vinegar/lemon juice/olive oil mixture over the sprouts.

7. Mix in ½ the pecans, the bacon, and scallions. Place slaw in a serving bowl and top with remaining pecans.

**Variations**—*Try some chopped up or shredded Granny Smith apples in this, some dried cranberries, or walnuts instead of pecans. If bacon is not your thing, just use the oil of your choosing, and omit the bacon.*

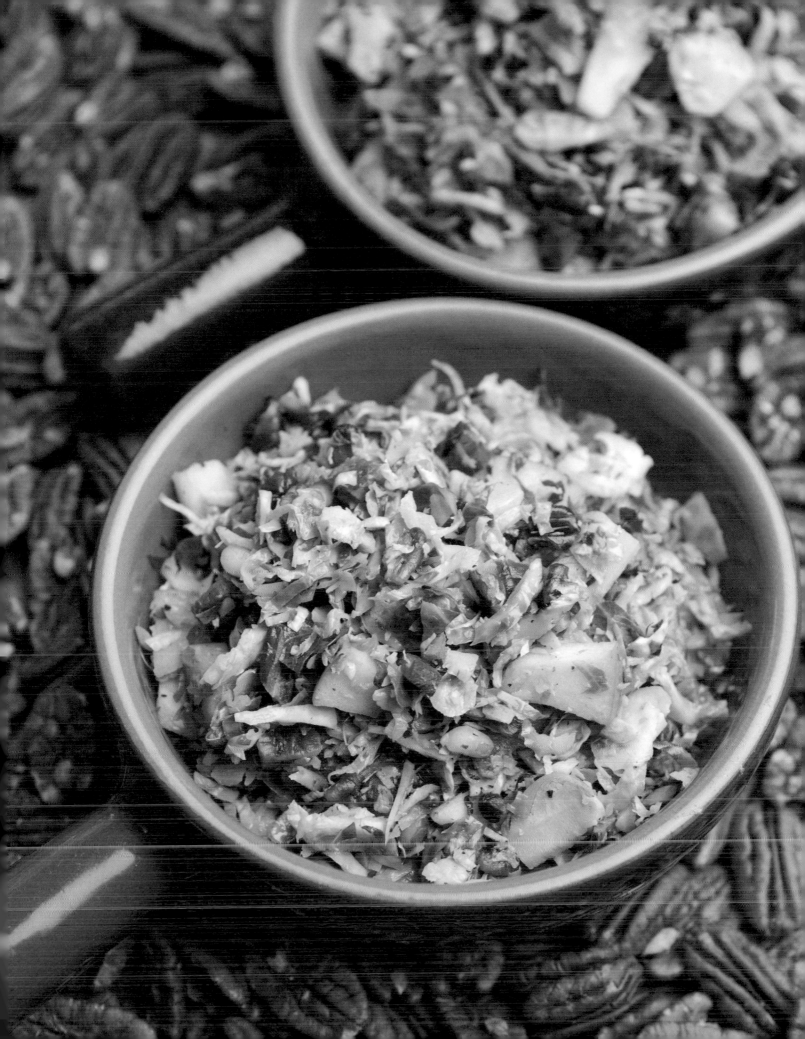

# grilled veggies

*These go well with just about anything, and are a great way to use all the fresh vegetables from our garden in the summertime. If you have a large crowd coming over, double or triple your recipe and consider serving the veggies whole. These keep extremely well in the refrigerator. We will chop up a cup or two of leftovers in with scrambled eggs in the morning for a quick and tasty breakfast.*

| | |
|---|---|
| 2 | large zucchini |
| 3 | large yellow squash |
| 3-4 | whole portobello mushrooms |
| 2 | red bell peppers |
| 1 | large red onion |
| ½ | (125 mL) cup olive oil |
| 1 | tablespoon cumin |
| 2 | teaspoons black pepper |
| 1 | teaspoon salt |

1. Have your grill pan ready on medium-high heat and make sure the surface is clean. Using paper towels, coat the surface with oil if needed.

2. Cut zucchini and squash lengthwise at about ¼-inch thickness. Cut sides off of your red peppers and slice your onion into rings (do not pull rings apart).

3. Using a pastry or grilling brush, coat both sides of veggies with olive oil.

4. Combine cumin, black pepper and salt in a small bowl and mix well. Sprinkle the spice mixture on all sides of the veggies.

5. Place onto your hot grill pan and cook for 2–3 minutes each side.

6. Cut veggies into chunks and combine in serving bowl.

**Plan Ahead**—*You can have all your veggies precut and in a ziplock in your refrigerator the night before. Just coat with olive oil and seasonings just before cooking.*

**Variations**—*Try all sorts of peppers to add heat or color. Mix some chimichurri (recipe page 92) in with the veggies to add even more flavor to things. Obviously, if you have an outdoor grill, go ahead and grill these veggies outdoor over a direct medium-high heat.*

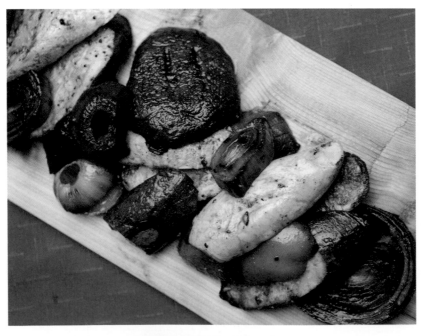

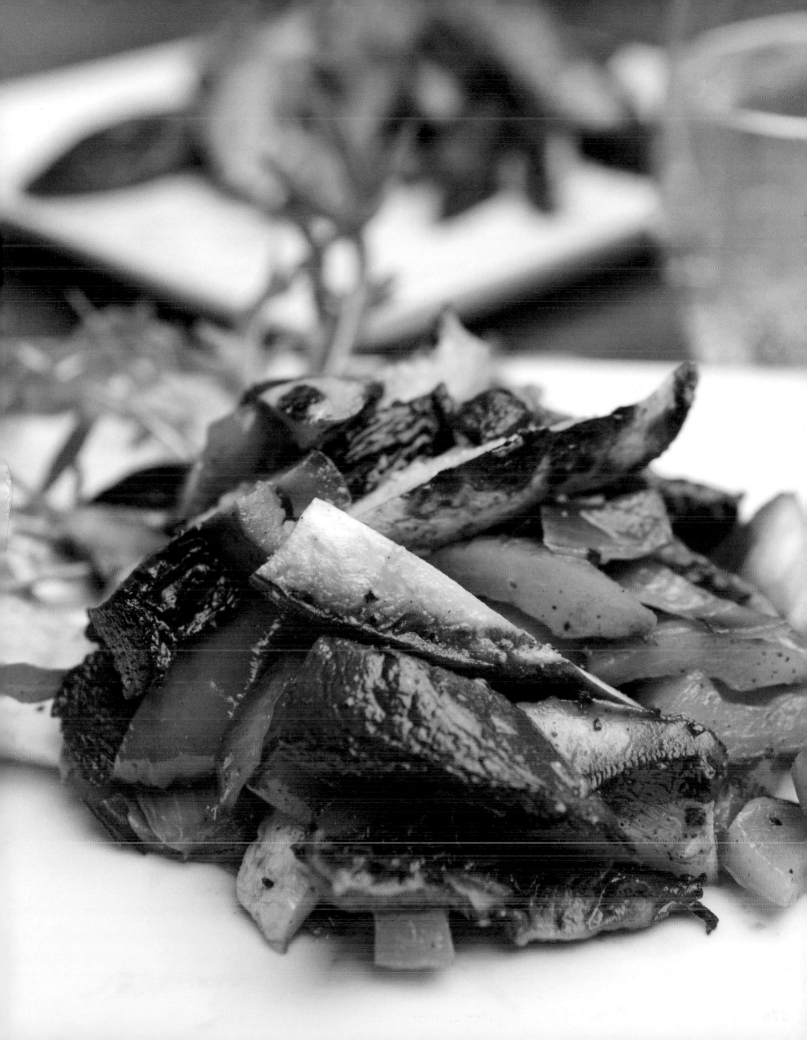

# fried okra

*Late summer at the Mayfield house would almost guarantee fried okra was on the table. Okra is as commonplace in the South as grits. You don't have to give up any flavor or texture to enjoy this classic adapted in this manner. If you're going to go to the trouble, double this recipe up and save some for later. It keeps extremely well for days in the refrigerator.*

| | |
|---|---|
| 2 | pounds (900 g) fresh okra |
| ½ | cup (75 g) coconut flour |
| 1 | teaspoon black pepper |
| ¼ | teaspoon garlic powder |
| ½ | teaspoon cayenne pepper |
| 1 | large egg |
| ¼ | cup (60 mL) coconut milk |
| 2 | cups (500 mL) coconut or olive oil |
| 1½ | cups (225 g) almond flour |
| 1 | teaspoon cumin |
| ¼ | teaspoon salt |

1. Cut okra into ½-inch pieces and place in a large bowl.

2. In small bowl, mix together coconut flour, black pepper, garlic powder, and cayenne pepper. Pour mixture over okra and coat well.

3. In same small bowl, whisk egg in with coconut milk. Pour egg/milk mixture over the okra and allow to soak for 3–5 minutes.

4. Heat oil in a medium skillet. You'll want the oil at around 350°F (175°C). Be sure to not let it get over 375°F (185°C).

5. Combine almond flour, cumin, and salt together on large plate. Dredge one piece of the soaked okra in the flour mixture, and test in the hot oil to ensure the oil is hot enough (it should sizzle immediately). If the oil is hot enough, dredge the rest of the okra in the flour mixture, and add in a single layer in the pan, Use a slotted spatula to flip okra over and remove from oil.

6. Place okra on newspaper or paper towels to soak up excess oil before serving.

**Tips & Tricks**—*Use a medium-sized frying pan. Any larger than that and your oil won't be deep enough. The oil should come halfway up the okra when you place in the pan.*

**Variation**—*Try this recipe with fried dill pickle slices for an amazing appetizer.*

**Ingredient note**—*Olive oil does not have a very high smoke point, and will in fact oxidize at higher temperatures. It's not the preferred oil here, so we suggest using coconut oil, though it may be off-putting to those who don't like the subtle coconut flavor.*

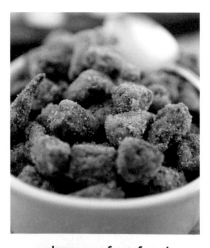

**paleo comfort foods**

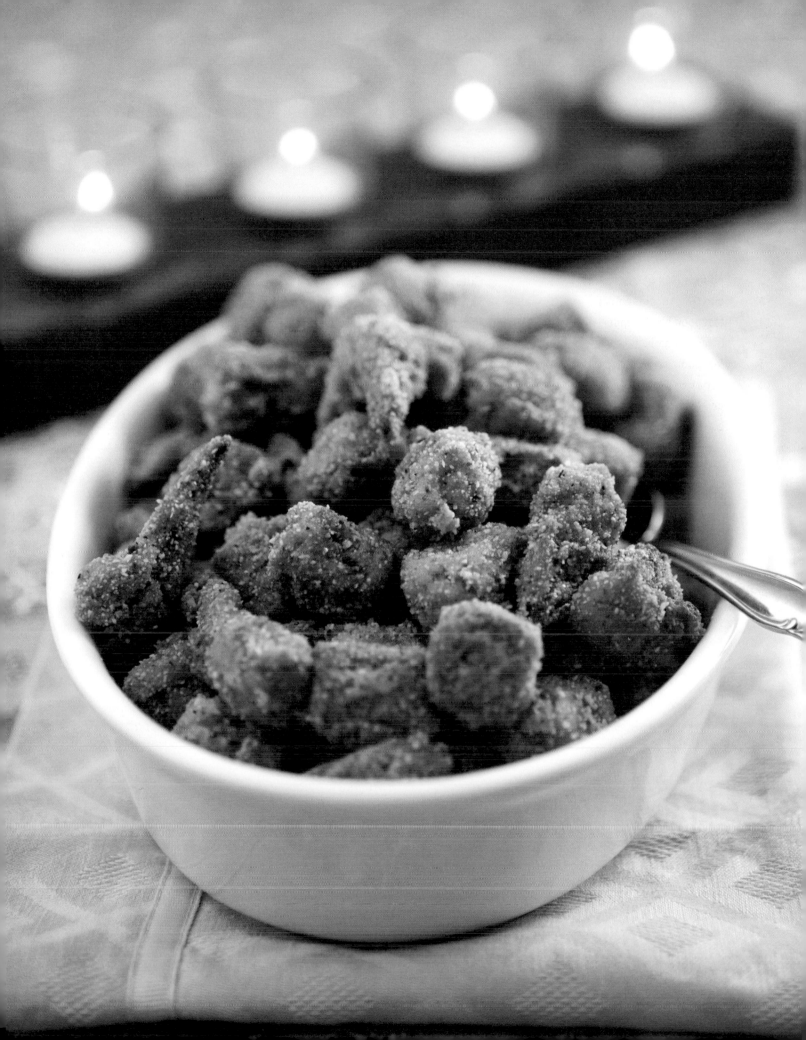

# mashed cauliflower

*True story: we served mashed cauliflower at our wedding reception. We didn't care if other people wanted mashed potatoes—this was our wedding! I gave our caterers my recipe for the mashed cauliflower, and they served it in these great pewter serving dishes. It was awesome, and I was thrilled to share this healthy mashed potato alternative on our big day. Friends and family still comment on how tasty they thought the mashed cauliflower was! Check our refrigerator at home, and on most days you are apt to find a container of mashed cauliflower. It's super-low-carb, goes great with everything from burgers to pot roast to grilled chicken, and is incredibly easy to make.*

*My secret? Cooking the cauliflower in a chicken stock adds depth to the flavor.*

| | |
|---|---|
| 1 | head fresh cauliflower |
| 1 | cup (250 mL) chicken stock |
| ¼ | teaspoon fresh cracked pepper |
| 2 | cloves garlic, crushed |

1. Cut your cauliflower head into small chunks of the florets and stem.

2. Place all ingredients in a medium saucepan or Dutch oven and bring to a boil.

3. Reduce heat to medium heat, and cover, allowing to cook for 20 minutes or so until the cauliflower is very tender and easily mashed with a fork. You may need to add more stock if everything is dried up . . . or if you have a lot of liquid still remaining, pour most of it off into a bowl and reserve. *Much* better to start with too little liquid than too much (you can always add more if needed). Cauliflower holds a ton of liquid, so start with less than you think necessary.

4. Carefully pour cauliflower and all ingredients into the bowl of a food processor, or keep in pan and use an immersion blender or hand mixer to mash. If the mashed cauliflower seems too dry, add in some of the reserved liquid or additional chicken stock.

**Tips & Tricks**—*While you could use a hand potato masher, it will not get the cauliflower super smooth. If you prefer chunky, this is absolutely the way to go!*

**Variations**—*There are so many ways you can tweak this recipe: add some roasted garlic and rosemary. Try some Hungarian smoked paprika. Or go with some crumbled-up bacon and fresh chopped chives. If you want a kick, opt for some horseradish or wasabi. Maybe a drizzle of olive oil and fresh chopped basil? Putting in a few tablespoons of butter helps make these really creamy. I've made the mash with a combination of turnips and cauliflower. The turnips add a little sweetness, and are super tasty!*

**Ingredient Notes**—*Pre-bagged fresh or frozen cauliflower works just fine for this one.*

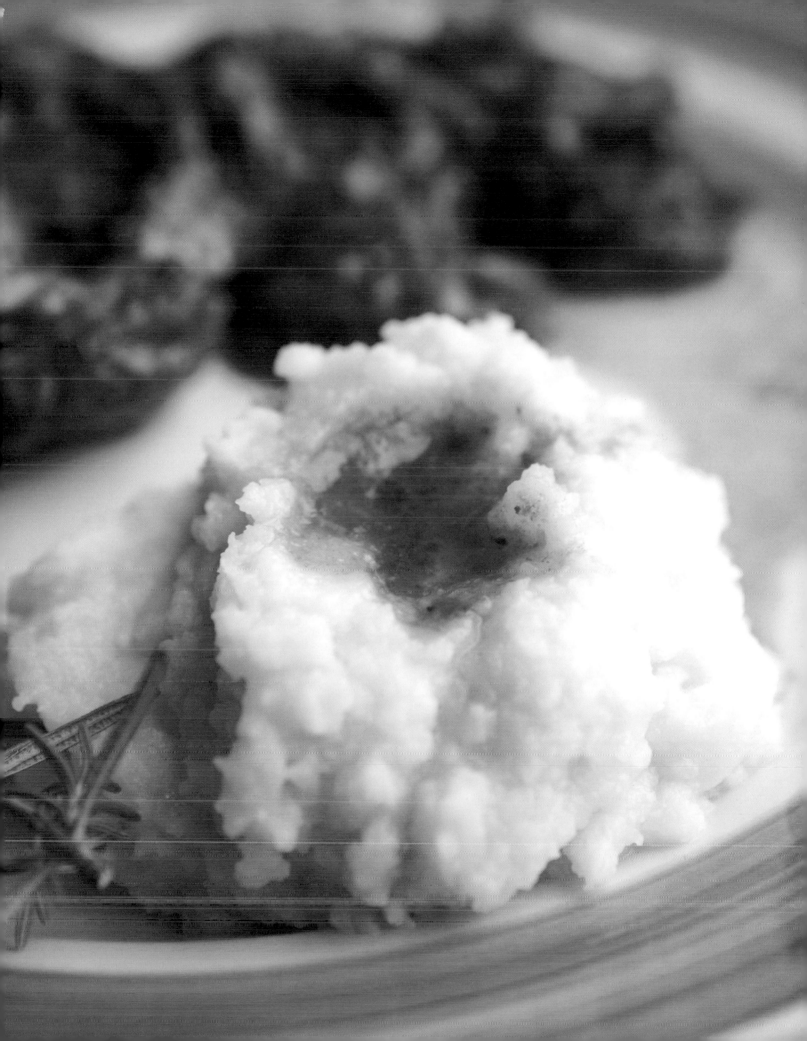

# collard greens

*This tasty and nutrient-dense Southern side is one that we enjoy throughout the fall. It's no surprise that collard greens are such a staple for New Year's Day. I remember Mom saying that eating collards on New Year's Day would bring you money all year long. That may not be true, but in any case, these cruciferous vegetables pack an amazing punch when it comes to lowering cholesterol and fighting cancer. Eating these on a regular basis is doing your body a ton of good.*

*You can play around with different spices and accompaniments. Spice them up by adding a jalapeño or crushed red pepper into the pot. Steaming them will actually maintain a higher nutrient content. However, I love that smoky taste that comes with the ham hock, and who doesn't love that flavor? Be sure not to overcook them. Cutting the strips the same size will allow them to cook evenly. If this is your first time cranking up collard greens, stay on the safe side and cook for 20–35 minutes. Overcooking them will bring on a sulfur-like smell and nobody wants that at the supper table.*

| | |
|---|---|
| 2 | bunches collard greens, washed and de-stemmed |
| 4 | strips bacon, cut into 1-inch (2 cm) squares |
| 1 | tablespoon garlic, minced |
| 1 | medium onion, sliced |
| 3 | quarts (3 L) water |
| 1 | teaspoon black pepper |
| 1 | ham hock, smoked |

1. Wash collard greens thoroughly. Remove the stems.

2. Once all leaves are removed and stems discarded take 6–8 leaves at a time and roll them up. Using a chef's knife, cut the rolls every inch or so. Once cut, put all the cuttings into a large bowl and set aside for later.

3. In a large stock pot, cook bacon until dark and crispy. Remove bacon and retain the drippings in the pot. Set bacon aside for garnishing later.

4. Sauté garlic and onion in drippings until onions are translucent. Now drop in the collards a handful at a time. Toss them with a long spoon until they have wilted to ½ their original size.

5. Add water, black pepper, and ham hock. Stir well and bring to a slight boil. Reduce heat and let simmer for 30–40 minutes or until tender.

6. Chop bacon into small bits. Remove the collards from pot and place in large serving bowl. Garnish with chopped bacon bits.

**Variations**—*Mustard Greens or even Kale can be used instead of the collard greens.*

**Tips & Tricks**—*Folding greens in half along the stalk allows you to remove leaves quickly by cutting on either side of the stem. If you don't have a large pot, add greens slowly. They should wilt and reduce in size quickly.*

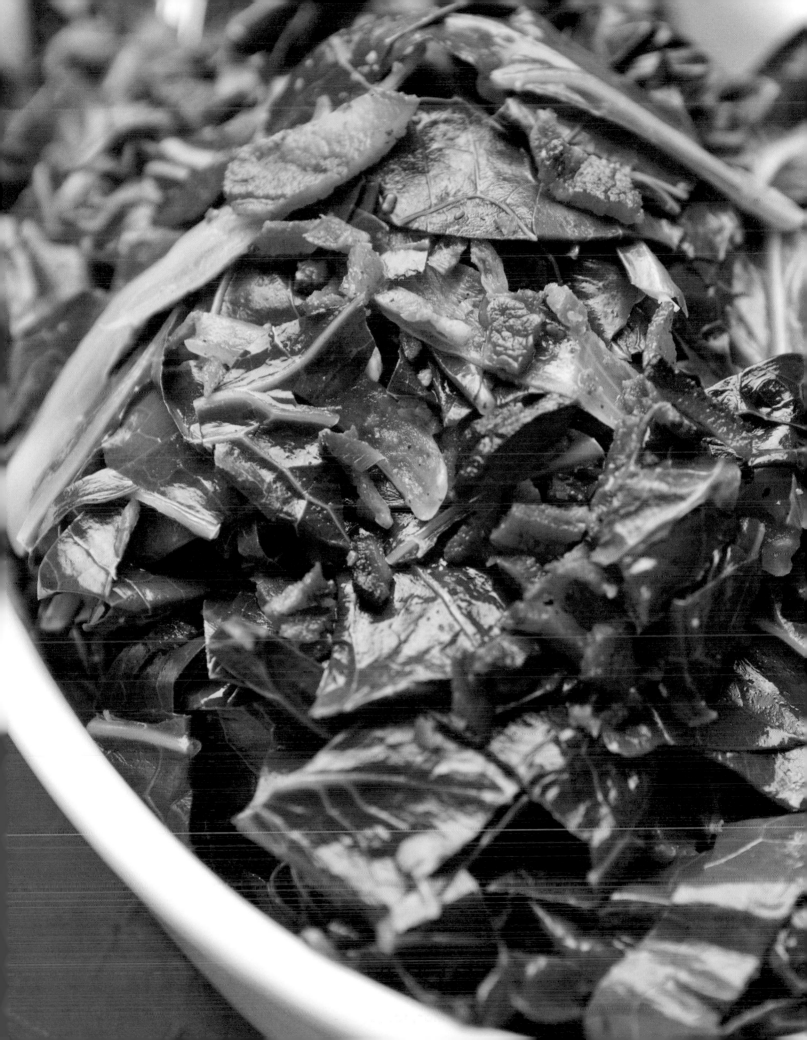

# creamed spinach

*Creamed spinach. But without the cream. There is still a slight lingering coconut flavor in this dish, which I'm sure might be off-putting to some, or sheer delight to others.*

*I will say that I love doing twists on this recipe, like adding in some chopped-up artichokes (think pseudo spinach-artichoke dip), drizzling with a little hot sauce, sprinkling on some cayenne pepper, or if I'm doing a dairy cheat, getting some parmesan cheese in there. So many options, and so full of vitamins and garlicky goodness.*

| | |
|---|---|
| 1 | pound (450 g) frozen spinach |
| ½ | cup (125 mL) coconut milk |
| 3 | cloves fresh garlic, minced |
| ½ | teaspoon coconut flour |
| 2 | teaspoons olive oil |
| 1 | shallot, minced |
| ½ | teaspoon paprika |
| ~ | salt and pepper, to taste |

1. Thaw spinach completely in a colander over the sink, and using your hands, squeeze out all remaining liquid.
2. Heat a small saucepan over medium heat.
3. Add the coconut milk and 2 teaspoons of the minced garlic (this will infuse the coconut milk with a bit of the garlic flavor).
4. Whisk in the ½ teaspoon coconut flour until slightly simmering. Remove from heat.
5. Meanwhile, heat olive oil in skillet over medium heat, and add shallot, remaining garlic and paprika.
6. Cook until shallots are just translucent, being careful not to burn the shallots or garlic.
7. Add spinach and coconut cream sauce, and simmer until everything is cooked through.
8. Serve immediately.

**Ingredient Note**—*If you have a bunch of fresh spinach, you can totally use that too. If using fresh spinach: preheat large pot of water. Once it reaches a boil, submerge spinach for about 60 seconds or until bright green. Using a slotted spoon, transfer spinach to a bowl of ice water (this process is called "blanching" and will preserve the bright green color). Drain spinach, squeezing out all residual moisture, and rough chop.*

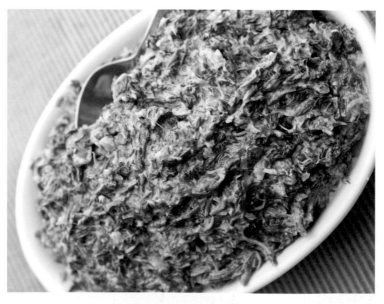

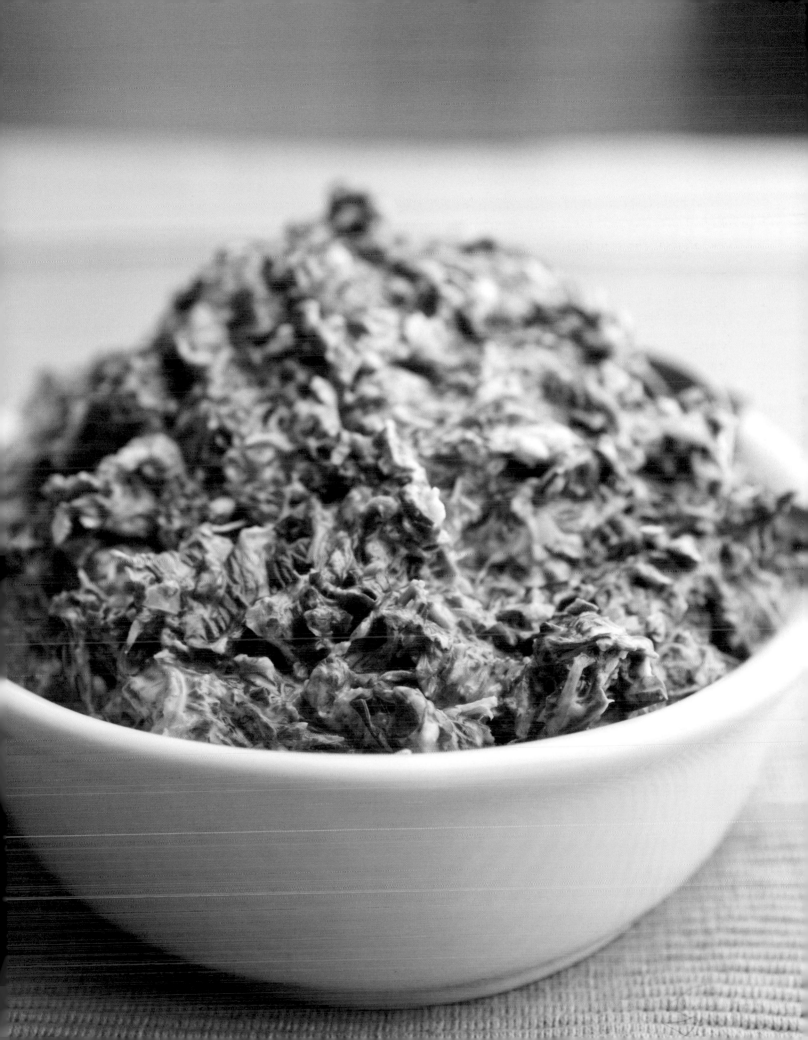

# sautéed apples

*I stumbled upon this recipe one morning trying to be creative. Julie and I had been super busy for several days and breakfast consisted of repeated trips to the frittata we had made a few days before. The refrigerator was pretty bare, and I wanted to mix things up a bit. Still pressed for time, I grabbed an apple off the counter and got to work. Honestly, though, how bad can butter and cinnamon taste? Well, when you combine them with tart apples, it tastes like dessert at breakfast. Truthfully, we add them as a side for any meal. This recipe goes really well with chicken and pork.*

| | |
|---|---|
| 3 | apples, cored and sliced |
| 1 | tablespoon butter (grass-fed, clarified is preferred) |
| 2 | teaspoons cinnamon |
| ½ | cup (50 g) pecans, chopped |

1. Bring frying pan to medium-high heat.
2. Toast pecans for 3–4 minutes and then add butter to the pan.
3. Add the apples and cinnamon.
4. Sauté for 5–7 minutes and serve.

**Variations**—*Peel the apples before cooking. Once they soften, mash them up for homemade apple sauce.*

**Ingredient Notes**—*Firm, slightly tart apples work best. We like to use Pink Ladies.*

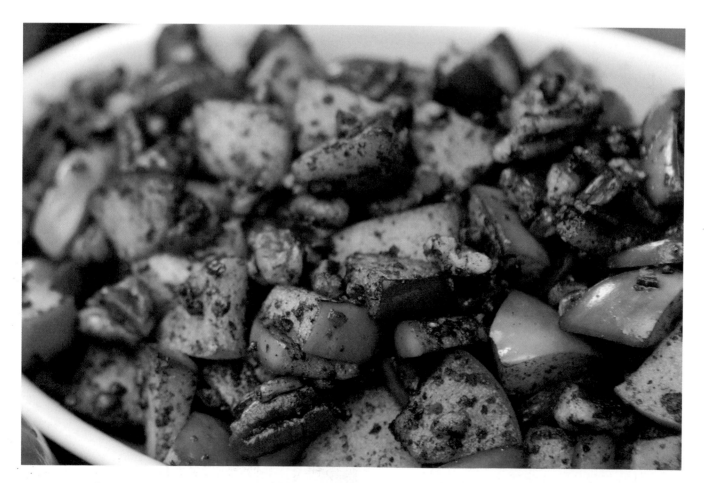

paleo comfort foods

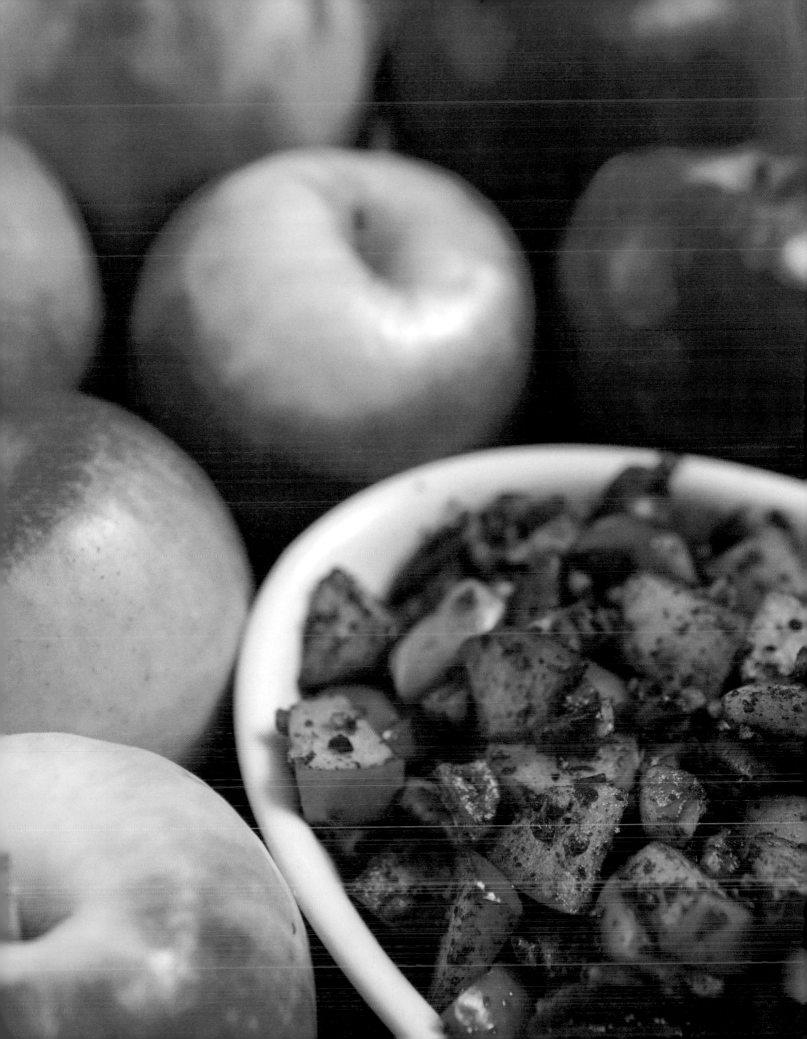

# scattered, smothered and chunked sweet hash

*Just about anyone in the South will recognize the black-and-yellow sign of a Waffle House from miles away. While yes, Waffle House is known for its waffles, perhaps better known to the masses are the variations on hash browns and the vernacular that accompanies them (the servers use diner lingo to call their orders). Scattered (scattered and fried on the griddle), smothered (with onions), covered (topped with a piece of cheese), chunked (with diced ham) . . . the list goes on and on. Here's our variation on hash browns with more paleo-friendly sweet potatoes that are "scattered, smothered, and chunked."*

| | |
|---|---|
| 2 | tablespoons coconut, avocado, or olive oil |
| 1 | sweet onion, diced |
| 1 | pound (450 g) sweet potatoes, peeled and shredded/grated |
| 1 | pound (450 g) cooked chicken or turkey sausage, cubed into small dice |
| 3 | teaspoons cumin |
| 1 | teaspoon cayenne pepper |
| ~ | salt and pepper to taste |

1. Heat a large sized skillet over medium heat and add in oil.

2. Sauté onion until translucent.

3. Stir in the potatoes, mixing to combine and cook until potatoes start to soften and then eventually brown.

4. Mix in the sausage, cumin, cayenne, salt, and pepper, and cook until sausages start to get a bit brown.

**Variations**—*While I personally love these hash browns with some chorizo or andouille sausage (I heart spicy!), it also tastes great with any of the Whole Foods or Trader Joe's chicken/turkey sausages. You could dice up some ham, or so many other protein options here. If you need extra protein with your hash, fry up or poach an egg and serve it on top. Or, just like Waffle House, cap them (mushrooms), pepper them (jalapeños), or get really crazy and top them (with chili!).*

**Tips & Tricks**—*The potatoes cook up and get crispy a lot faster if your par-cook them in the microwave first (heat for about 3–4 minutes in a microwave safe bowl or dish).*

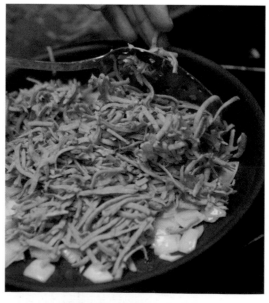

paleo comfort foods

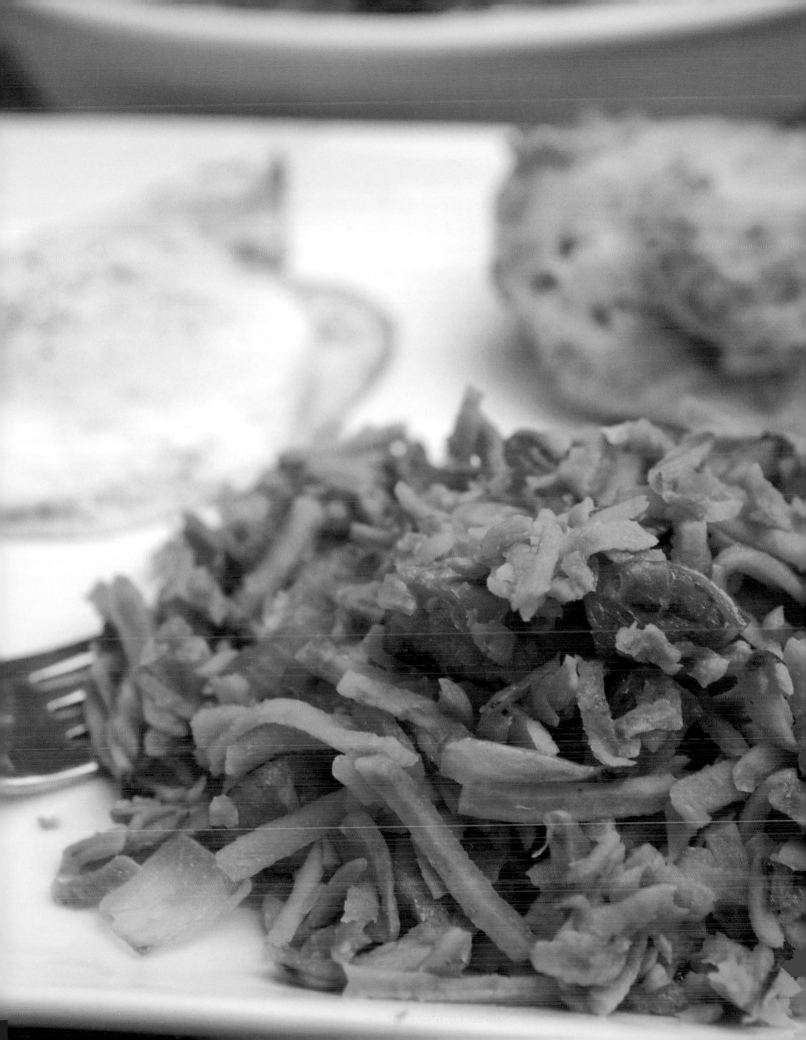

# the tastiest slaw ever

*This slaw will go well with just about any fish you want to serve. The host of various flavors in this are a great accompaniment to most anything with fins. We especially like this slaw with our Fish Tacos (see page 264).*

*Red cabbage and the optional shredded carrots give this dish lots of color and it looks great on any picnic table.*

*Feel free to double up on this recipe. It keeps well in the refrigerator and it travels well to work or your next potluck supper. The use of red cabbage will fill you with anthocyanins. When it comes to fighting inflammation, these compounds rank high.*

| | |
|---|---|
| 2 | teaspoons red wine vinegar |
| 2 | tablespoons olive oil |
| ~ | juice of 2 limes |
| ½ | teaspoon garlic, minced |
| ⅛ | teaspoon black pepper |
| 2 | cups (200 g) red cabbage, thinly sliced |
| 2 | cups (150 g) romaine lettuce, chopped |
| 1 | mango, peeled, pitted and chopped |
| 1 | cup (150 g) cucumbers, peeled, seeded and cut into strips |

1. Combine vinegar, olive oil, lime juice, garlic, and black pepper in a small bowl.
2. In large bowl and mix all other ingredients.
3. Mix well and pour liquid over the slaw, tossing to mix.
4. Cover and chill for at least 1 hour.

**Variations**—*Add a chopped jalapeño for a kick, ½ cup carrots for more color, or tablespoon of honey for more sweetness. Shred cabbage in a food processor for different texture.*

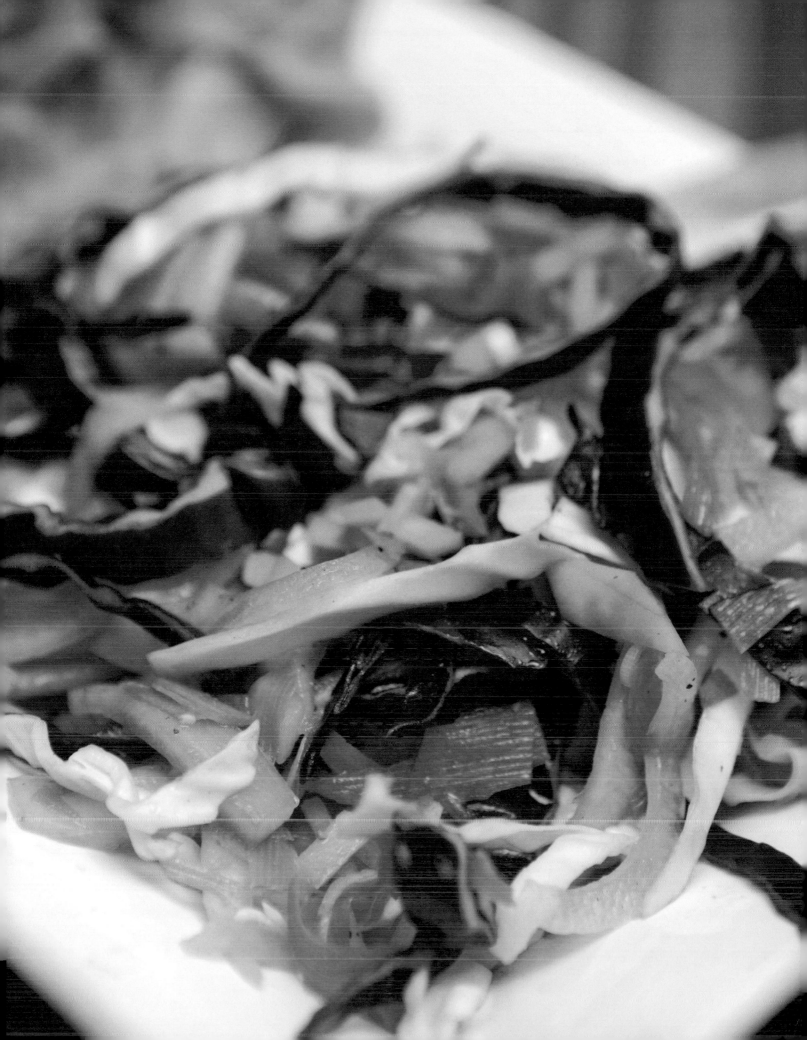

# oven-roasted okra

*Are you getting tired of okra yet? We aren't. As Southern as you may be, I'll bet you have never had "just okra." We hadn't until Julie's brother Andy gave us two tickets to Outstanding in the Field. Please go Google them now. Jim Denevan has put together the most amazing experience. Jim pairs local farmers with local chefs throughout the country to bring restaurant patrons to the source of their food. As opposed to "Farm to table," this organization brings the table to the farm.*

*Our dinner was at Love Is Love Farm in Douglasville, Georgia. We toured the farm at the side of Joe Reynolds and Judith Winfrey, the couple hired to manage the farm. They were the masterminds behind some pretty incredible vegetables, and simply the nicest people. That evening, we were treated to our first-ever spiced oven-roasted okra at the talented hands of Chef Kevin Gillespie (Top Chef finalist). No slimy texture as can sometimes be the case with okra! The following week, we tried our own variation of these tasty morsels, and the recipe has been a staple in our house ever since.*

*The only sad part about the day was that it was rather rainy outside, and within forty-eight hours of this amazing farm tour and dinner, the very land we toured under umbrellas was five feet underwater with the worst flooding that had hit Atlanta in over 100 years.*

*We are happy to report that Judith and Joe are back on their feet, now managing Gaia farms in Atlanta, and they are still producing some of the most amazing vegetables in the greater Atlanta area. For a unique "table on the farm" experience, check out the listings for Outstanding in the Field and try to get out to support some of these awesome farmers growing your food!*

---

| | |
|---|---|
| 1 | pound (450 g) okra (whole), washed |
| ¼ | cup (60 mL) olive oil |
| 2 | tablespoons cumin |
| 1 | teaspoon salt |
| 1 | teaspoon black pepper |
| ¼ | teaspoon cayenne pepper |

1. Preheat oven to 400°F (205°C).
2. Toss okra in olive oil to coat and place onto a sheet pan in a single layer.
3. Combine all dry spices and sprinkle over okra, mixing well.
4. Bake for 5–7 minutes and turn over onto the other side. Place the okra back in the oven for another 3–5 minutes or until pods are softened.

---

**Ingredient Notes**—*When shopping for good okra, take your thumb and pop the small tip off the okra. If it pops off, the okra is good. If it bends and doesn't snap, then you know it is a bad one.*

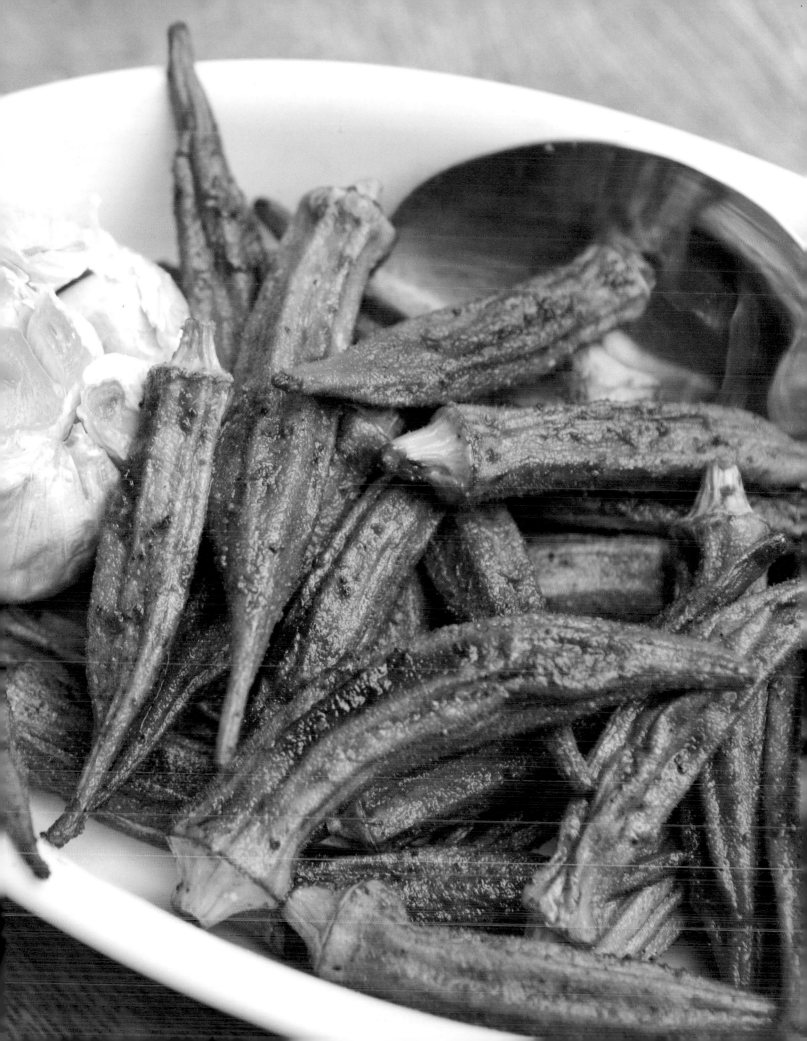

# fried green tomatoes

*No, not the movie. Although I'm certain Kathy Bates and crew would approve of this recipe. You can bet that we will be cooking this one up from mid-summer all the way through fall. There are at least fifteen tomato plant varieties in the ground at our house in the summer. It is nice to be able to snag a few that aren't quite yet ripe and turn them into something tasty—or at least save the green tomatoes from our labradoodle, Phoenix, who thinks the green tomatoes look a lot like tennis balls.*

*My favorite is poaching an egg and placing right on top of some fried green 'maters for a breakfast bonanza of flavor.*

| | |
|---|---|
| 4 | medium green tomatoes |
| 1½ | cups (225 g) almond flour |
| 2 | teaspoons black pepper |
| ½ | teaspoon salt |
| 1 | teaspoon chipotle powder |
| ¼ | teaspoon garlic powder |
| 1 | large egg |
| ½ | cup (125 mL) olive or coconut oil |

1. Slice tomatoes about ¼ inch (½ cm) thick.
2. Combine all the dry ingredients in bowl and mix well.
3. Beat egg in separate bowl. Drop the tomato slices (one at a time) in the egg batter to coat both sides (use a fork to lift in/out).
4. Place tomato slices into the bowl of the dry mixture and coat both sides. Gently shake off the excess flour and set aside until ready to cook.
5. Heat oil in medium-sized cast-iron skillet or frying pan over medium-high heat.
6. Once the oil is hot, use a fork, to place the tomato slices gently into the oil. Work in batches so as not to overcrowd the pan.
7. Turn the tomatoes over when the sides begin to brown slightly (about 2 minutes) and cook for another 2–3 minutes Remove from the frying pan and place on a plate with some newspaper or paper towels to soak up extra oil (you can add paper towels on top as you go).
8. Repeat process until you have cooked all the tomatoes. Serve hot!

**Variation**—*These can be served solo with a little Chipotle Dipping Sauce (page 94) on the side or as an appetizer.*

**Ingredient Notes**—*Green tomatoes should have a slight give in them. I find the best ones have a hint of color at the blossom end.*

**Tips & Tricks**—*You can keep your batches of just-cooked fried green tomatoes warm by placing them on a sheet pan in the oven at 250°F (130°C). To ensure they stay crispy, place them on a heat-proof cooling rack on the sheet pan.*

paleo comfort foods

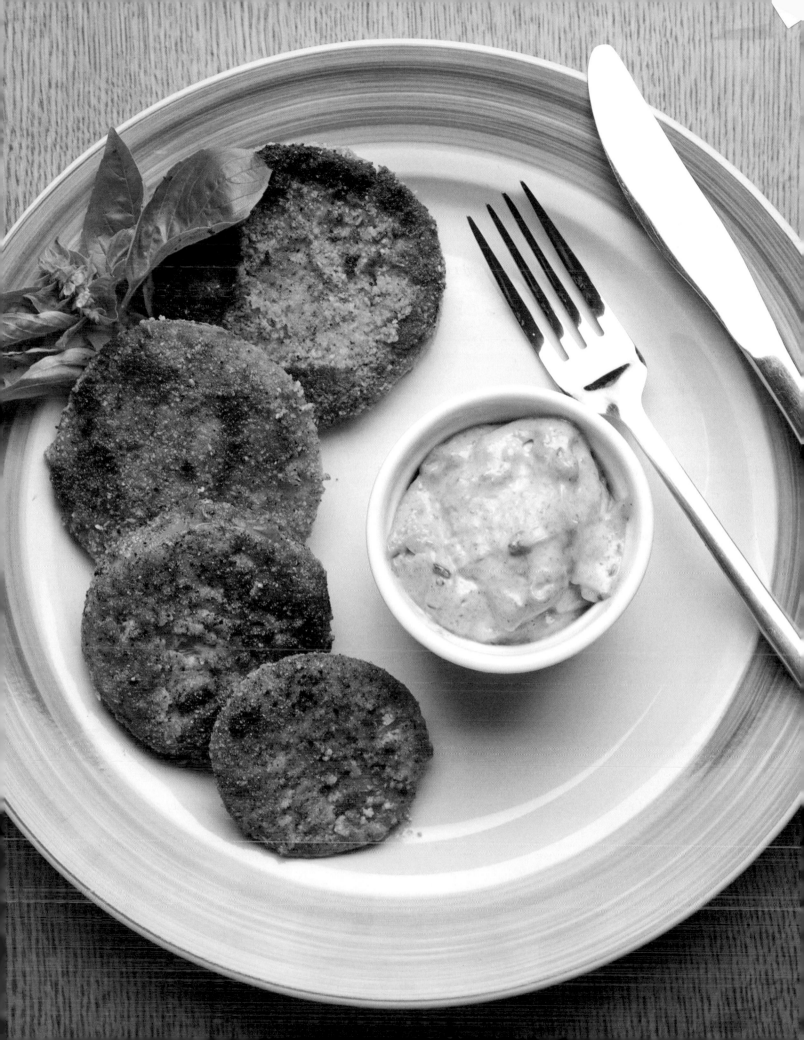

# tart cranapple sauce

*Growing up, Thanksgiving at our house meant the only acceptable way to serve cranberry sauce was from a can. You know the one. That gelatinous mold of cranberries sweetened with enough sugar to overtake the turkey's tryptophan side-effects. As I got older, and experienced different variations on cranberries (cranberry salad, cranberry molds, cranberry chutney, you name it), I preferred the tarter stuff to the usual super sweet from my youth.*

*This is not your "cranberry stuff from a can," as it's not super sweet, but it plays up the tartness of the cranberries. It's fresh, delicious, and perfect with that tender piece of turkey.*

| | |
|---|---|
| 12 | ounces (340 g) fresh cranberries, picked over for mushed ones |
| 2 | apples, peeled and sliced into small bites |
| ~ | zest of 1 lemon |
| ~ | zest of 1 orange |
| ¾ | cup (180 mL) fresh squeezed orange juice |
| ¼ | cup (60 mL) water |
| ¼ | cup (60 mL) honey, more or less to taste |
| 1 | cinnamon stick |

1. Place all ingredients in a medium saucepan, and while stirring, bring to boil.

2. Reduce heat to a simmer and allow to simmer for 10–15 minutes or until the sauce thickens some. Remove cinnamon stick.

3. Refrigerate sauce until ready to serve. As it cools it will thicken some. Serve cold!

**Variations**—*Some folks like nuts and celery added to their cranberry sauce. Whatever makes you happy! Omit the honey if you prefer.*

**Plan Ahead**—*Making this sauce a day or two ahead of time will make your Thanksgiving preparations that much easier!*

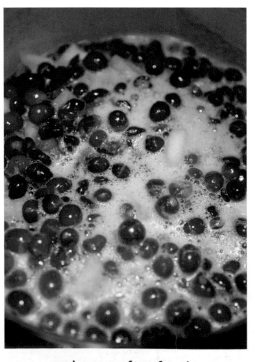

paleo comfort foods

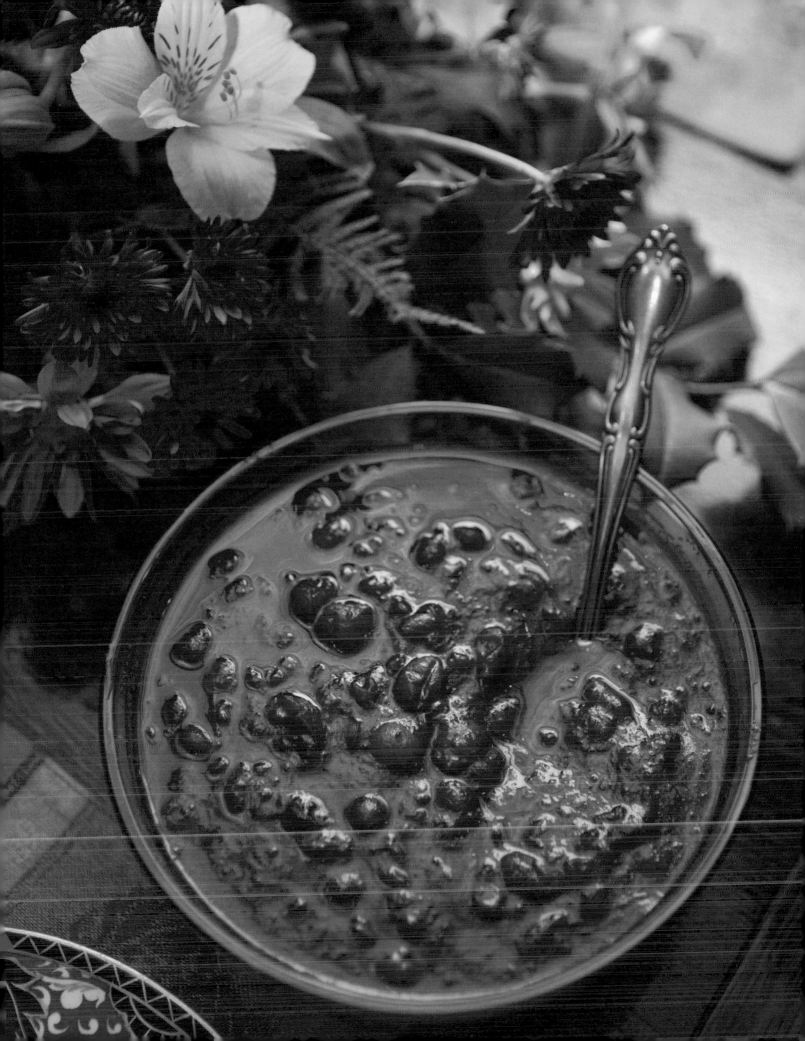

# sweet potato spears

*I remember the first time Julie made these for me, accompanied with her Chipotle Dipping Sauce. I thought, how can sweet potatoes taste good with chipotle sauce on them? You'll have to see for yourself. Trust me that you will not be disappointed. They also plate very well if you're trying to impress a guest or two. My brother, who still hasn't jumped on the band wagon, is constantly asking for this recipe to be cooked up when we're in Tennessee visiting.*

| | |
|---|---|
| 4 | medium-sized sweet potatoes, cut lengthwise into spears |
| ¼ | cup (60 mL) olive oil |
| 2 | teaspoons cumin |
| ½ | teaspoon salt |
| ½ | teaspoon pepper |
| ½ | cup (60mL) Chipotle Dipping Sauce (recipe page 94) |

1. Preheat oven to 400°F (205°C). Cover two cookie sheets with aluminum foil.

2. Toss sweet potatoes with olive oil, cumin, salt, and pepper and spread out evenly on cookie sheets, making sure not to crowd the spears.

3. Turn potatoes once or twice during baking. Bake 30–40 minutes or until potatoes are done and slightly crispy.

4. Serve with Chipotle Dipping Sauce.

**Tips & Tricks**—*These go great with just about whatever condiment suites your fancy. For some time-saving tricks, have the potatoes already cut into wedges, and in a container filled with water in the fridge. When you are ready to cook them, pour off the water, dry the spears, then season and cook. While we don't call for peeling the sweet potatoes, feel free to do so if that is your preference.*

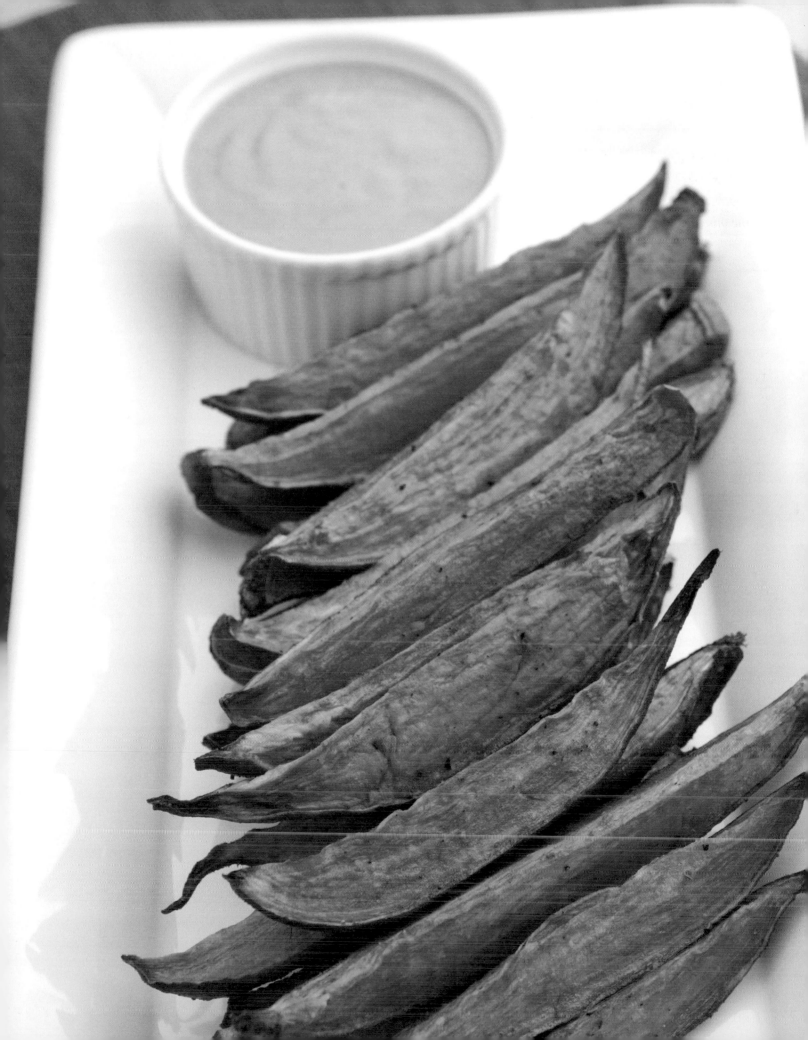

# dirty cauliflower "rice"

*Dirty rice is most commonly thought of as Cajun in origin (though it is very common throughout the entire South). Why is this rice called dirty? The rice in this dish gets an almost dirty color from the giblets, some people thinking the little bits of giblets resemble little clumps of dirt.*

*I have to be the first to admit that I am not a super fan of offal (offal most commonly refers to the inner parts of animals—intestines, organs, etc.). That being said, I did love my mom's fried chicken gizzards growing up (gizzards are the second stomach found in birds and other animals that lack teeth).*

*You can absolutely make this recipe without the giblets, however, it won't have quite the same taste. Furthermore, if you ever buy a whole turkey/chicken, please don't throw the giblets away (packaged inside the poultry cavity). Feed them to your pets or make gravy out of them—just don't let them go to waste!*

| | |
|---|---|
| 2 | tablespoons olive oil |
| 4 | cloves garlic, minced |
| 1 | cup (150 g) white onion, diced |
| 2 | celery stalks, chopped |
| 1 | cup (175 g) green pepper, diced |
| ~ | salt and pepper to taste |
| 3 | cups (700 g) cauliflower, riced with your food processor or box grater |
| 1 | teaspoon fresh thyme |
| 1 | bay leaf |
| ¼ | teaspoon cayenne pepper |
| ½ | teaspoon cumin |
| ½ | pound (230 g) pork sausage meat |
| ½ | pound (230 g) chicken giblets |
| 1 | bunch green onions, chopped |
| 2 | cups (500 mL) chicken stock |

1. Heat olive oil over medium heat in large skillet.

2. Add garlic, onions, celery, and green pepper, and sauté until soft.

3. Stir in cauliflower rice, adding in thyme, bay leaf, cayenne, and cumin.

4. Meanwhile, brown sausage in a separate skillet. Strain off excess fat, and add sausage to rice.

5. In a medium sauce pot, cover giblets and half of the green onions with water and cook over medium heat about 30 minutes. Strain and allow to cool, then chop into very small pieces.

6. Combine giblets and remaining green onions with rice mixture, adding in the chicken stock.

7. Allow to simmer over medium-low heat, stirring frequently, for 30 minutes or so or until flavors meld and the liquid has cooked off.

**Variations**—*You can have all kinds of fun with this recipe. Add in some tomato paste and cumin to make this a bit more like Spanish rice, mix in diced chicken instead of or along with the giblets and sausage, and make a meal out of it! Get creative and have fun!*

**Ingredient Notes**—*Giblets is a term for the offal of a fowl. These are the edible organs and typically include the heart, liver, gizzard, and visceral organs.*

paleo comfort foods

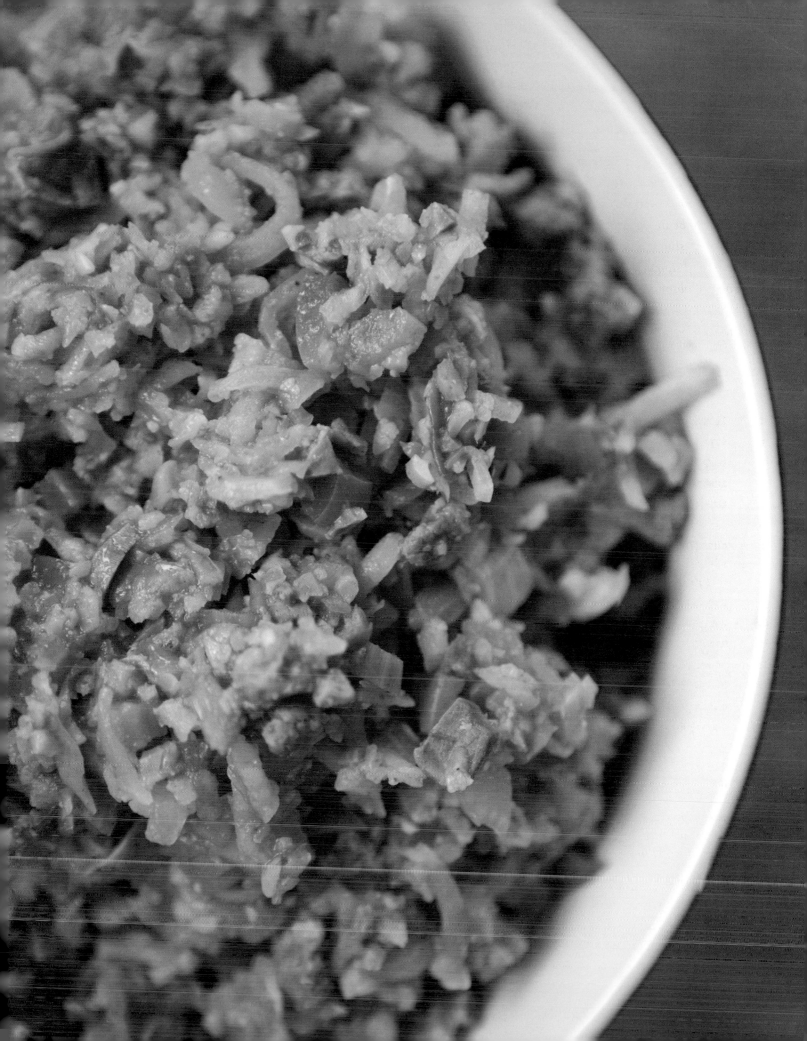

# momma's slaw

*This is a backyard barbecue staple. If you want to add that traditional yellow hue to it, throw a tablespoon of yellow mustard into the slaw. Your friends won't know any better.*

*Yes, we have two slaw recipes in this book. It's just one of those dishes that keeps well, travels well, and goes great with so many dishes. Enjoy!*

| | |
|---|---|
| 1 | head green cabbage, finely shredded |
| 2 | large carrots, shredded |
| 1 | cup (250 mL) Paleo Mayonnaise (recipe page 100) |
| ¼ | cup (40 g) onion, grated |
| 2 | tablespoons white vinegar |
| 1 | tablespoon dry mustard |
| 1 | teaspoon black pepper |
| ½ | teaspoon celery salt |
| 1 | tablespoon honey (optional) |

1. Combine cabbage and carrots in a large bowl.

2. In separate bowl, whisk together mayonnaise, onion, vinegar, mustard, black pepper, and celery salt.

3. Pour mixture over your cabbage and carrots and mix well.

4. If you feel it needs a little more sweetness than the carrots deliver, add the honey and mix well.

**Tips & Tricks**—*The food processor makes this recipe a snap, as it does all that chopping and shredding for you. If you'll be serving this outdoors, just remember to keep the slaw refrigerated to avoid the possibility of food-borne illnesses!*

**Variations**—*Use apple cider vinegar instead of the white vinegar, or add some shredded radishes.*

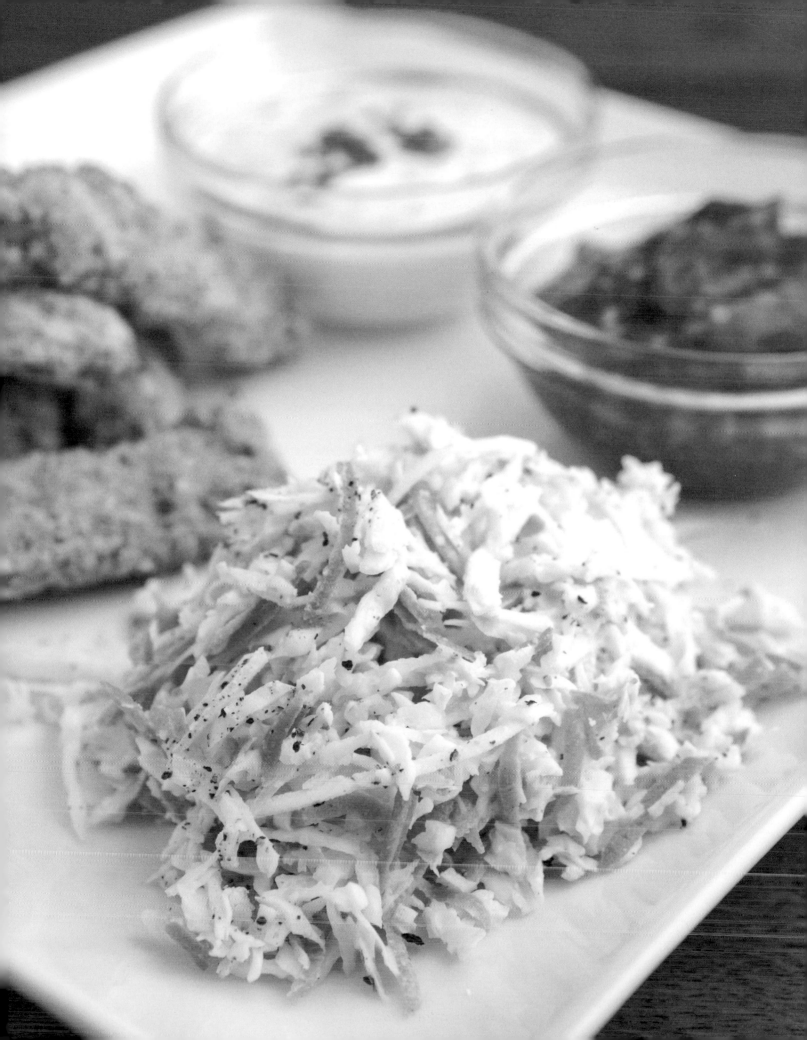

# okra stew

*There is no telling how many times I've treated myself to okra stew. This one is a favorite of my Dad, especially when Mom is out of town, perhaps because it is so easy to prepare! It is thick and hearty and goes great with any meal. We especially enjoy this one with chicken or steak in the fall.*

| | |
|---|---|
| 1–1¼ | pounds (500 g) fresh okra |
| 1 | teaspoon black peppercorns |
| ½ | teaspoon cumin seeds |
| ¼ | teaspoon salt |
| ½ | teaspoon oregano |
| 1 | teaspoon dried thyme |
| 1 | tablespoon olive oil |
| 2 | cloves garlic, minced |
| ½ | red bell pepper, chopped |
| 1 | large onion, chopped |
| 28 | ounces (825 mL) whole canned tomatoes |
| 1 | cup (250 mL) chicken stock |

1. Trim stems off the okra and cut crosswise into halves.
2. Combine peppercorns, cumin seeds, salt, oregano and thyme in a coffee grinder or mortar and pestle to grind.
3. Over medium-high heat, sauté in olive oil the garlic, red pepper, and onion until they begin to soften (about 5 minutes).
4. Add in the okra, tomatoes, chicken broth, and spices. Stir to combine well.
5. Keep on medium heat for 20–25 minutes or until okra is tender enough to pierce with a fork.

**Ingredient Notes**—*If you don't have peppercorns or cumin seeds lying around, just use the ground version.*

**Variations**—*Add a diced jalapeño to the sauté for some added heat.*

**Hint**—*This recipe freezes well.*

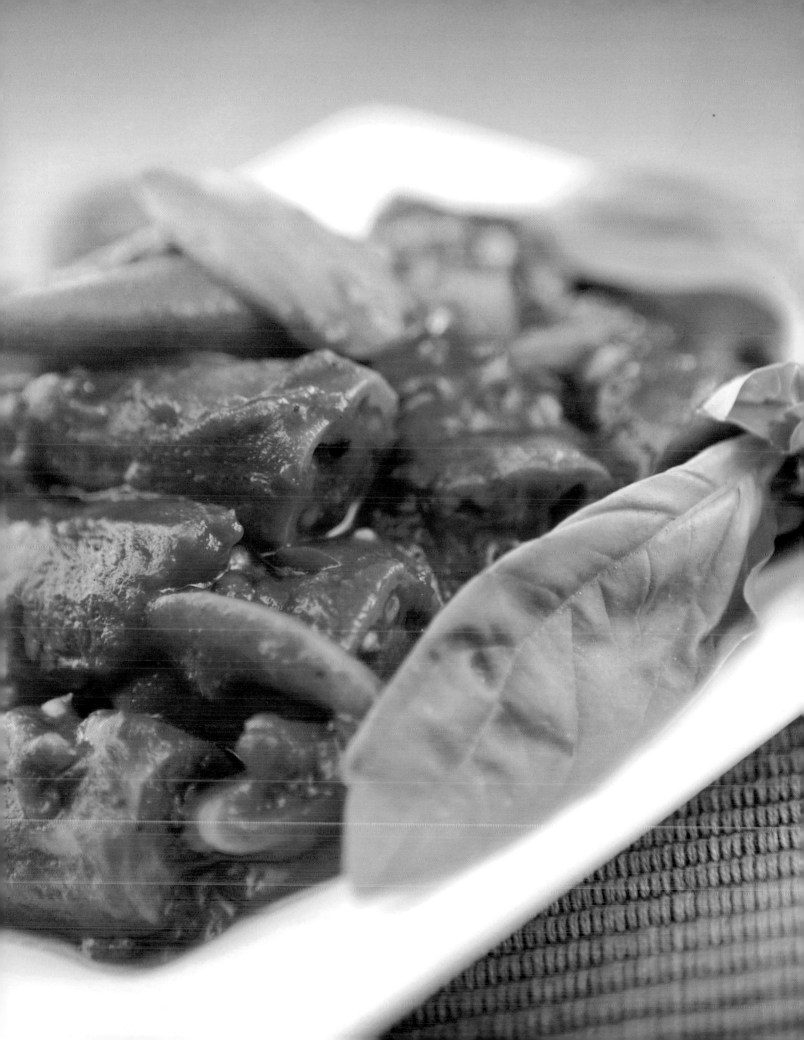

# paleo grits

*The movie My Cousin Vinnie says it best: "No self-respecting Southerner uses instant grits."*

*Yep, grits are a cornerstone for any Southern breakfast. The wonderful thing about these paleo grits is that there is very little difference in prep time between this gem and the normal fare. You can serve these with darn near anything. Julie gets credit for perfecting this one after I gave it a go for a Shrimp and Grits recipe one evening. Good news for you, that recipe is included in this book (recipe page 256).*

| | |
|---|---|
| 4 | cups (700 g) cauliflower, riced |
| 1 | cup (150 g) almond meal |
| 3 | cups (750 mL) chicken stock |
| ~ | salt and pepper, to taste |

**1.** Mix cauliflower, almond meal, and chicken stock over medium heat in large sauce pan.

**2.** Cover and reduce heat to medium/medium-low, simmering for 20 minutes—stirring every 5 minutes or so—until the liquid is absorbed.

**3.** Season with salt and pepper to taste.

**Tips &Tricks**—*To rice cauliflower, shred it in a food processor or with a box grater.*

**Variations**—*Throw in a small can of diced pickled jalapeños for some extra flavor. If dairy is in your life, add in some shredded sharp Cheddar cheese or shredded Parmesan cheese. While certain recipes in this book do call for blanched almond flour, this is one where we think the almond meal works best!*

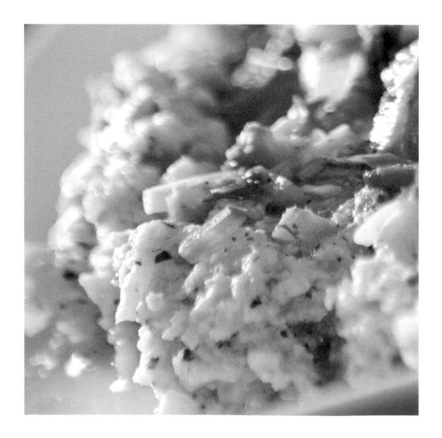

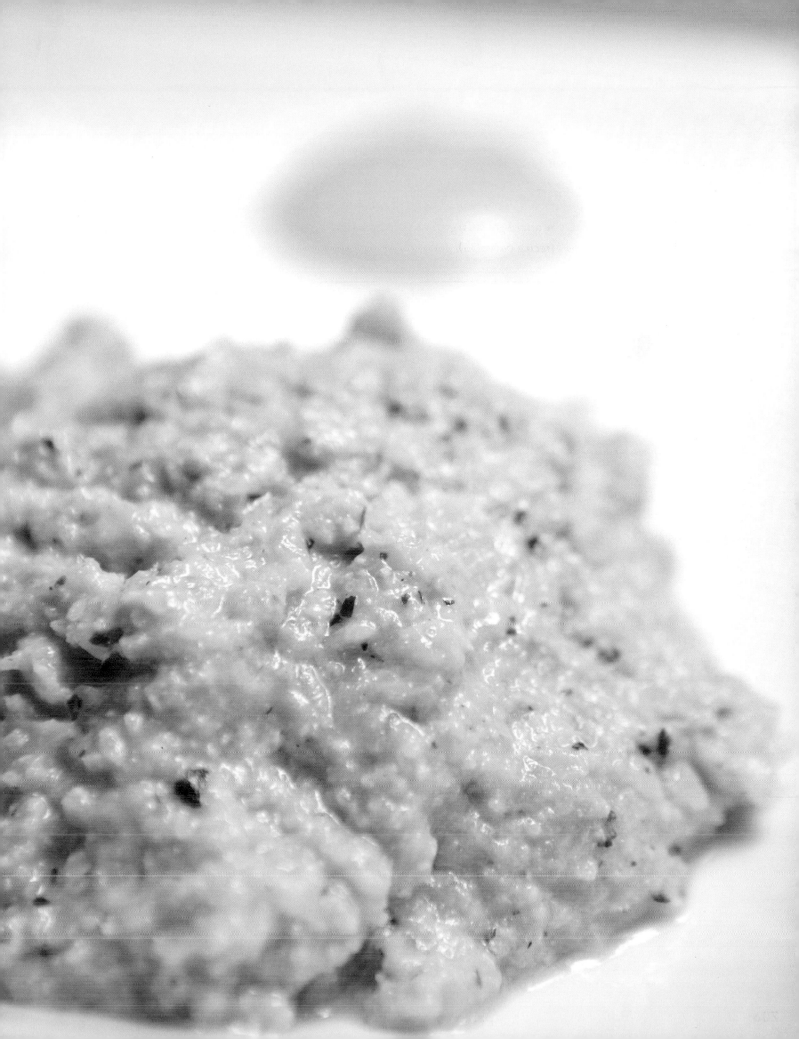

# sweet potato casserole

*We see this delicious dish served up with turkey and dressing all the time. Don't reserve this dish for only Thanksgiving and Christmas, as it can make its way to the table year round. No need for all that brown sugar to hide the natural sweetness of the sweet potato. Sweet potatoes are easy to find and can sit on your kitchen counter for days until you are ready to rock. Just please, no marshmallows on top!*

| | |
|---|---|
| 2 | pounds (900 g) sweet potatoes |
| ¼ | cup (60 mL) coconut milk |
| 2 | large eggs, lightly beaten |
| 1 | teaspoon vanilla extract |
| 1 | tablespoon coconut oil or butter |
| 2 | teaspoons cinnamon |
| 1 | teaspoon nutmeg |
| 1 | teaspoon lemon zest |
| ~ | salt and pepper, to taste |
| ½ | cup (50 g) chopped pecans |

1. Peel sweet potatoes and cut into equal-sized cubes. Place all in large sauce or stock pot, cover with water, and boil until potatoes are very tender.
2. Preheat oven to 350°F (175°C).
3. Drain potatoes and return to pot. Using a handheld mixer, blend in coconut milk.
4. Add eggs, vanilla, oil (or butter), cinnamon, nutmeg and lemon zest.
5. Place sweet potato mixture into 9" x 9" (22cm) Pyrex pan, or oval baker.
6. Sprinkle crushed pecans on top.
7. Bake 20–30 minutes, or until golden brown on top.

**Variation**—*If you don't like the lemon zest, just leave it out. I think it happens to really brighten the flavors.*

**Hint**—*You can freeze this recipe with a protein and make a great portable meal.*

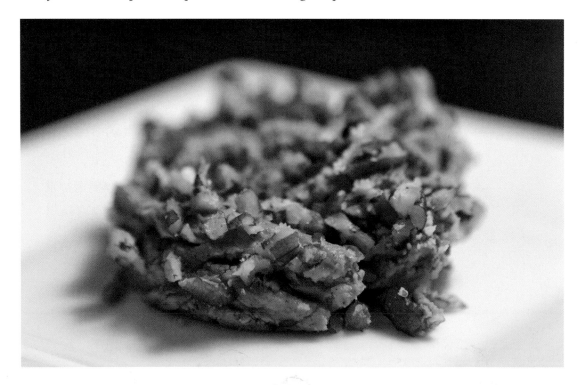

paleo comfort foods

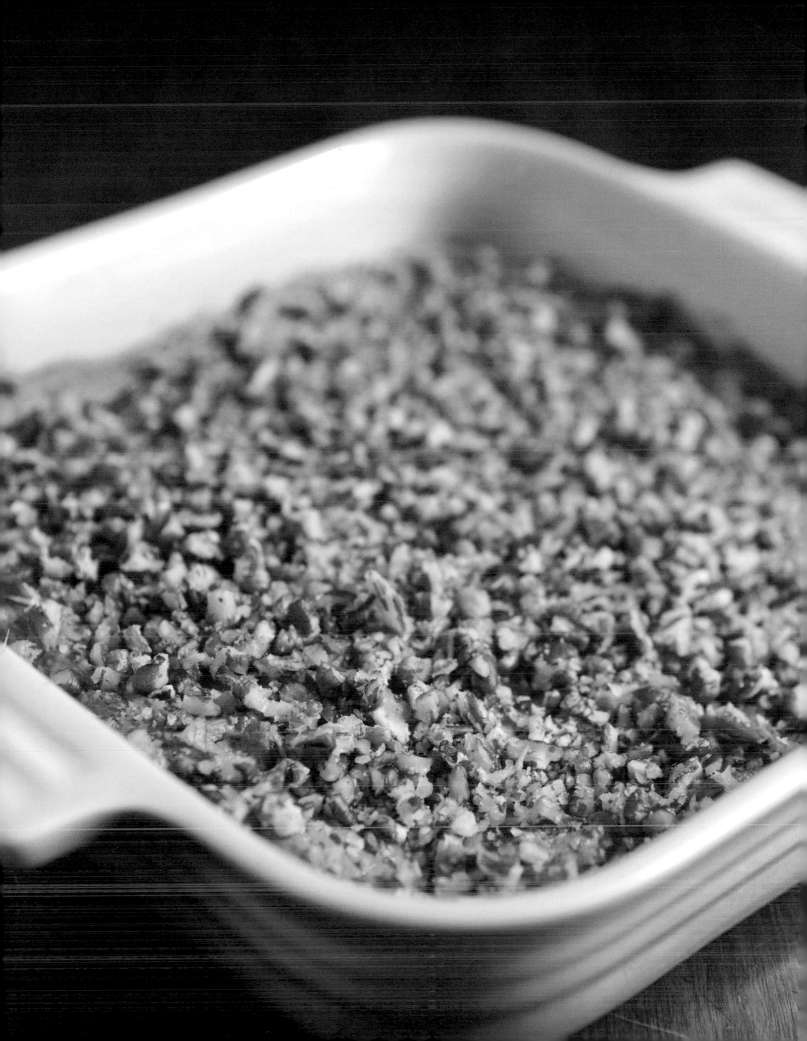

# sautéed green beans

*To bean or not to bean? Yes, beans are technically a legume, but the green beans here are super low in lectins compared to other beans in the family, as it's primarily the non-starchy pod that we eat. We limit our occasional legume exposure to just green beans, fresh sugar snaps or snow peas. Perhaps that is because my Mom has been canning green beans for as long as I remember, and she is always bringing us a jar here and there.*

| | |
|---|---|
| 1 | pound (450 g) green beans, trimmed |
| 1 | clove garlic, finely chopped |
| 1 | tablespoon clarified butter |
| ~ | zest of 1 lemon |
| ~ | salt and fresh ground pepper, to taste |
| ¼ | cup (25 g) slivered or sliced almonds, toasted |

1. Sauté green beans and garlic in skillet with clarified butter.
2. When the beans begin to become slightly tender, add the lemon zest and salt/pepper to taste.
3. Throw in the almonds a few minutes before serving to warm them a bit.

**Ingredient Notes**—*Only try this recipe with fresh green beans . . . NOT frozen.*

**Variations**—*For a little change of pace, toss in some cherry tomatoes or sun-dried tomatoes for color and additional flavor. Orange zest also goes great with this!*

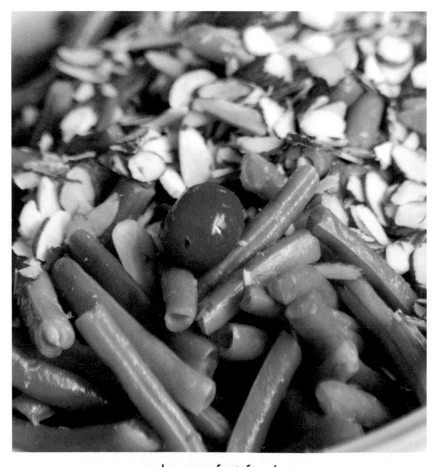

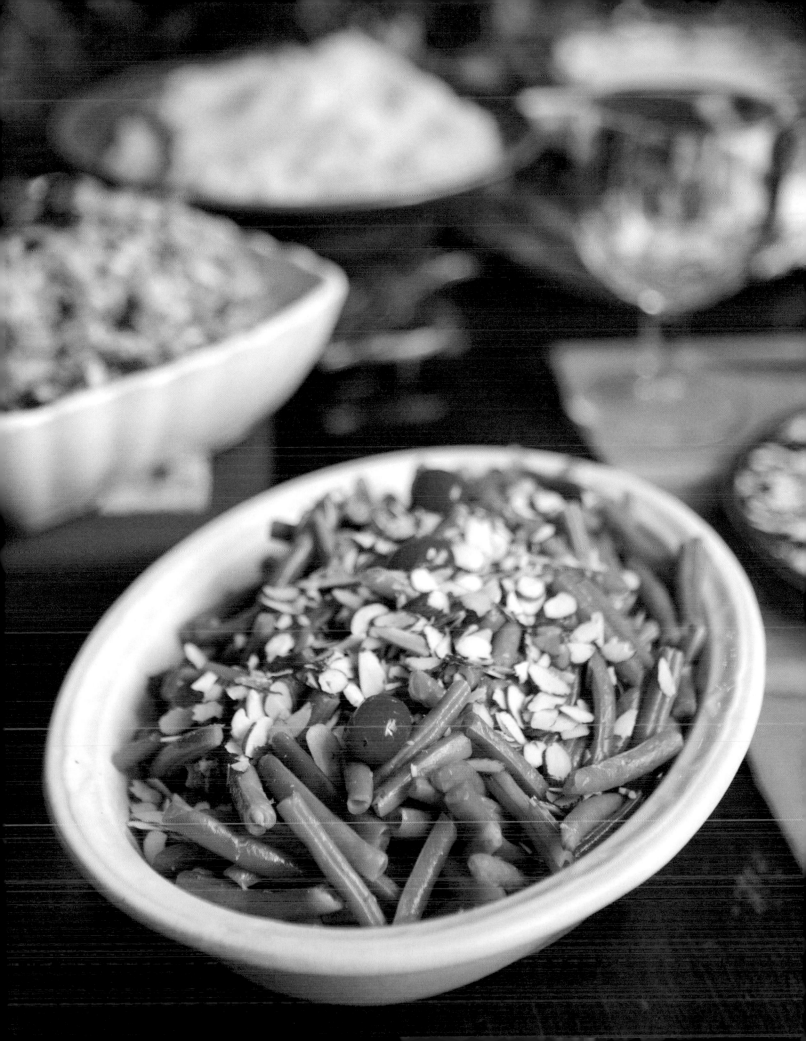

# pesto spaghetti squash with tomatoes

*Yet another use for the plentiful basil and tomatoes from the garden. If you have never grown basil at home, try it this summer, as it's such a wonderful herb to have on hand in those summer months.*

*This recipe is a play on pesto, which conventionally involves basil, olive oil, garlic, pine nuts, and Parmesan cheese. I love Parmesan as much as the next person, but this interpretation ditches the dairy and still comes out incredibly flavorful.*

| | |
|---|---|
| 1 | spaghetti squash |
| 1 | cup (25 g) fresh whole basil leaves (packed) + ¼ cup (6 g) more—chiffonade |
| ¼ | cup (25 g) walnuts |
| ⅓ | cup (80 mL) good-quality olive oil |
| 2 | whole cloves garlic + 1 additional clove, minced |
| ~ | salt and fresh ground pepper, to taste |
| 1 | tablespoon clarified butter |
| 2 | cups (400 g) assorted fresh tomatoes, chopped |
| ¼ | cup (25 g) toasted pine nuts (optional) |

1. Preheat oven to 375°F (190°C).
2. Cut the spaghetti squash in half, removing all seeds. Place facedown into a large baking dish, and pour water in the dish so it comes about halfway up the pan.
3. Bake for about 30–40 minutes (you want to slightly undercook the spaghetti squash).
4. Meanwhile, in a food processor, combine 1 cup (25 g) of the basil leaves along with the walnuts, olive oil, 2 cloves of garlic, and salt and pepper to taste. Process until smooth.
5. When spaghetti squash is done, scrape the insides of the squash with a fork to remove the insides of the squash. Set aside.
6. Heat a large skillet over medium heat, and add the butter. Once melted, add the 1 clove of minced garlic.
7. Stir in the spaghetti squash, along with the pesto. Gently fold in the tomatoes, fresh basil, and pine nuts (if desired).
8. Cook until everything is well-incorporated and the spaghetti squash is cooked to your preferred doneness.

**Tips & Tricks**—*To really preserve the bright green color of the basil in the pesto, shock the leaves for about 30 seconds in boiling water, then submerge in an ice water bath. This preserves that bright green color.*

**Variations**—*If you are lacto-paleo, go ahead and top with some Parmesan cheese. To make a complete meal out of this, stir some grilled shrimp into this spaghetti, as it makes for a really filling and fresh meal. If you don't want to use walnuts at all, feel free to use pine nuts in the pesto (however, they do come at a much higher price point than walnuts).*

**Plan Ahead**—*If pressed for time, go ahead and halve the spaghetti squash, remove the seeds, place facedown in a glass baking dish with some water, and cook for 5–7 minutes in the microwave. This will par cook the spaghetti squash, keeping it nice and al dente prior to sautéing it with the pesto and tomatoes.*

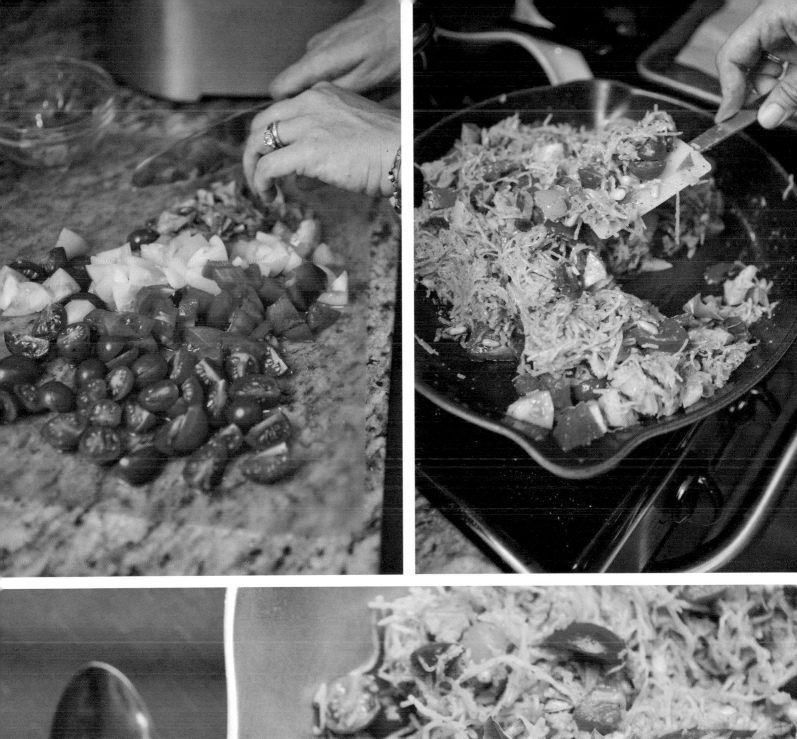
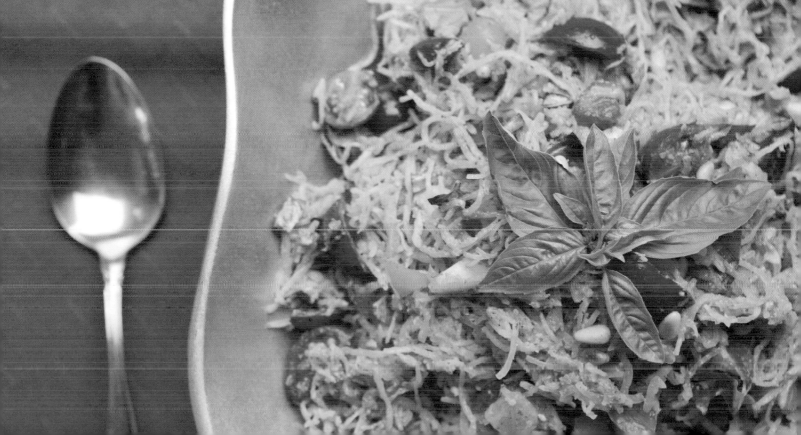

# squash casserole

In the South, squash casserole is most often made with loads of cream, and topped with Ritz crackers for crunch. Some recipes call for adding cream of chicken or mushroom soup to give the casserole that creamy flavor and texture. With this variation, coconut milk makes a great substitute for the cream, and the pecans add a fantastic crunch that is sure not to disappoint!

| | |
|---|---|
| 2 | pounds (1 kg) yellow squash, sliced into rounds |
| 1 | onion, thinly sliced |
| ¾ | cup (180 mL) coconut milk |
| ½ | cup (75 g) almond meal |
| ¼ | teaspoon smoked paprika |
| ½ | cup (50 g) pecans, coarse chopped |

1. Preheat oven to 350°F (175°C).
2. Place squash and onions in a medium-sized sauce pan.
3. Fill the pan with enough water to cover the vegetables.
4. Cover the pan, and place on stove over medium to medium-high heat, cooking until vegetables are translucent and soft.
5. Drain the vegetables of the water, and place back in sauce pan.
6. Mix the coconut milk, almond meal, and paprika into the squash/onion mixture, and stir until well combined.
7. Place the mixture into a casserole dish, and sprinkle the top with the pecans.
8. Bake for approximately 20 minutes or until mixture is very bubbly and somewhat thickened and pecans are golden brown.

**Variation**—*Pecans not your thing? Go ahead and top with any chopped nuts of your choosing. When your summer garden is running over with squash and/or zucchini, use a combination in this recipe if you'd like.*

**Hint**—*This freezes and stores quite well, and it's a favorite of ours for leftovers!*

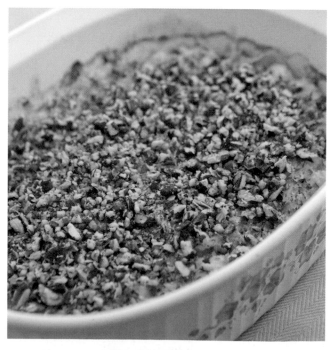

paleo comfort foods

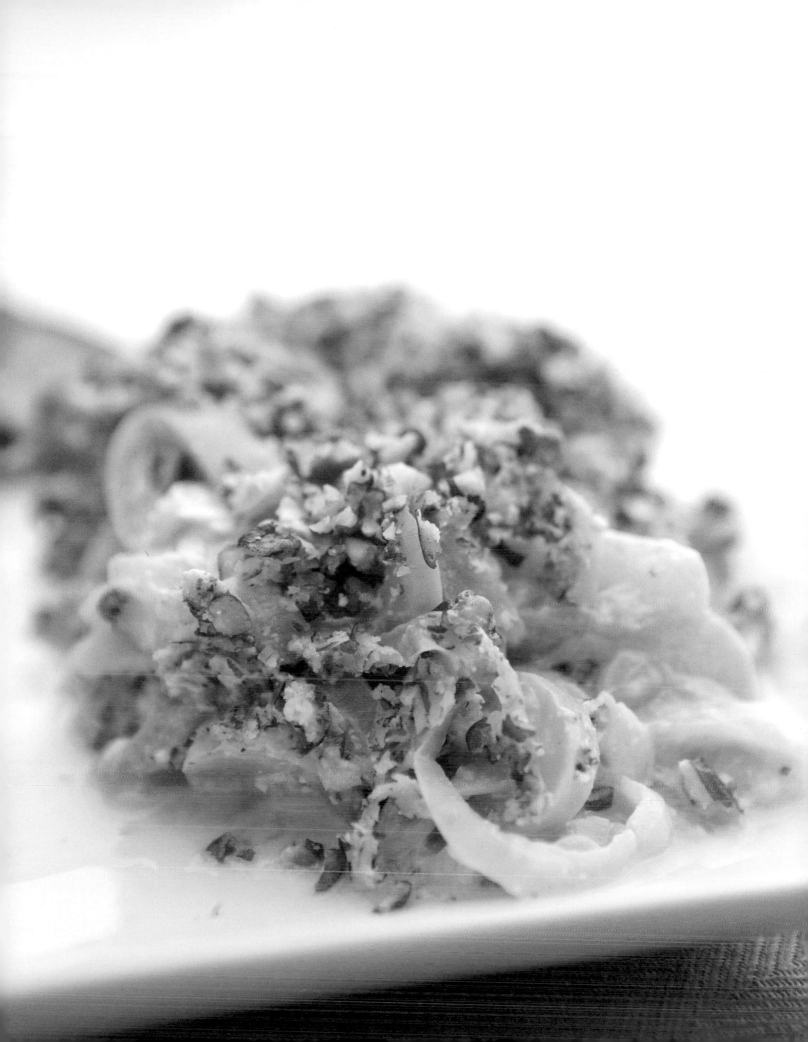

# oven-roasted broccoli or cauliflower

*Oftentimes, simplicity is best. This is one such recipe that plays on simplicity. I've had many a "I can't stand broccoli or cauliflower" sort become a convert with this recipe. You won't end up with mushy broccoli or cauliflower this way, and the caramelization along with the serious garlic flavor is pure tastiness.*

| | |
|---|---|
| 3-4 | large broccoli crowns |
| 3 | tablespoons extra virgin olive oil |
| ~ | salt and pepper to taste |
| 5–6 | cloves fresh garlic, minced |

1. Adjust your oven rack to lowest position, and place a large rimmed baking sheet on rack, and heat oven to 500°F (260°C).
2. Cut each crown into 4 to 6 big wedges.
3. Place broccoli in a large bowl and drizzle with oil. Toss well until evenly coated. Sprinkle with salt and pepper along with garlic, and mix to combine.
4. Working quickly, remove the baking sheet from the oven. Carefully transfer broccoli and all oil and garlic to the baking sheet and spread into even layer, placing flat sides down.
5. Return baking sheet to oven and roast until stalks are well browned and tender and florets are lightly browned, 9 to 11 minutes.
6. Transfer to serving dish and serve immediately.

**Variation**—*If you're using cauliflower for this recipe, set your oven to 450-475 (230-245). A nice sprinkling of cumin or any of your favorite seasonings adds some great flavor.*

**Ingredients**—*If you're rushed for time, buy one of those bags of broccoli or cauliflower florets. If you're using cauliflower for this recipe, set your oven to 450–475F° (230–245C°).*

**Tips & Tricks**—*The cauliflower usually cooks best if you first cover it with aluminum foil for about the first 5–10 minutes of cooking, then flip pieces over and cook another 5 or so until done.*

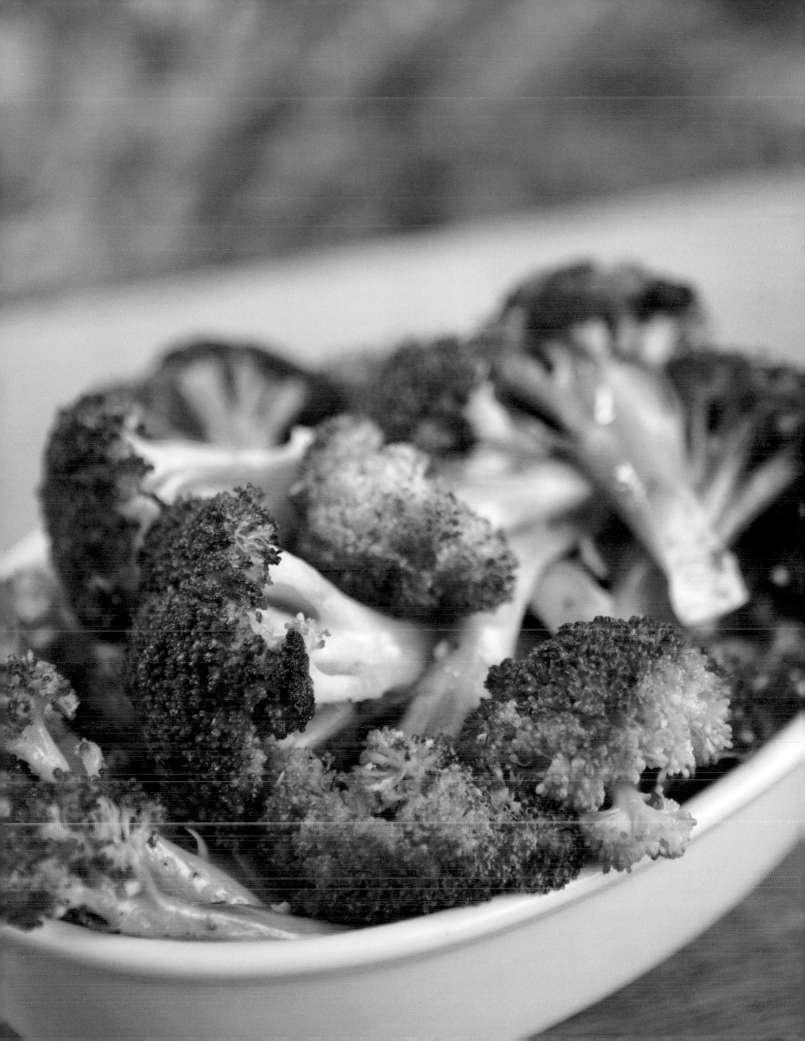

# carrot timbales

*Bugs Bunny would love this recipe. Carrots pack the highest punch when it comes to pro-vitamin A carotenes. They help fight cardiovascular disease and cancer. Who doesn't love the portability of this vegetable? That said, carrots deserve to be cooked from time to time just like all the other veggies.*

*Curious as to what the word "timbale" actually means? Aside from it being a Cuban and Latin American percussion instrument, when it comes to food it means "various ingredients cooked in a round mold." Go on and call your next item cooked in a ramekin or other round mold a "timbale"—you'll sound super fancy.*

| | |
|---|---|
| 2 | tablespoons coconut oil or grass-fed butter |
| 1 | pound (450 g) carrots, peeled and thinly sliced |
| 1 | clove garlic, minced |
| ¼ | teaspoon salt |
| ½ | teaspoon sweet paprika |
| 1 | pinch nutmeg |
| ½ | teaspoon fresh thyme, minced |
| ⅓ | cup (80 mL) coconut milk |
| 2 | large eggs |
| 2 | teaspoons Italian parsley, to garnish |

1. Heat oil in a heavy saucepan.

2. When oil is hot, add carrots and garlic and toss to coat. Cook covered, over medium-low heat until tender, about 30 to 40 minutes, stirring occasionally. Cool for 5 minutes.

3. Preheat oven to 325°F (165°C). Lightly grease or spray six ½-cup (125 mL) ramekins or other oven-friendly cups. Set aside.

4. Scrape carrots into bowl of food processor. Add salt, paprika, nutmeg, thyme and coconut milk and puree until smooth.

5. Add in eggs and purée for 1 minute or until mixture is well combined.

6. Spoon carrot purée into ramekins until they are almost full.

7. Place timbales into a roasting pan. Pour boiling hot water into roasting pan until it comes ½ way up the sides of the ramekins.

8. Place in oven and bake for 40–45 minutes.

9. Unmold gently by running a knife around sides of ramekins. Serve warm or slightly chilled garnished with parsley.

**Variations**—*For slightly different flavor, garnish your timbales with some finely chopped chives or scallions, or consider adding some curry powder, turmeric, or ginger for a more exotic taste.*

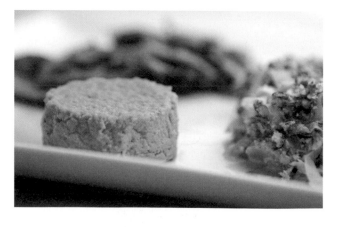

paleo comfort foods

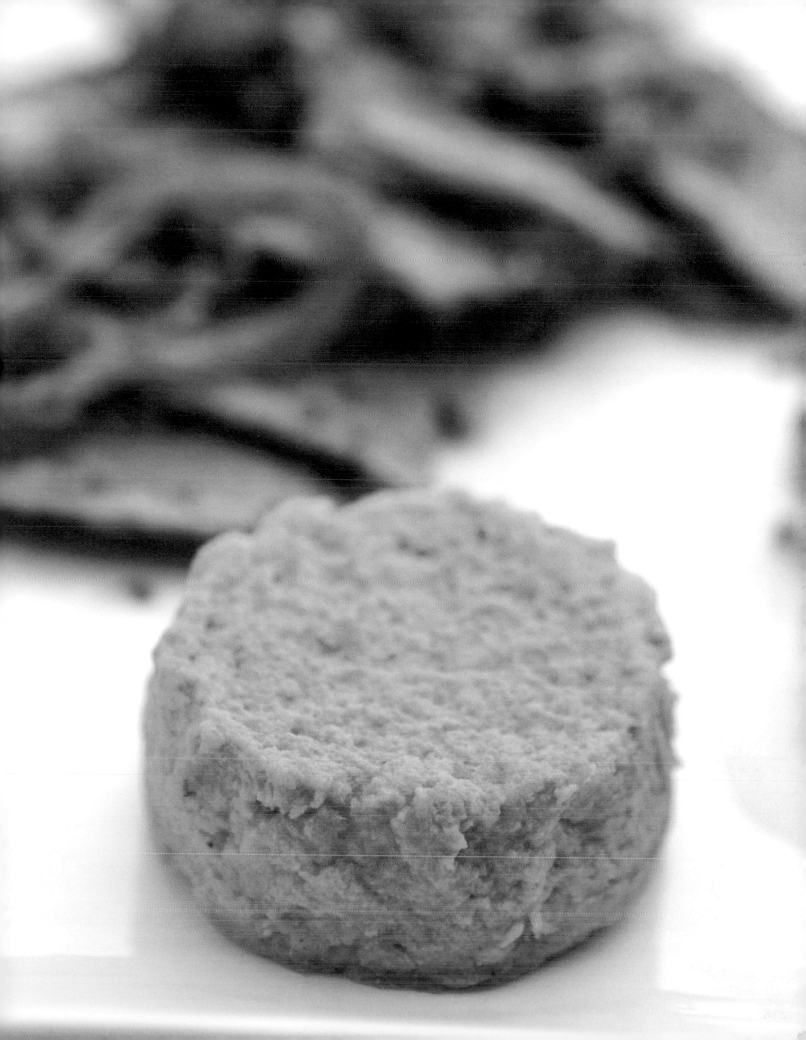

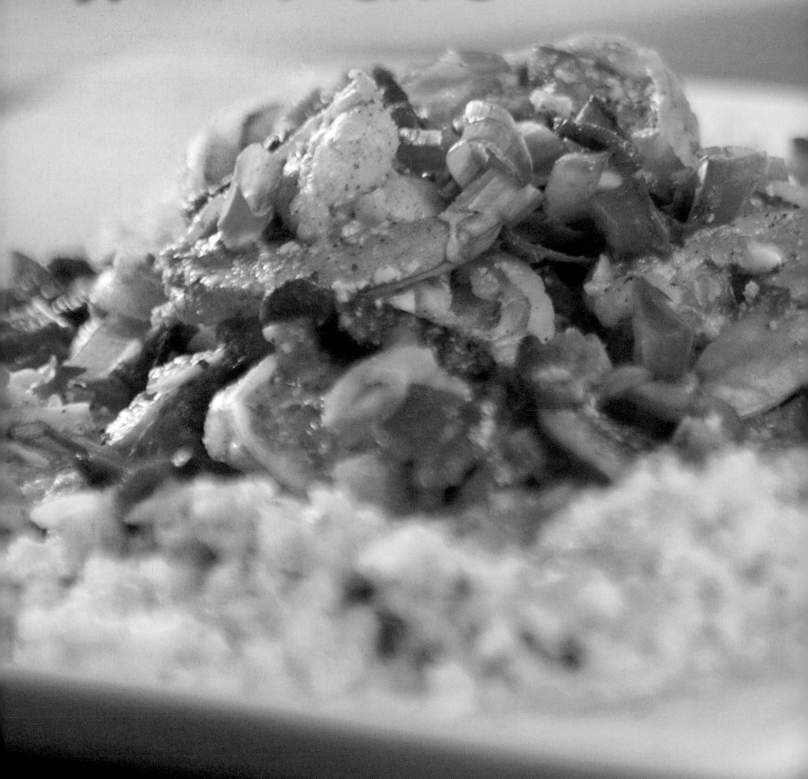

# Main Dishes

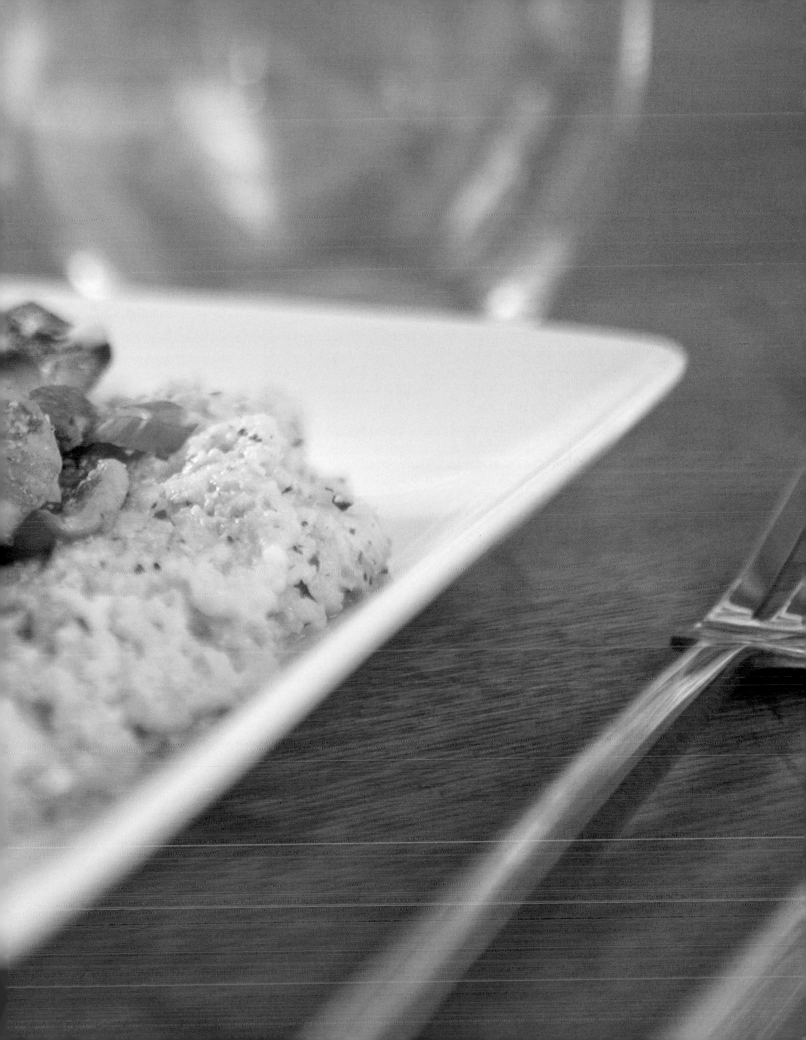

# breakfast egg muffins

*Aesthetically, you'll want to serve these muffins shortly after removing from the oven. They will shrink up a bit and loose some of their fluffy texture once they sit out too long—kind of like soufflés!*

*These are a perfect on-the-go meal or snack. They also work great if you have a few folks coming by for breakfast. Accent them with a little sausage, bacon and fruit and you have a "finger food" breakfast for folks that keeps clean up nice and quick.*

*The jalapeños are optional if you want a kick. I suggest having some guacamole or salsa handy to top these. Feel free to add your favorite omelet ingredients to the frying pan and sauté them in with the onions to make these your own.*

| | |
|---|---|
| 1 | tablespoon olive oil |
| 1 | large sweet onion, finely chopped |
| 1 | green bell pepper, finely chopped |
| 1 | red bell pepper, chopped |
| 1 | jalapeño pepper, finely chopped (optional) |
| 12 | large eggs, whisked |
| ½ | teaspoon black pepper |
| ¼ | teaspoon salt (optional) |

1. Preheat oven to 350°F (175°C).

2. Sauté onions in olive oil over medium-high heat for 2-3 minutes. Add peppers and continue cooking for another 2-3 minutes.

3. While peppers are cooking, whisk eggs in a large bowl.

4. Once onions/peppers are cooked, remove from heat and let cool for a few minutes. Dump in egg mixture and stir well, sprinkling in the salt and pepper.

5. Coat a large muffin pan with olive oil spray or coconut oil. Using a ¼-cup (60 mL) measuring cup, fill each muffin cup.

6. Place in oven for 10–15 minutes. Remove them once the tops get high, fluffy and golden brown. Pop them out with a butter knife or thin spatula.

**Plan Ahead**—*To make this really quick and easy, sauté veggies the night before. Keep them in the refrigerator and simply stir them into your eggs when you're ready to make the muffins.*

**Variations**—*For some added protein, sauté some of your favorite sausage or some ground turkey or beef, and mix into the egg mixture, about ½ - ¾ pound (225-350g) would be sufficient.*

**Hint**—*These also freeze incredibly well.*

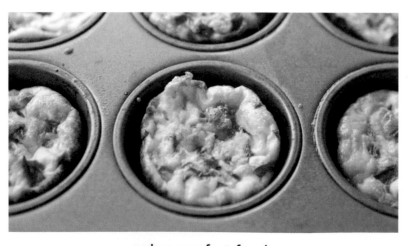

paleo comfort foods

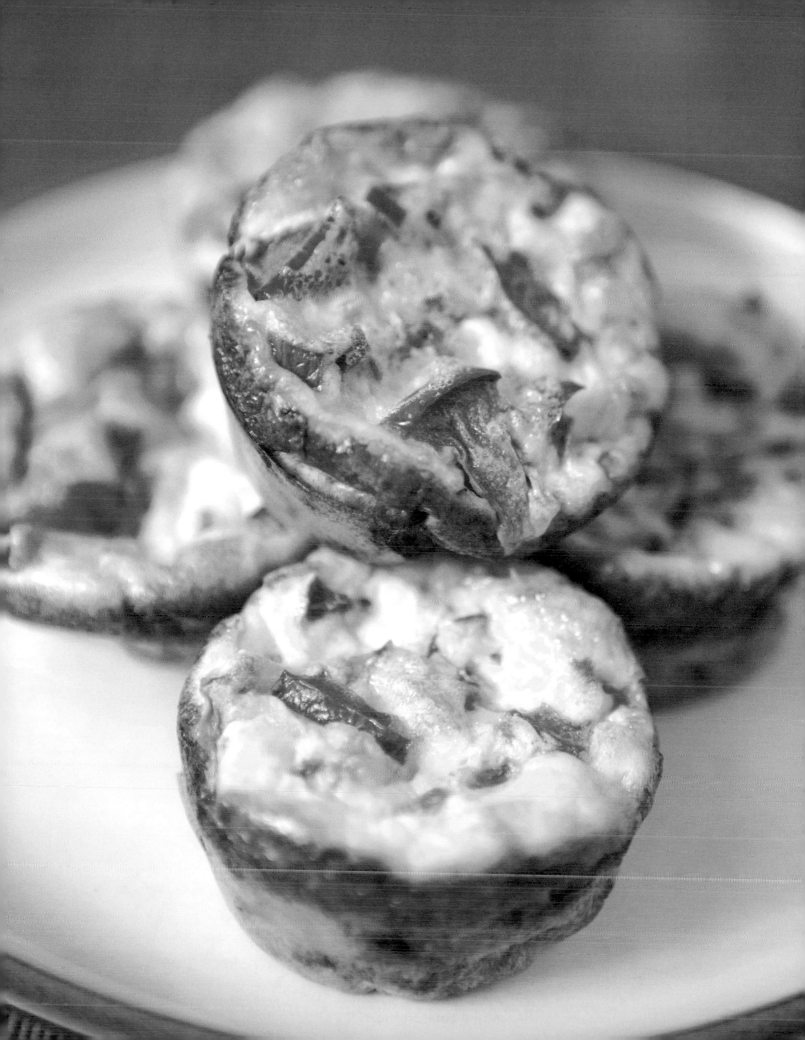

# green eggs and turkey

*We absolutely love frittatas. This is one of our go-to recipes and is great for when a crowd is coming over. Feel free to mix up ingredients if this one starts to bore you. One thing we always do is make a few different sauces to pour over them. Look no further than the pages of this book for tasty salsas, Chunky Guacamole (page 74) or Chipotle Dipping Sauce (page 94).*

| | |
|---|---|
| 2 | pounds (900 g) ground turkey |
| 1 | teaspoon black pepper |
| ½ | teaspoon salt (optional) |
| 1 | tablespoon coconut oil |
| 2 | cups (300 g) onions, chopped |
| 4 | cups (700 g) broccoli florets, chopped |
| 2 | cups (700 g) artichoke hearts, chopped |
| ~ | a couple handfuls fresh spinach, roughly chopped |
| 1 | teaspoon smoked paprika |
| 3 | tablespoons fresh basil, chopped |
| 12 | large eggs |

1. Preheat oven to 350°F (175°C).

2. In a large skillet, brown turkey meat with salt and pepper. Drain liquid off and spread turkey meat into bottom of greased 9 inch x 13 inch (23 cm x 33cm) baking dish.

3. Using the same skillet, heat coconut oil over medium heat. Add onions and stir, cooking onions until translucent.

4. Add broccoli, artichoke, spinach, and paprika and cook until broccoli is tender and spinach has wilted. Add basil and remove from heat.

5. Whisk eggs in bowl.

6. Pour vegetable mixture over turkey meat, then pour eggs over veggies and meat.

7. Bake for about 45 minutes or until eggs are cooked through.

**Variation**—*Use ground sausage instead of turkey to change up the flavors in your frittata.*

**Tips & Tricks**—*If you find you are pressed for time and chopping a bunch of vegetables is not your thing, pay a little extra and get the pre-chopped veggies at the store. If your skillet is ovenproof, go ahead and cook all the components as directed above, then remove to a bowl. Grease your skillet with some coconut oil or other fat of your choosing, and pour in all vegetables, turkey and eggs into the skillet. Bake as you would a rectangular frittata, and slice into wedges (like a pie!).*

**Hints**—*This recipe freezes well. We like to cool our frittata for a day and vacuum seal individual portions.*

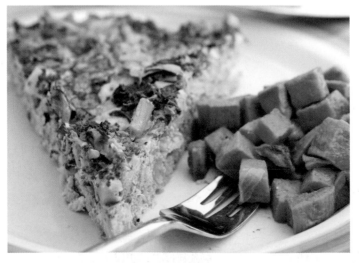

paleo comfort foods

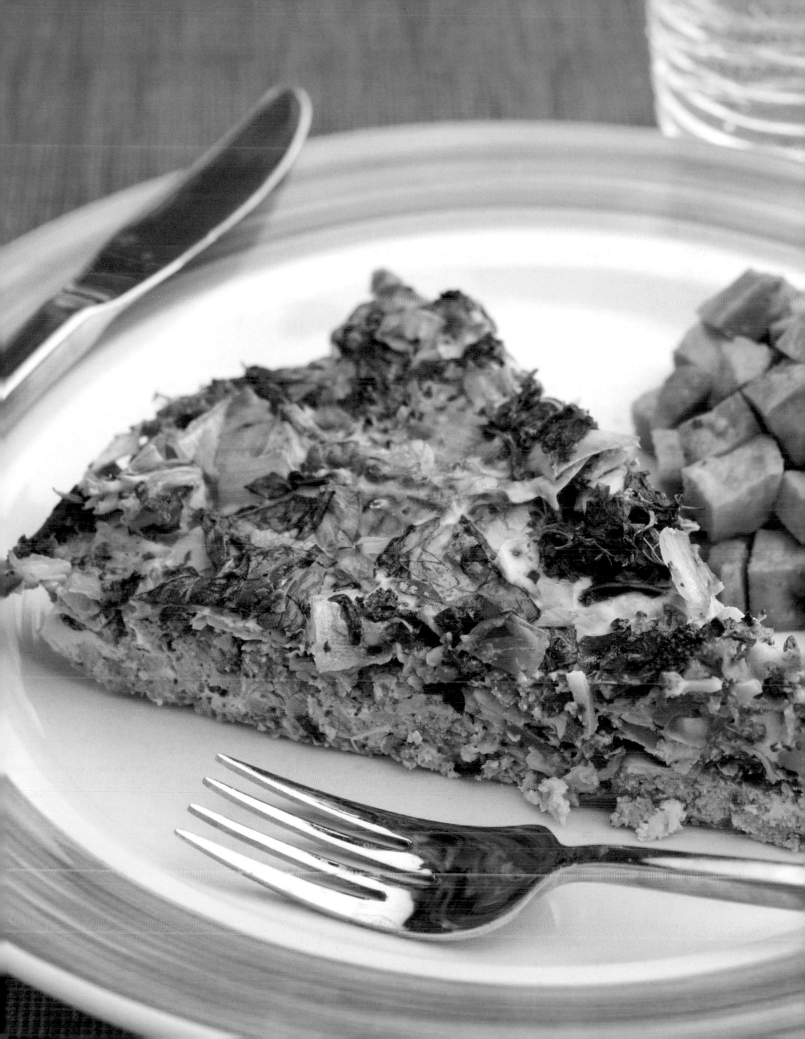

# sawmill gravy (& biscuits)

*Sure, this recipe probably wouldn't pass muster with Paula Deen, but I'm okay with that. The good news is that this recipe uses coconut milk instead of cow's milk. Coconut is pretty awesome and somewhat unique (compared to other fat sources) in that it is comprised mostly of medium-chain triglycerides. Go and Google MCTs and coconut if you're itching for more information.*

*Biscuits and gravy is pretty much a Southern staple, and you're incredibly likely to find this recipe on most restaurant menus. While our version is not the kind of meal you want for every breakfast, it's a good alternative to the everyday habit of eggs.*

| | |
|---|---|
| 1 | pound (450 g) ground pork or turkey sausage |
| 1 | tablespoon almond flour |
| 1 | tablespoon arrowroot powder |
| 1 | can coconut milk |
| 2 | teaspoons sage |
| 1 | teaspoon paprika |
| ½ | cup (125 mL) chicken stock (if needed) |

**Basic Biscuits (recipe page 116)**

1. Sauté sausage in large skillet until completely cooked. Remove sausage from pan, saving about 2 tablespoons of the drippings from the sausage. Keep these drippings in the pan.

2. Add the almond flour and arrowroot powder to the skillet, and whisk with the sausage fat over medium-low heat, until a paste is formed, working to scrape up some of the sausage drippings.

3. Pour in about ¼ of the coconut milk, the sage, and paprika at this point, and bring to medium heat, stirring often and scraping up the browned sausage bits.

4. Add remaining coconut milk, stirring as you go, and bring to light simmer. Add sausage back in, and simmer until gravy reaches desired thickness

5. If gravy becomes too thick, thin out with some of the chicken stock.

6. Pour over biscuits sliced in half and serve.

**Variations**—*Nobody says you have to serve this gravy over biscuits. We love pouring it over scrambled eggs or steak. Play around with what you like it on.*

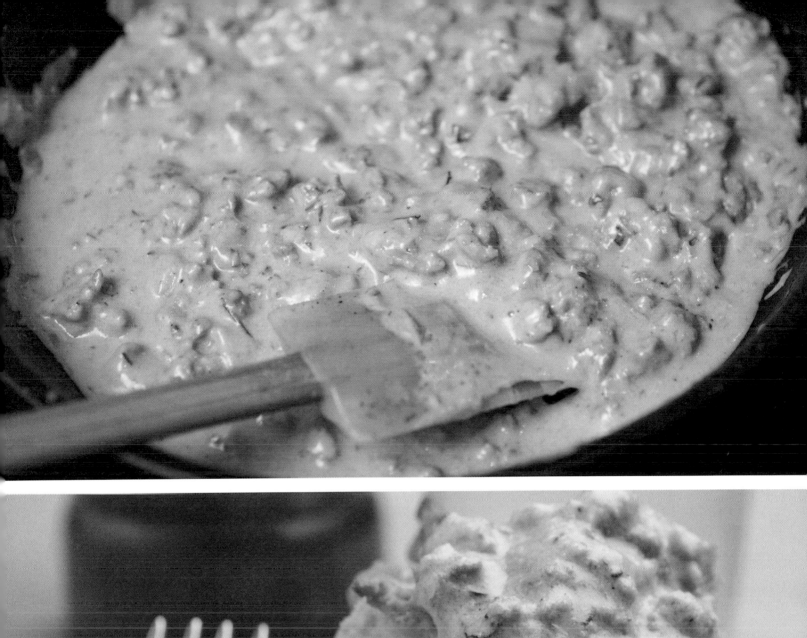

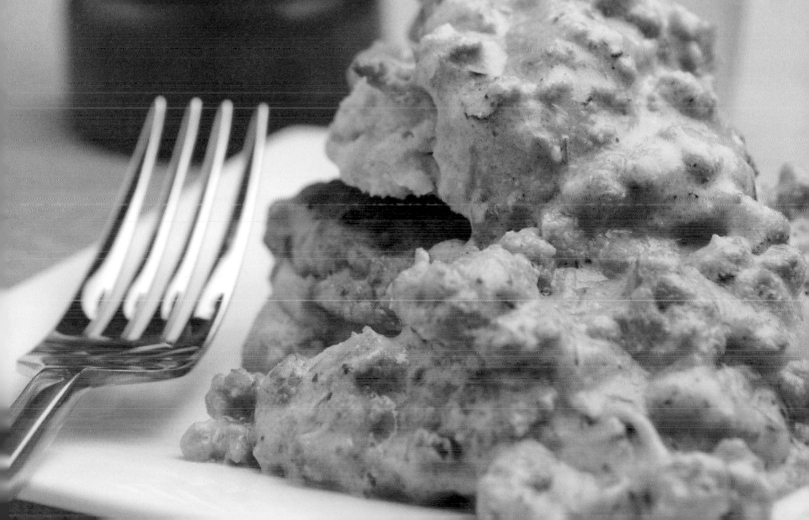

# ham & egg cups

*Travel friendly and super tasty, these treats often accompany me to the office or gym. They refrigerate well for days so they are a nice breakfast bite when you're in a real pinch for time. We recommend finding a quality deli or butcher in your area when shopping for your ham. In our quest to find really solid ham, Julie and I discovered an amazing Eastern European meat market only a few miles from our house. We go there all the time now to get various sausages and meats for recipes like this one. If you're in the Atlanta area, we highly recommend Patak Meat Products.*

| | |
|---|---|
| ½ | cup (50 g) mushrooms, finely chopped |
| ½ | cup (75 g) shallots, finely chopped |
| 12 | large eggs |
| 12 | slices ham |

1. Preheat oven to 350°F (175°C).
2. Sauté shallots and mushrooms in skillet with butter.
3. Coat muffin pan with olive oil spray or other oil and place ham slices in cups. You may want to cut a sliver in each ham slice to allow it to fold over itself when placed in the round muffin cup.
4. Spoon out the sautéed mushroom/shallot mixture into each cup.
5. Crack individual eggs into the ham cups.
6. Cook for 15-16 minutes or until edge of ham is slightly crisp.

**Variation**—*To add some color and extra flavor, garnish with fresh chopped chives or cracked pepper.*

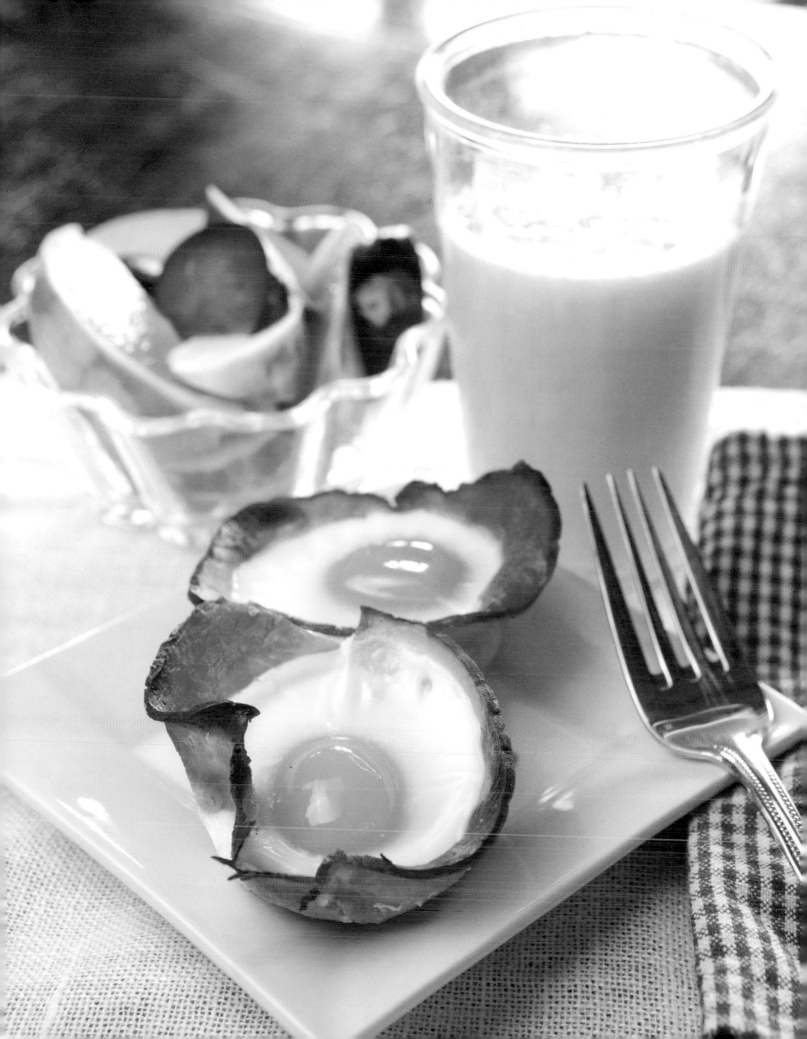

# crustless quiche

*When I'm in a rush, I love being able to grab one of these slices for breakfast and knowing that I'm going to get a good amount of carbs, protein, and fat in one sitting. The first time I made one of these I used my 14-inch All Clad fry pan, sautéed up the veggies, added in the eggs, and finished it in the oven. Mind you, for that original recipe, I think I only used about half the eggs, which still filled up the pan quite a bit . . . so I figured I needed to switch to a rectangular baking pan to really make this work.*

*This recipe stems from a recipe Charles' mom passed along to me, which involved some Cheddar and cottage cheese, which I have since omitted (though if you are doing dairy you can certainly add these back in). I do love the colors of the vegetables in with the eggs, and there are so many variations you can do with this!*

| | |
|---|---|
| 12 | large eggs |
| ½ | cup (75 g) almond flour |
| 1 | teaspoon baking powder |
| ½ | cup (120 g) butter, melted |
| 1 | cup (150 g) onions, chopped |
| 1 | cup (30 g) spinach, rinsed |
| ½ | cup (90 g) red bell pepper, diced small |
| ½ | cup (90 g) green bell pepper, diced small |
| ¼ | teaspoon black pepper, freshly ground |

1. Preheat oven to 350°F (175°C).

2. In a large bowl, whisk eggs together until slightly foamy. Stir in the almond flour and baking powder.

3. In a large sauté pan, melt the butter, then add in the onions and spinach, cooking until onions are translucent. Mix in the peppers and any other vegetables of your choosing.

4. Stir the veggie/butter mixture into the eggs, and pour the contents into a 9 inch x 13 inch (23 cm x 33 cm) baking dish, and top with pepper.

5. Bake for 45 minutes or until cooked through.

**Variations**—*You can alter this some by marinating some steak (of your choosing) in Chipotle Dipping Sauce (adobo sauce, see recipe on page 94) and browning that in the pan to mix in with the eggs. Or, mix in some sausage to the eggs, and top the frittata with some, as pictured.*

**Tips & Tricks**—*Just like the Green Eggs and Turkey recipe, you can cook this in a large, ovenproof stainless steel skillet, cooking the eggs in with the veggies until they start to firm up, then placing in the oven to finish. Many chefs prefer to really cook the eggs on the stovetop, then just finish the eggs under the broiler. As you wish! Given the size of this dish, we recommend halving the recipe if you opt for baking it in the skillet. Pieces of this quiche store beautifully in the freezer and will keep for several weeks.*

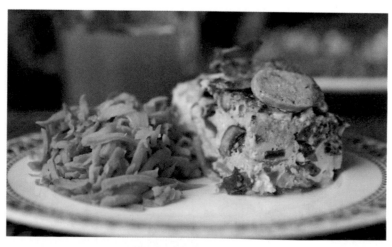

paleo comfort foods

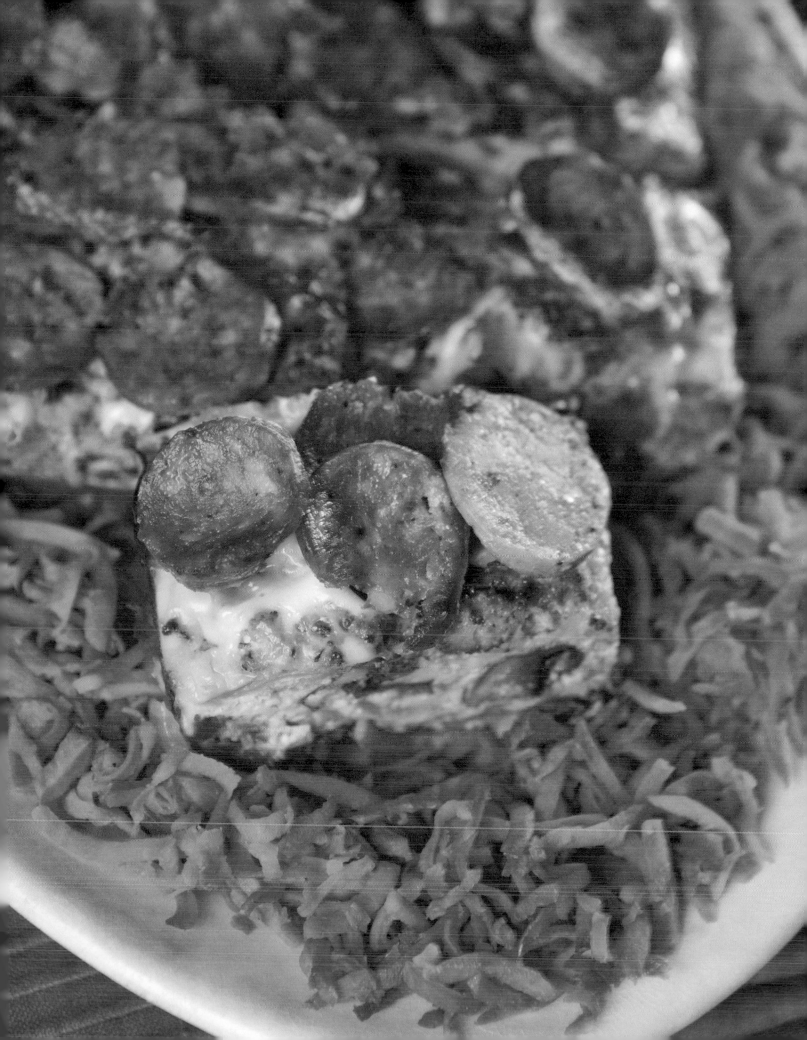

# leftover chicken scramble

*There always seems to be leftover chicken. Whether you are grilling in the back yard or cooking up a cooler full of chicken for your tailgate, be sure to keep those leftovers handy. This little breakfast number is fast, easy and super flavorful. Besides, nobody likes eggs every day. Since the meat is already cooked, this recipe takes very little time to prepare. Let's be honest, following that Saturday tailgate you need something fast, easy, and full of flavor to rid your head of that post–game day hangover. Too many skinny margaritas anyone?*

*We love to make our own broccoli slaw. If you have been wondering what to do with those big broccoli stalks all these years, now you have the answer. This recipe is almost certain to grace our stovetop if we have had broccoli in previous days. Just save the stalks in the refrigerator until you are ready to shred them. To do so, just cut off the rough exterior of the stalks, then either using your box grater or food processor, shred the stalks.*

| | |
|---|---|
| 2 | tablespoons coconut oil |
| 1 | clove garlic, minced |
| 1 | cup (150 g) onion, chopped |
| ½ | cup (75 g) green or red pepper, chopped |
| 3 | cups (500 g) broccoli slaw |
| 3 | cups (600 g) tomatoes, chopped |
| 1 | pound (450 g) chicken, cooked and cut into small chunks |
| 1 | teaspoon black pepper |
| 1 | teaspoon cayenne pepper |

**1.** Heat coconut oil in medium skillet over medium heat and sauté garlic, onions, and peppers until onions are translucent.

**2.** Add broccoli slaw and tomatoes and cook for 5 minutes or until slaw is somewhat softened.

**3.** Add the chicken, black and cayenne peppers.

**4.** Stir and reduce heat to simmer for another 10 minutes stirring occasionally.

**Variation**—*This scramble works great with any leftover meats.*

**Tips & Tricks**—*Broccoli slaw can be bought pre-bagged and is found at most supermarkets. It's a great source of some low-density carbohydrates.*

**Hint**—*Scrambles like these freeze really well and make for a great on-the-go breakfast.*

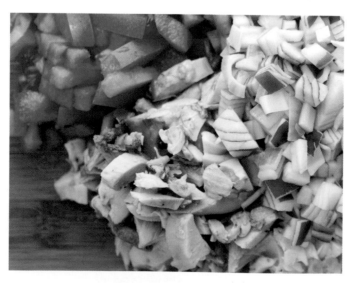

paleo comfort foods

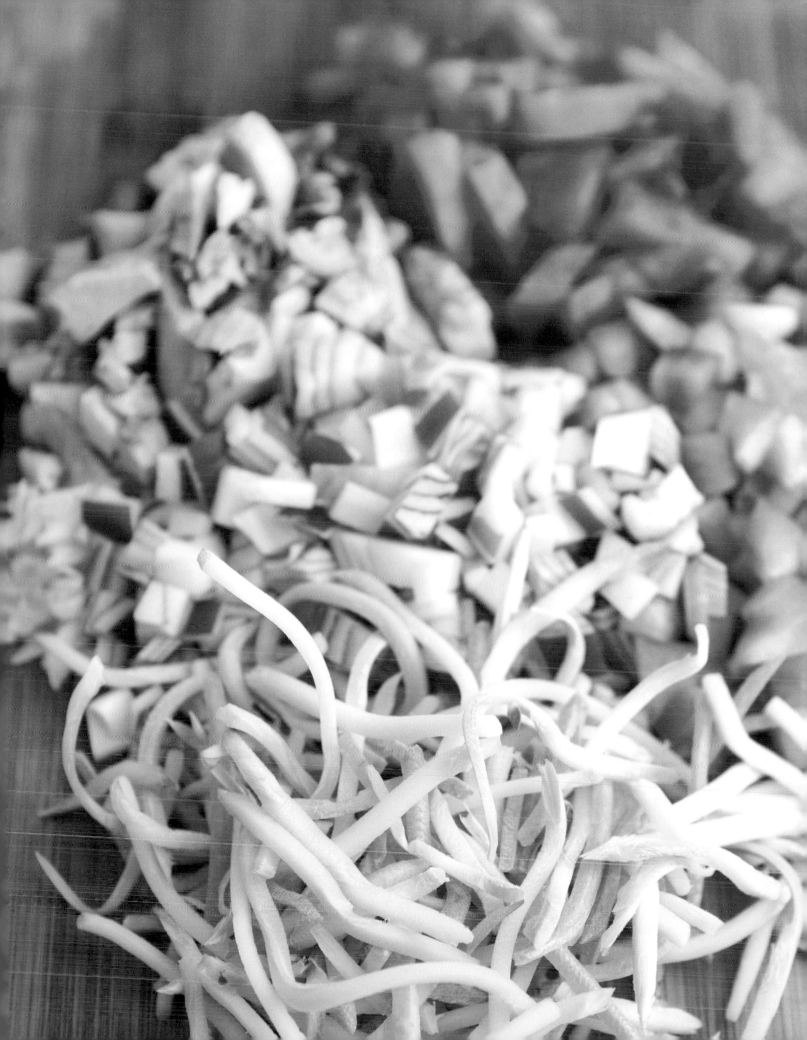

# chicken breasts
# with mushroom sauce

*I've said it before and I will say it again: mushrooms—with all their earthiness—are great comfort food for me. I love experimenting with different mushroom types, and tossing them into everything from eggs to burgers to sauces. Shiitakes are indeed a favorite of mine, and though part of their name sounds like a less-than-flattering four-letter word, their taste (to me) is very far from that and this recipe is proof positive.*

*A word on using alcohol in cooking: I know that sherry and really any kind of alcohol is Neolithic and would not have been available to a caveman. Why sherry is okay (for our standards) in this recipe: before the sherry is reduced, it comes out to about 2 teaspoons per serving. Once the sherry is cooked, it loses most (not every single little ounce though) of its alcohol content (which evaporates), and what's left is the nutty flavor of the sherry—a flavor I have a hard time replicating with something else. However, feel free to substitute with additional stock if you are a no-sherry kind of person or cooking with alcohol is something you choose not to do.*

| | |
|---|---|
| 1½ | pounds (700 g) chicken breasts |
| ½ | cup (75 g) almond flour |
| ½ | teaspoon tarragon |
| ½ | teaspoon onion powder |
| ½ | teaspoon garlic powder |
| ¼ | teaspoon paprika |
| ¼ | teaspoon black pepper |
| 1 | tablespoon olive oil |
| 1 | tablespoon clarified butter |
| 2 | cloves garlic, minced |
| 1 | cup (125 g) shiitake mushrooms, de-stemmed and sliced |
| ¼ | cup (60 mL) dry sherry |
| ¾ | cup (180 mL) chicken stock |
| 2 | teaspoons fresh chives, chopped |

1. Preheat the oven to 375°F (190°C).

2. If chicken breasts are exceptionally thick, pound to about ¾ inch (1.75 cm) thickness.

3. On a large plate, combine almond flour with tarragon on through black pepper. Dredge chicken breasts in seasoned flour and shake off excess.

4. Preheat large stainless steel skillet over medium-high heat. Add in olive oil and once oil is slightly smoking, gently place chicken breasts in skillet. Sear for 4–5 minutes per side, or until browned. Remove chicken and place on sheet pan or other oven-proof dish and place in oven. Bake for 10–12 minutes or until chicken is cooked through.

5. Reduce skillet heat to medium. Add butter to skillet, scraping up the browned bits from the chicken. Stir in the garlic and sauté until fragrant (but not burned), then stir in mushrooms. Sauté for 1–2 minutes, then add in sherry and chicken stock. Let simmer until reduced slightly and mushrooms are cooked. Add in chives just before serving.

6. Serve mushroom sauce over chicken.

**Ingredient Notes**—*If you are going with the sherry, make sure it is "real" Sherry. Preferably from Spain. Do not use cooking wine. Most cooking wines are loaded with salt.*

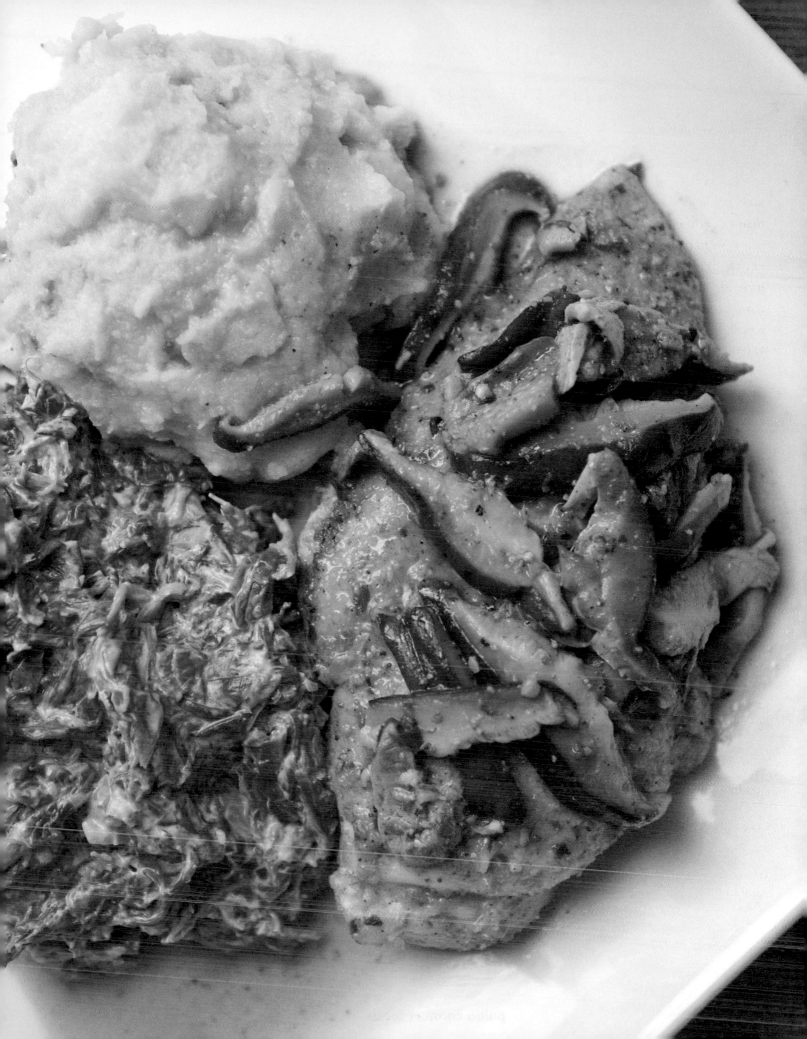

# country captain chicken

*The history of Country Captain absolutely fascinates me. Do some searching around the Internet, and you'll spend hours upon hours reading about this dish and folks like Cecily Brownstone, President Franklin D. Roosevelt, and even the U.S. Army making Country Captain one of its Meals Ready to Eat (MRE) flavors (I'm kind of scared to see all that might be in it!). Some argue Country Captain was first introduced to the United States in the mid 1800s in my home city (Philadelphia), while others say that a captain involved in the spice trade in India brought it in via Charleston or Savannah. Whatever you believe, one thing is true: this dish is a staple in the South. I absolutely love the way Sam Sifton of the* New York Times *described this dish in a 2009 article: "Made correctly, it captures exactly that moment of excitement you can feel when first arriving in the region from far away: a sense that everything really is different in the South, that it is the one last, true regional culture in the United States." Philly may have cheese steaks, but the South does have a culture all its own and Country Captain is one such example.*

*As I'm a fan of "one-dish meals," the original recipe in no way called for broccoli—I just wanted some additional carbs.*

*Adapted from Cecily Brownstone's recipe.*

---

| | |
|---|---|
| ¼ | cup (40 g) almond flour |
| 1 | teaspoon salt (optional) |
| ¼ | teaspoon black pepper |
| 1 | teaspoon dried thyme |
| 3 | pounds (1.5 kg) chicken, thighs and breasts work best |
| 2 | tablespoons olive oil or grass-fed clarified butter |
| 1 | onion, diced |
| 1 | green pepper, diced |
| 2 | cloves garlic, minced |
| 1 | tablespoon curry powder |
| 1 | quart (1 L) tomatoes |
| 3 | cups (500 g) broccoli (optional) |
| 3 | tablespoons currants |
| 3 | tablespoons almonds, blanched and toasted |

1. Preheat oven to 350°F (175°C).

2. Combine the almond flour, salt, pepper, and thyme in a large bowl or dish. Dredge the chicken in the flour mixture and set aside.

3. Heat a large Dutch oven or braiser over medium heat, add the chicken and brown on all sides. Remove from pan and set aside.

4. Reduce heat to medium low, and add the onions, green pepper, garlic and curry powder, stirring to scrape up browned bits. Add the chicken back to the pan along with the tomatoes and broccoli, stirring to combine.

5. Cover and cook for 25–30 minutes, then add currants, stir, and place back in the oven for another 5–10 minutes or until chicken is cooked through.

6. Serve topped with almonds.

---

**Variation**—*Don't tell Ms. Brownstone (rest her soul), but I find the recipe is super tasty even without the currants. Feel free to omit if you'd like, or if you can't find currants, use some golden raisins.*

**Ingredient Notes**—*Saying "curry" is a bit like saying "sauce." There are so many variations to it. If you aren't making your own curry powder, find one you like. I particularly like the Penzey's Maharajah curry powder.*

**Hint**—*If kept in air-tight container, these freeze for a few months just fine.*

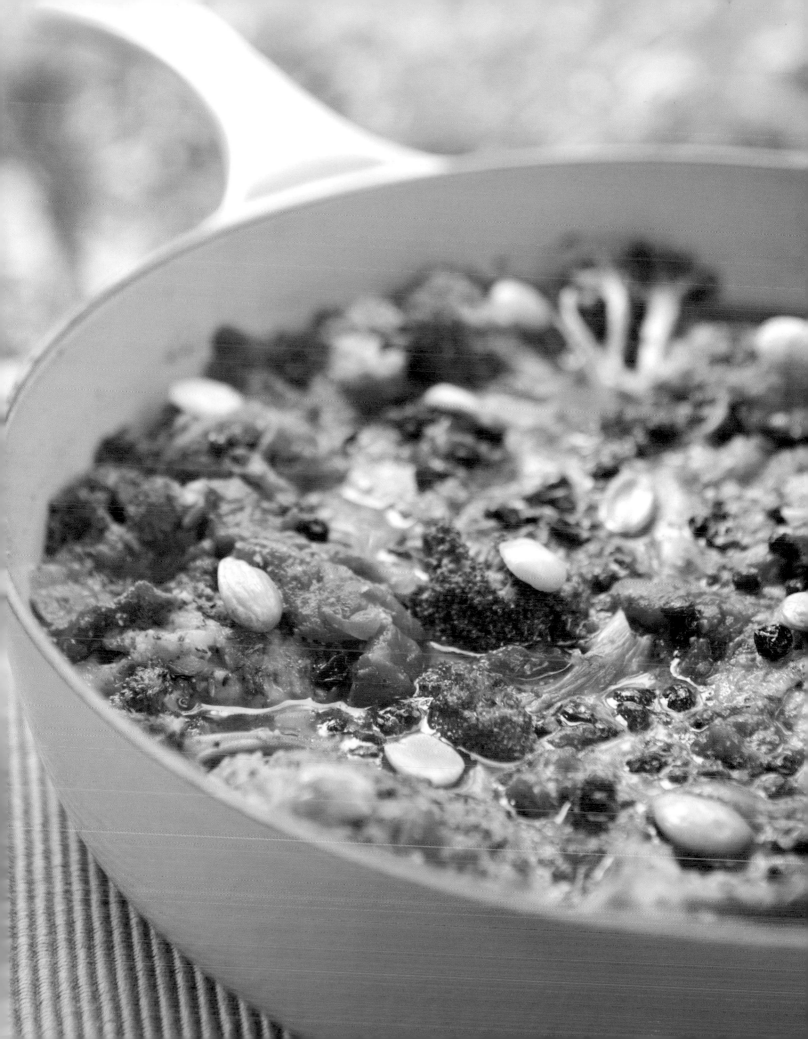

# chicken enchiladas

*Let it be known that to say I (Julie) love Mexican food might actually be an understatement. Since converting to a paleo way of eating, Mexican food at our house and out at restaurants has usually meant fajitas in some way, shape, or form, minus the beans and rice, and no tortillas. This has meant redefining tacos somewhat, and figuring out that the insides of the taco are incredibly tasty when wrapped in lettuce. However, I just couldn't figure out enchiladas—at least still calling them enchiladas. Lettuce when cooked is pretty gnarly, and a lot of other veggie matter just falls apart and can't hold the insides.*

*And then, when perusing the Tropical Traditions website, I saw them. And by them, I mean some coconut flour tortillas. And the enchiladas became a reality.*

*When I first made this dish, I worried that the coconut flavor from the coconut flour in the tortillas would over-power the enchiladas (which isn't really such a bad thing when you think about it). The amazing part is that you really hardly taste the coconut. These enchiladas make me happy.*

| | |
|---|---|
| 1 | tablespoon coconut oil |
| 1 | poblano pepper, chopped |
| 2 | cloves garlic, minced |
| 1 | medium onion, chopped |
| 2 | teaspoons cumin |
| 2 | teaspoons chili powder |
| 1 | pound (450 g) cooked and shredded chicken breast |
| 3 | cups (750 mL) enchilada sauce (or refer to the Red Chile Sauce on page 106) |
| 6–8 | Coconut Flour Tortillas (recipe on page 118) |

**1.** Preheat oven to 350 °F (175 °C). Meanwhile, heat a large skillet over medium-high heat. Add in the coconut oil. Once the oil is hot, add the pepper, garlic, and onion. Sauté until onions are tender and translucent. Add in cumin, chili powder, chicken, and about ½ cup of the enchilada sauce. Reduce heat and simmer to cook off any runny liquid that may exist.

**2.** Pour a small amount of the enchilada sauce into the bottom of a small baking dish.

**3.** Carefully take one tortilla at a time and fill with some of the chicken mixture, rolling and placing seam side down in the dish.

**4.** Repeat with all the tortillas until the pan is full. Pour the remaining enchilada sauce over and bake for about 10 minutes.

**Variation**—*Pork, beef and shrimp are all super tasty substitutes for chicken, or you can use a green chili or tomatillo sauce if you prefer that over red. If you are a person allowing dairy into your life, this is a great time to use cheese.*

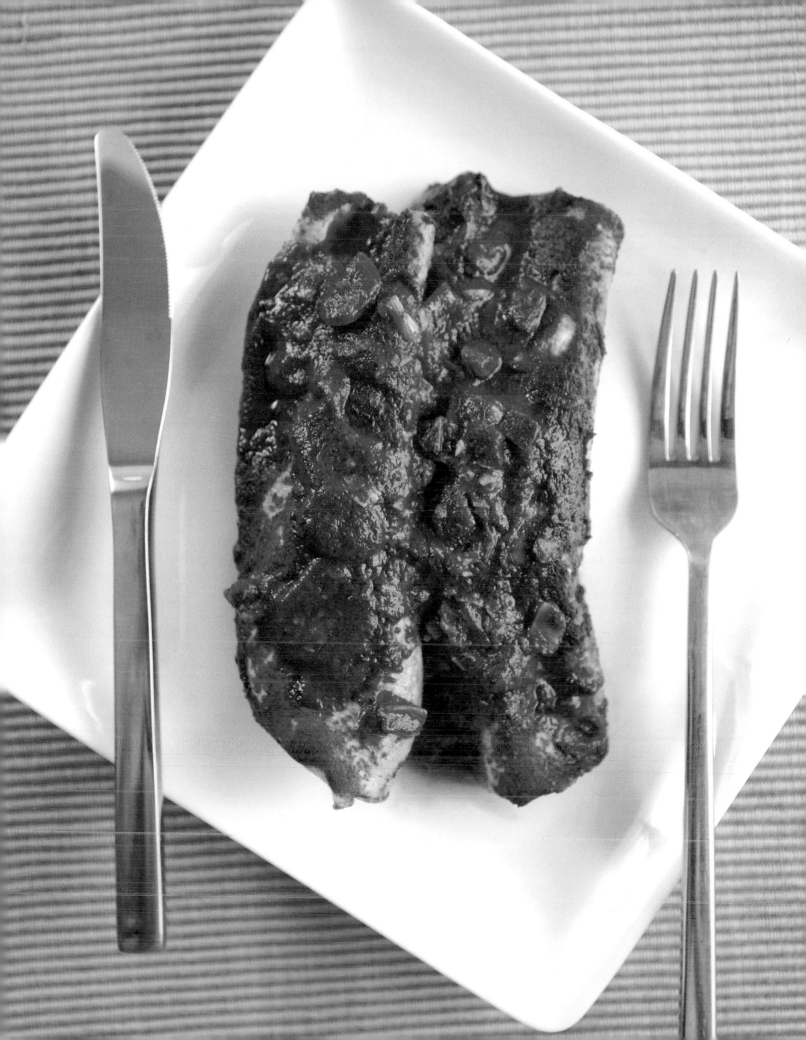

# dry-brined big bird

*Turkey will come across your radar at minimum once a year. We gave this recipe a try this Thanksgiving when we spent four days in Tennessee and told my Mom to stay out of the kitchen. You should have seen her. She didn't know what to do with herself the entire time we were there. Funny thing was that while we were cooking our turkey in the oven, my Dad was outside cooking 86 turkeys for his Sunday school class's Thanksgiving fundraiser. Needless to say, we had plenty of bird on the table. While we all love the smoked turkeys, my dad went on record saying this preparation was one of the best turkeys he had ever eaten.*

*Troll through the Internet and you will find many different ways to brine a turkey. Why do we like this dry brine? Sometimes it's a real challenge to find a cooler or other insulated vessel to put a turkey and all that brining liquid into. And it would likely drive our dogs crazy. Dry brining is great because it uses the moisture content of the turkey itself. The salt pulls the moisture out of the turkey on the first day of dry brining, then mixes with some of the salt, then is reabsorbed into the turkey, making for a really tender but not mushy meat.*

| | |
|---|---|
| 1 | 10- to 20-pound (5–9 kg) fresh or frozen whole turkey, neck and giblets removed from cavity |
| 2–4 | tablespoons kosher salt |
| 1 | tablespoon black pepper |
| 2 | small onions, quartered |
| 2 | medium apples, peeled and cored, cut into medium slices |
| 1 | bunch fresh thyme |
| ½ | bunch flat-leaf parsley |
| ½ | cup (110 g) butter |
| 1 | cup (250 mL) water |
| 1 | cup (250 mL) white wine |

## 72 hours before cooking

**1.** Rinse the turkey under cold water and pat dry. Rub with kosher salt including into cavities where possible.

**2.** Wrap the bird in a large plastic bag and place in the refrigerator, taking time to massage salt into skin on day 2.

## 24 hours before cooking

**3.** Turn the turkey over in the refrigerator.

## A few hours before cooking

**4.** Remove the turkey from the bag and pat dry. Place in a roasting pan and allow to come to room temperature. Sprinkle half the black pepper into chest cavity adding half the onions/apples and all of the thyme/parsley. The remaining onions/apples can go in the neck cavity. Tie the legs up with twine and tuck the neck skin under.

**5.** Rub as much of the bird with butter as possible (under skin and onto thighs). Sprinkle remaining black pepper on exterior of bird and place in 450°F (235°C) oven for about 30 minutes.

**6.** Remove from oven and reduce heat to 350°F (175°C). Cover breast and wings with one big sheet of foil. Pour water and white wine into roasting pan and return to oven for about 2–3 hours or until an instant-read thermometer inserted into the breast reads 170°F (75°C). Good rule of thumb is to cook 15 minutes per pound of bird.

**Variation**—*Mix in some aromatics with the salt, such as lemon zest, rosemary, or your favorite herbs and spices. This will infuse the turkey with those tasty flavors.*

paleo comfort foods

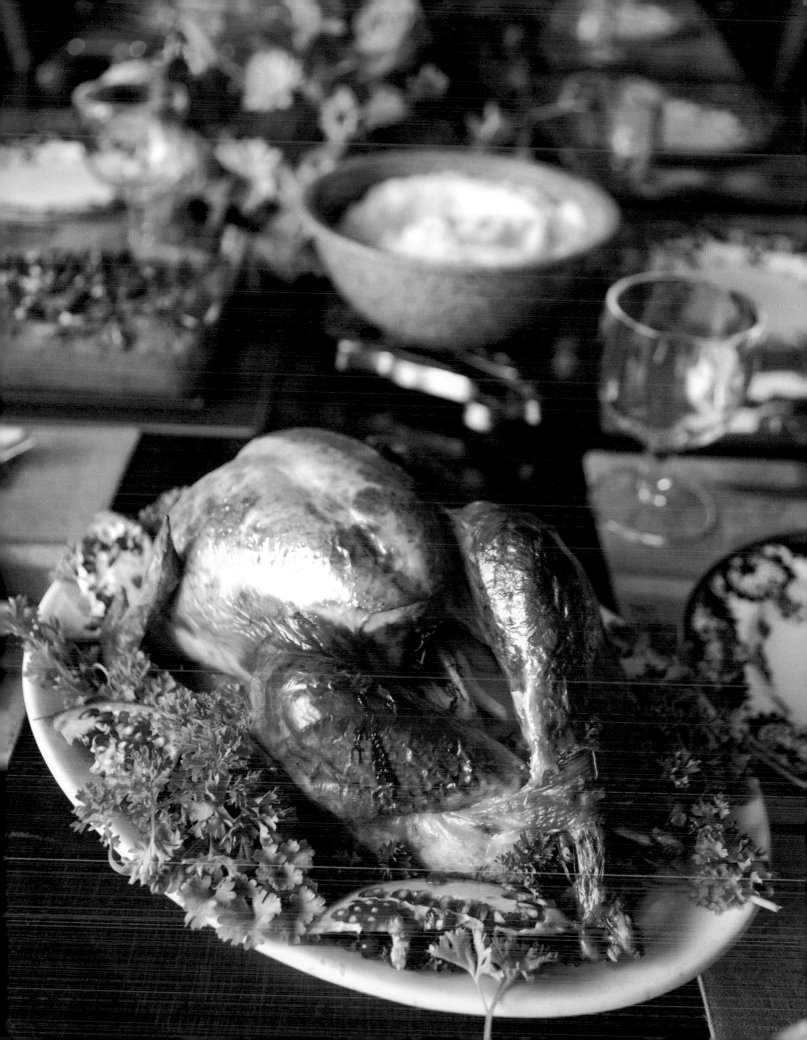

# pot of chicken pie

*There is just something special about chicken. It seems to have its toe in so many comforting recipes. Chicken pot pie has to be near the top of most folks' comfort food lists. Something about the word "pie," I guess. The crust may crack and separate a bit, depending on the size of your baking dish. Don't fret, the flavors and textures will still be there waiting on your fork.*

## For the topping

| | |
|---|---|
| 2 | cups (300 g) almond flour (blanched is preferred) |
| ½ | cup (125 mL) olive oil |
| 1 | teaspoon baking soda |
| ½ | teaspoon salt |

## For the filling

| | |
|---|---|
| 2 | tablespoons olive oil |
| 1 | tablespoon garlic, minced |
| 1½ | cups (225 g) onion, chopped |
| 3 | cups (300 g) mushrooms, coarsely chopped |
| 1 | cup (100 g) carrots, chopped |
| 1 | cup (100 g) celery, chopped |
| 2 | cups (350 g) broccoli florets, chopped |
| 2 | pounds (900 g) cooked chicken breasts, chopped in small pieces |
| 2 | cups (500 mL) chicken stock |
| 1 | teaspoon parsley |
| ½ | teaspoon black pepper |
| 1 | tablespoon coconut flour |

**1.** Oven should be preheated to 350°F (175°C).

**2.** Mix almond flour, olive oil, baking soda, and salt in small bowl. To make your crust, roll out the dough on wax paper into a sheet large enough to cover the casserole dish of your choosing.

**3.** Place in refrigerator until you are ready to cover your other ingredients.

**4.** Heat 2 tablespoons of olive oil in large skillet and sauté garlic and onion. Once they have softened, add mushrooms and cook for a few minutes.

**5.** Add carrots, celery, and broccoli and continue to cook for another 5 minutes. When they begin to cook through, add the chicken, stock, parsley, and pepper.

**6.** Add coconut flour to thicken mixture and let simmer for 10 minutes.

**7.** Pour all ingredients into casserole dish and place dough over top. Bake for 25–30 minutes.

**Plan Ahead**—*Having your meat already cooked helps expedite this recipe. Otherwise you'll need to bake the chicken for 45–50 minutes before creating the filling.*

**Variations**—*Try using turkey or duck breast to change the flavor and texture of this classic.*

**Hint**—*This recipe freezes very well.*

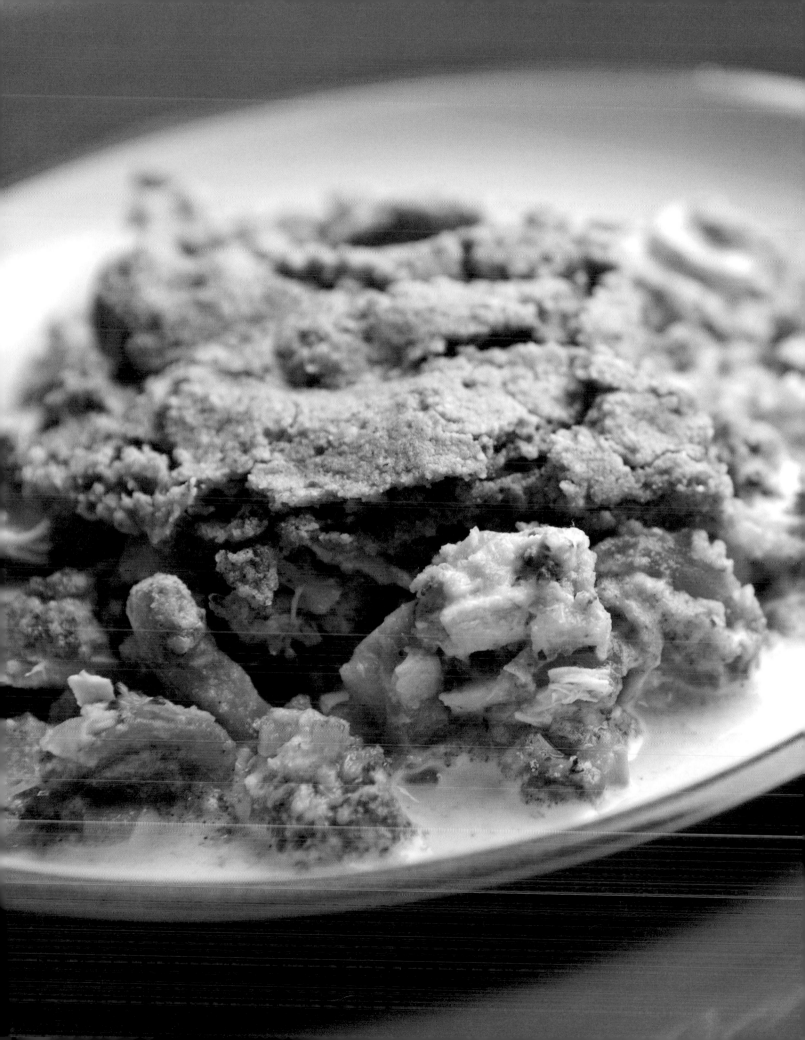

# fried chicken

*For many people we know, it doesn't get any more comforting than fried chicken. This recipe is pretty darn easy and you can add whatever you want to the dry mixture for seasoning. You will want to use a slotted spatula or tongs to move the chicken around, and try to only turn once in the frying pan. The more you handle the pieces of the chicken, the more fried goodness will be left in the pan.*

| | |
|---|---|
| 1 | cup (250 mL) coconut oil |
| 2 | large eggs |
| 1 | cup (150 g) almond flour |
| 1 | teaspoon paprika |
| 1 | teaspoon garlic powder |
| ½ | teaspoon salt |
| ½ | teaspoon black pepper |
| ½ | teaspoon dried thyme |
| 1 | teaspoon chipotle powder (optional) |
| 2 | pounds (900 g) chicken—thighs, drums, breasts |

1. Heat oil in large frying pan to 350°F (175°C).
2. Whisk eggs in medium sized bowl.
3. Combine all dry ingredients in large bowl and mix well.
4. Dip chicken in whisked eggs.
5. Coat/cover chicken with dry mixture and place in hot oil. Allow both sides to brown (about 2 minutes on each side).
6. Place drying rack on sheet pan and assemble chicken on the rack so there is space between all pieces.
7. Place in 400°F (205°C) preheated oven for 10–15 minutes. Remove and get ready for some good eating.

**Tips & Tricks**—*Line your sheet pan with aluminum foil to make clean up a bit easier. You can also try brining the chicken the day before to enhance flavor.*

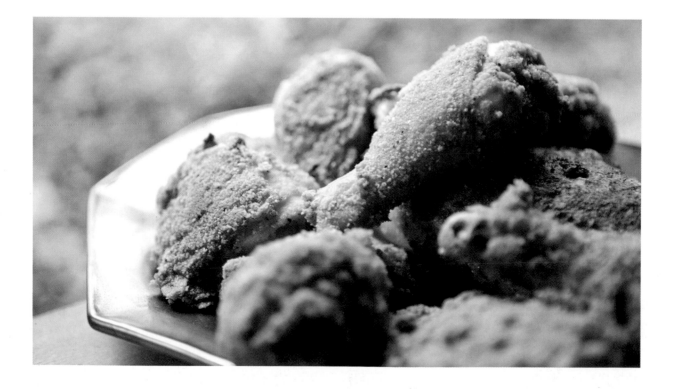

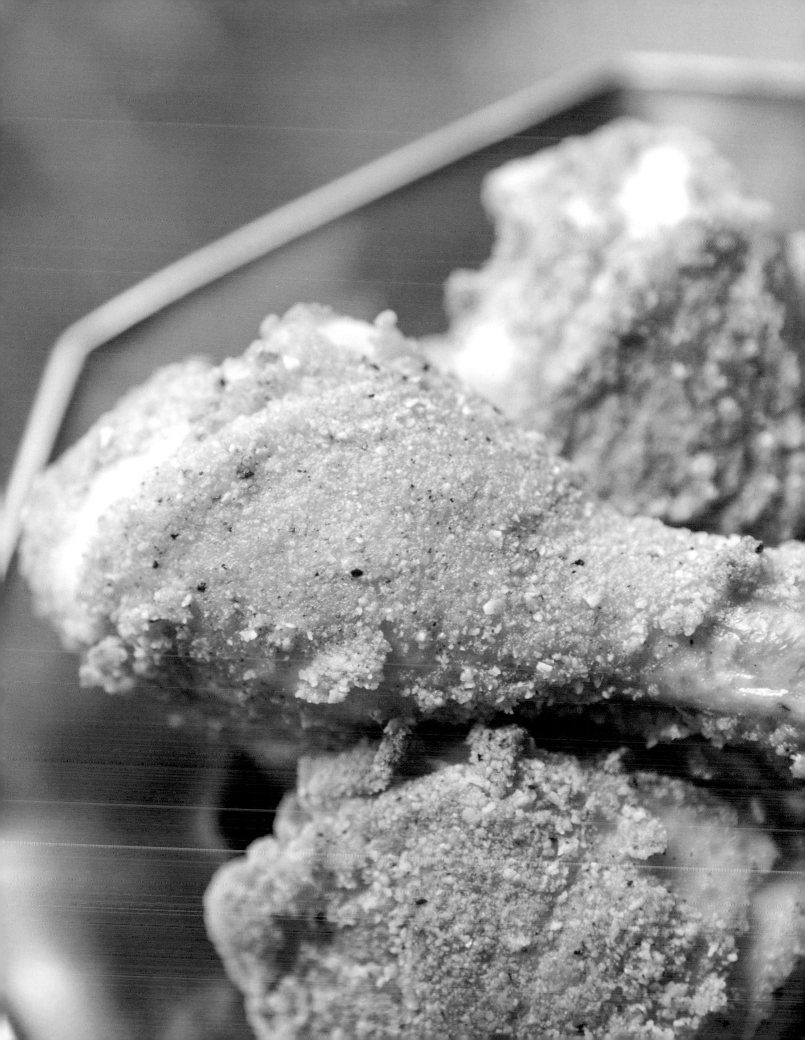

# julie's barbecue chicken

*A few things to remember about chicken, barbecue, and grilling: always use tongs to handle your meat, store-bought sauce isn't worth the gas you used to go pick it up, and it is really hard to screw up BBQ Chicken.*

*This recipe calls for using the same cuts of chicken. This assures that everything will be cooked on the same time-line. Chicken with the bone in it generally takes a bit longer to cook.*

*That said, feel free to play around with this recipe. You will find another recipe in our book for a different barbecue sauce. Consider them interchangeable and yourselves lucky to get a two-fer.*

---

| | |
|---|---|
| ½ | gallon (2 L) water |
| 2 | tablespoons kosher salt |
| ¼ | cup (60 mL) honey |
| 2 | cloves garlic, smashed |
| 6 | pounds (3 kg) chicken leg/thigh quarters, skin on |
| 1 | 6-ounce (180 mL) can tomato paste |
| 1½ | cups (375 mL) chicken broth |
| 3 | cloves garlic, minced |
| ½ | cup (75 g) shallots, finely chopped |
| 1 | tablespoon Dijon mustard |
| 2 | tablespoons apple cider vinegar |
| 1 | tablespoon olive oil |
| 1 | tablespoon honey |
| 1 | teaspoon prepared horseradish |
| 1 | teaspoon salt |
| 2 | teaspoons black pepper |
| 2 | teaspoons ground cumin |
| ½ | teaspoon cayenne pepper |

## Brine the chicken

1. Mix water, salt, honey, and smashed garlic in large plastic sealable bag.

2. When combined, place chicken in bag, seal, and place in refrigerator for 1–2 hours (25 minutes will do if you're in a hurry).

## Make the sauce

3. In medium sauce pan, combine remaining ingredients. Whisk thoroughly to combine and place on low heat. Cover and allow to simmer for 30–40 minutes.

## Cook the chicken

4. When your sauce has almost reached the thickness desired, preheat the grill. Set aside half of the sauce to serve with chicken and the other half will be brushed on while cooking. Preheat oven to 350°F (175°C).

5. Remove chicken from brine and pat dry with a paper towel. Be sure your grill surface has been properly coated to prevent sticking. The ideal temperature for the grill is around 375°F (190°C).

6. Arrange chicken on grill for direct heat and cook 6–8 minutes before flipping. Flip chicken over, and using a grill brush, smother chicken liberally with barbeque sauce. Cook for another 6-8 minutes and remove to sheet pan lined with foil.

7. Using a grill brush, smother every inch of the chicken with sauce and place in oven for another 15 minutes or until internal temperature of chicken reaches 160°F (70°C). You'll want to baste chicken one more time while they are in the oven.

---

**Tips & Tricks**—*Avoid using the oven by simply cooking chicken on grill for 15 minutes each side.*

**Plan Ahead**—*You can brine your chicken overnight and have the barbeque sauce made in advance.*

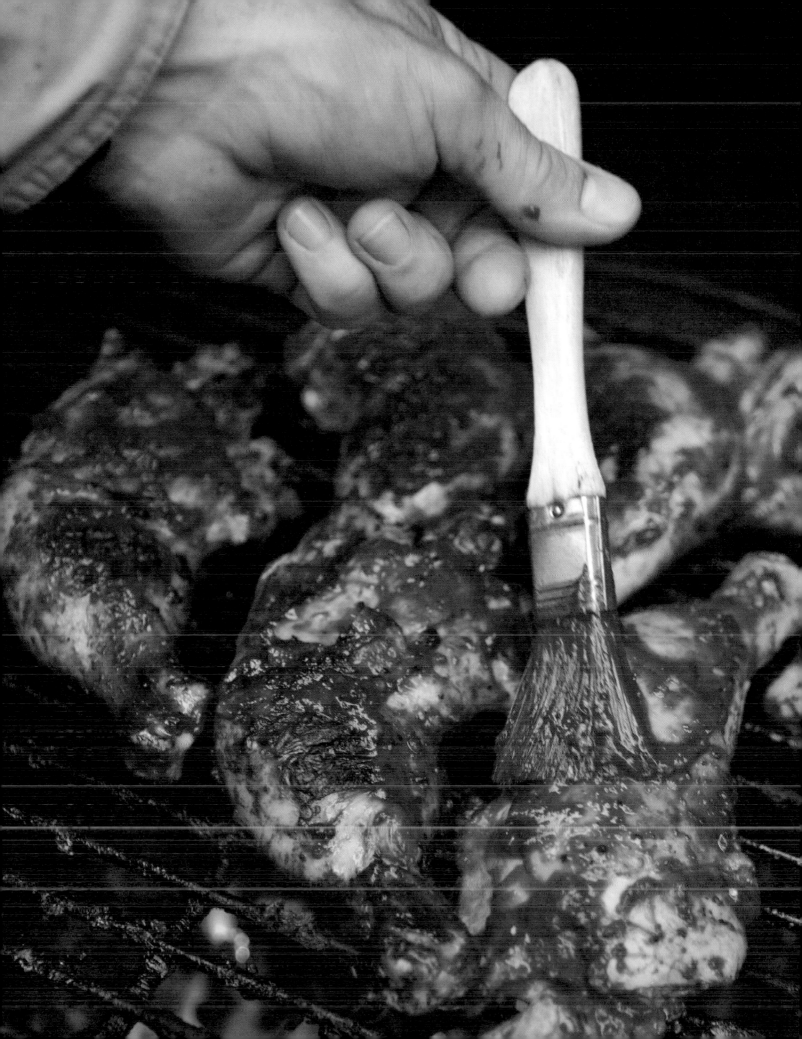

# coq au vin
# casserole of chicken in red wine

*The first time I made coq au vin for one of my Le Creuset cooking demonstrations, I was convinced that I was either going to burn my eyebrows off or injure some innocent bystander. Flambéing is dramatic, and always gets my heart racing with that noise it makes as it ignites. Yet the drama is part of the fun, as you always get some "oohs" and "aahs" when people see those flames shoot up in the air. This recipe is adapted from Williams-Sonoma and the queen of coq au vin, Julia Child.*

| | |
|---|---|
| 4 | tablespoons clarified butter |
| 6 | slices thick-cut bacon, cut into 1-inch (2 cm) pieces |
| 2 | cups (200 g) pearl onions or sliced yellow onions |
| 4 | skin-on chicken breasts and 4 skin-on chicken thighs, or an assortment of chicken that equals about 4 pounds (2 kg) |
| 2 | tablespoons almond flour |
| 2 | tablespoons warm brandy |
| 2 | cups (500 mL) pinot noir or other medium-bodied red wine |
| ½ | tablespoon tomato paste |
| 2 | cloves garlic, minced |
| 4 | sprigs fresh thyme |
| 4 | sprigs fresh flat-leaf parsley |
| 1 | bay leaf |
| ~ | salt and freshly ground pepper |
| 2 | cups (250 g) button mushrooms, halved |

1. In a large Dutch oven over medium/medium-low heat, melt 3 of the tablespoons of butter.

2. Add the bacon and onions, stir, and cook until bacon is somewhat browned and crispy (about 10 minutes). Transfer the bacon and onions to a plate and set aside.

3. Bring the heat up to medium high, and add the chicken, turning as needed to ensure all sides brown. Sprinkle the almond flour on the chicken, and turn, cooking until golden brown. Remove the Dutch oven from the stove, pour in the brandy over the chicken and let get hot for a moment, and immediately ignite with a long match. The flames will subside in a few seconds.

4. Stir the bacon and onions back into the chicken, and place back on the stove over medium heat. Add in 1 cup (250 mL) of the wine, and scrape up any of the fond (brown bits) that may be on the bottom of your pan.

5. Add in the rest of the wine and all the remaining ingredients except the mushrooms and 1 remaining tablespoon of butter. Stir and bring heat to low. Cover and let simmer for 45–60 minutes or until chicken is cooked through.

6. About 20 minutes before the chicken is done, in a small sauté pan melt the butter and sauté the mushrooms until golden brown. Add these to the chicken.

7. This part is optional, but highly recommended: using tongs or a slotted spoon, remove the chicken, mushrooms, onions and bacon to a platter. Raise the heat in the pan up to high, bring to a boil, and cook until liquid has thickened slightly and is reduced by about half. Return the chicken, mushrooms, onion and bacon back to the pan, heat through for a few minutes, and serve.

**Tips & Tricks**—*Please use caution with the brandy, and don't decide that you're going to up the amount of alcohol to some crazy amount (more alcohol = more of a bonfire effect), and please don't pour directly from the bottle. This is a serious hazard and could cause the flames to ignite the contents of the bottle. As stated with other recipes that use alcohol in cooking, if you prefer not to use, that is just fine too (but it won't taste quite the same). Replace the wine and brandy with some chicken stock and add just a touch of balsamic vinegar for some tangy flavor.*

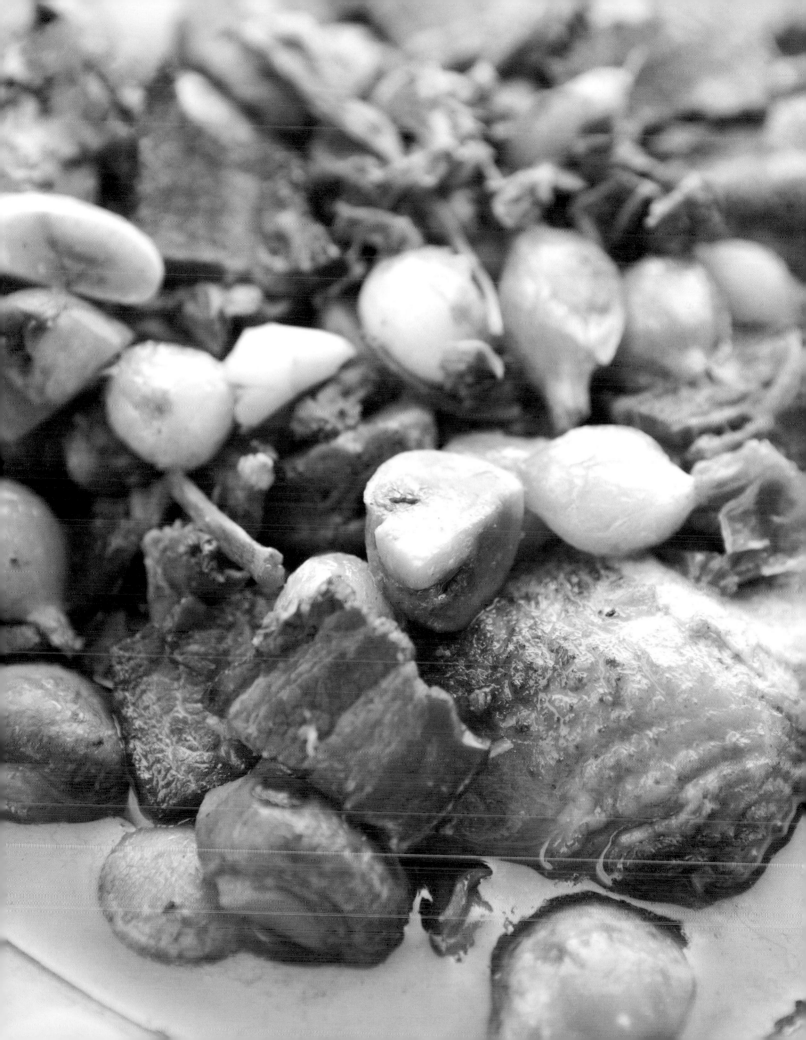

# basic, almost foolproof grilled chicken

*If you were to poll people who have embarked on a paleo path and ask them "what protein source do you most often eat?" chances are chicken would be at the top of the list.*

*There are hundreds if not thousands of ways to prepare chicken, which makes life all that more interesting. Yet, despite hundreds and thousands of chicken recipes, this recipe is one that never bores or disappoints me.*

*The most enlightening bit about this recipe: how to make grilled chicken at home and not dry it out. The secret really is finishing it in the oven.*

*This is also the best and easiest way to make grilled chicken for the masses. I made this once for a big dinner at one of the BTB instructor's homes, and it turned out perfectly. Fortunately, it was before we drank too much wine and headed out for '80s night. That's a recipe for disaster . . . this is a recipe for success!*

| | |
|---|---|
| 2 | pounds (900 g) chicken breasts |
| 4 | cloves garlic, chopped |
| ~ | zest of 1 lemon |
| 2 | tablespoons fresh rosemary |
| 3 | tablespoons olive oil |
| ½ | teaspoon sea salt (optional) |
| ½ | teaspoon black pepper |

1. Trim the chicken of any excess fat, and if both breasts are still attached by the cartilage in the middle, simply cut that out. If the breasts have the tenderloins still intact, go ahead and remove those and save for a future use.

2. In a large bowl, combine the garlic, lemon zest, rosemary, olive oil, salt, and pepper. Stir to combine thoroughly.

3. Add in the chicken, using your hands to make sure the marinade thoroughly covers all parts of the chicken. Allow to marinate at least 30 minutes. Longer is preferred, as the flavors will really permeate the chicken that much more.

4. Preheat oven to 400°F (205°C).

5. Heat a large cast-iron grill pan over medium-high heat. Once very hot, place chicken breasts smooth side down on pan. Do not even think about touching the chicken to turn until nice and caramelized and the chicken releases easily from the pan. If it resists releasing, it is not ready to be flipped. If your grill pan was nice and hot (as it should be) this should only take about 3–5 minutes per side.

6. Remove the chicken from the grill pan, and place on a sheet pan and into the oven for 12–15 minutes to finish cooking. You will know your chicken is done when juices run clear.

7. Allow breasts to rest for 5–10 minutes, then slice against the grain and serve.

**Variations**—*This marinade is awesome on lamb, beef, even shrimp. If you want to use this on shrimp, only marinate for about 30 minutes, as beyond that it tends to get too overpowering for your shrimp. You can also grill these outside if you prefer, still finishing the breasts in the oven to retain that juicy-ness.*

**Plan Ahead**—*The marinade can be made a few days beforehand, though you will want to bring it to room temperature when you are ready to use.*

paleo comfort foods

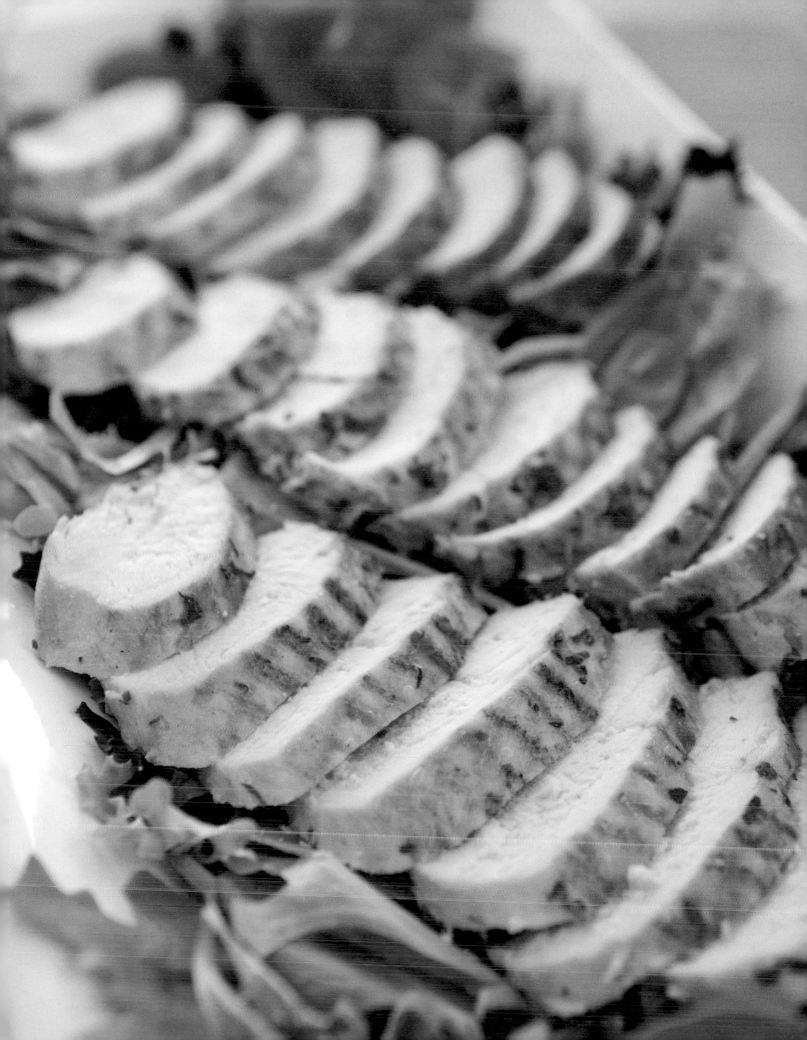

# turkey loafing

*This is our take on meatloaf, again one of those all-time ultimate comfort foods. Most family recipes for meatloaf involve similar basics, though quite a few home recipes call for added breadcrumbs and store-bought ketchup. Much like burgers, this Turkey Loafing recipe is one that you can make your own in so many ways.*

| | |
|---|---|
| 2 | medium sweet onions, chopped |
| 1 | red bell pepper, chopped (optional) |
| 1 | teaspoon kosher salt |
| 1 | teaspoon black pepper |
| 1 | teaspoon thyme |
| 1 | teaspoon garlic powder |
| 2 | tablespoons coconut oil |
| 1 | tablespoon tomato paste |
| ½ | cup (125 mL) chicken stock |
| 1 | tablespoon Worcestershire sauce |
| 2 | large eggs |
| 4 | pounds (1.8 kg) ground turkey |
| 1 | cup (250 mL) Cave Ketchup (recipe page 102) |

1. Preheat oven to 325°F (165°C).

2. Sauté onions, red pepper (optional) and all spices with coconut oil over medium heat until onions become translucent, about 10 minutes. Remove from heat, and stir in tomato paste, stock, and Worcestershire sauce.

3. In large bowl, crack eggs over your turkey and fold in the onion mix once it has cooled.

4. Form the meat mixture into whatever shape suits your fancy, but the traditional loaf will cook evenly. Place on sheet pan or casserole dish, no greasing required.

5. Pour your ketchup over the top and bake for about 90 minutes. You'll want the internal temp at 160°F (70°C) degrees to know that it has cooked all the way through.

**Variations**—*Use ground beef, bison, or venison. You can also replace ketchup with BBQ sauce.*

**Hint**—*Freeze this with some Mashed Cauliflower (page 180) for great portable meals.*

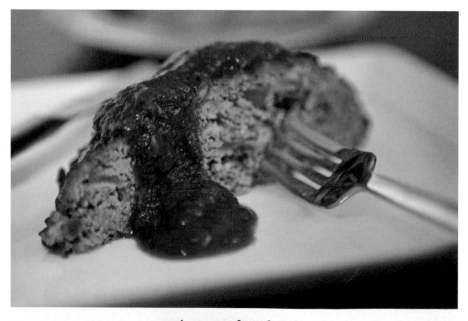

**paleo comfort foods**

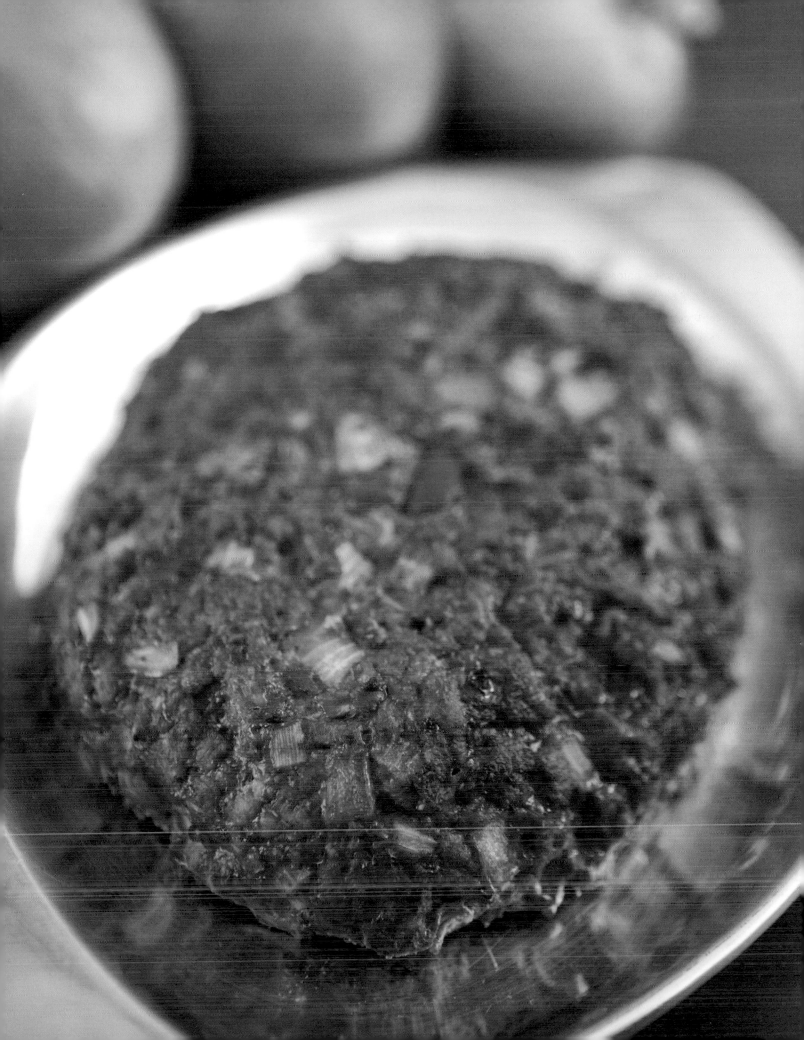

# mushroom stuffed quail with dijon sauce

*There are few outdoor experiences quite like quail hunting. Quail hunting season opens in early winter and goes through February in Georgia. Thanks to the amazing work by such organizations like Quail Unlimited, you can find all sorts of places to hunt birds. Like most outdoor sporting activities, the real fun for me is in observing the pageantry that takes place in nature. I'm getting a little too poetic here. Bottom line, if you have never watched a good group of bird dogs work, put that on your bucket list. I've been on some pretty amazing hunts in my day. In addition, you will be hard pressed to find a greater adrenaline rush than the one that comes when you jump a covey of wild quail. You have about 1 second to aim and fire if you're lucky.*

| | |
|---|---|
| 4 | quail |
| 1 | tablespoon olive oil |
| 1 | cup (125 g) assorted mushrooms (shiitake, cremini, porcini, etc.), chopped |
| 1 | small shallot, minced |
| ½ | cup (75 g) cauliflower, grated |
| 2 | teaspoons fresh thyme |
| 2 | tablespoons pecans, chopped |
| ~ | salt and pepper to taste |
| 1 | teaspoon smoked paprika or Creole seasoning |
| 1 | cup (250 mL) chicken stock or white wine |
| 2 | teaspoons Dijon mustard |

1. Debone the quail.
2. Preheat oven to 400°F (205°C).
3. To make the stuffing, heat a skillet over medium heat. Add the oil, then the mushrooms and shallots, stirring often until mushrooms are softened.
4. Stir in the cauliflower, thyme, pecans and salt and pepper. Cook until cauliflower is slightly softened.
5. With the quail skin side down, place some of the stuffing mixture on the meat, folding the quail around the stuffing.
6. Place in a small baking dish breast side up. Repeat with remaining quail, and sprinkle the paprika over each bird.
7. Bake in the oven for 5 minutes, then reduce heat to 350°F (175°C) and finish for 10 minutes or until the meat is cooked through (being careful not to overcook quail).
8. Remove quail from pan. While pan is still hot, add in chicken stock (or wine), stirring to dig up any of the browned bits in the pan. Pour this into a small sauce pan set over medium-low heat. Whisk mustard into liquid mixture until well combined. Serve quail with sauce poured over.

**Tips & Tricks**—*While you can certainly leave all the quail bones intact, I find that it presents a little bit nicer and is a ton easier to eat if the rib cage, wish bone and breast cartilage are removed.*

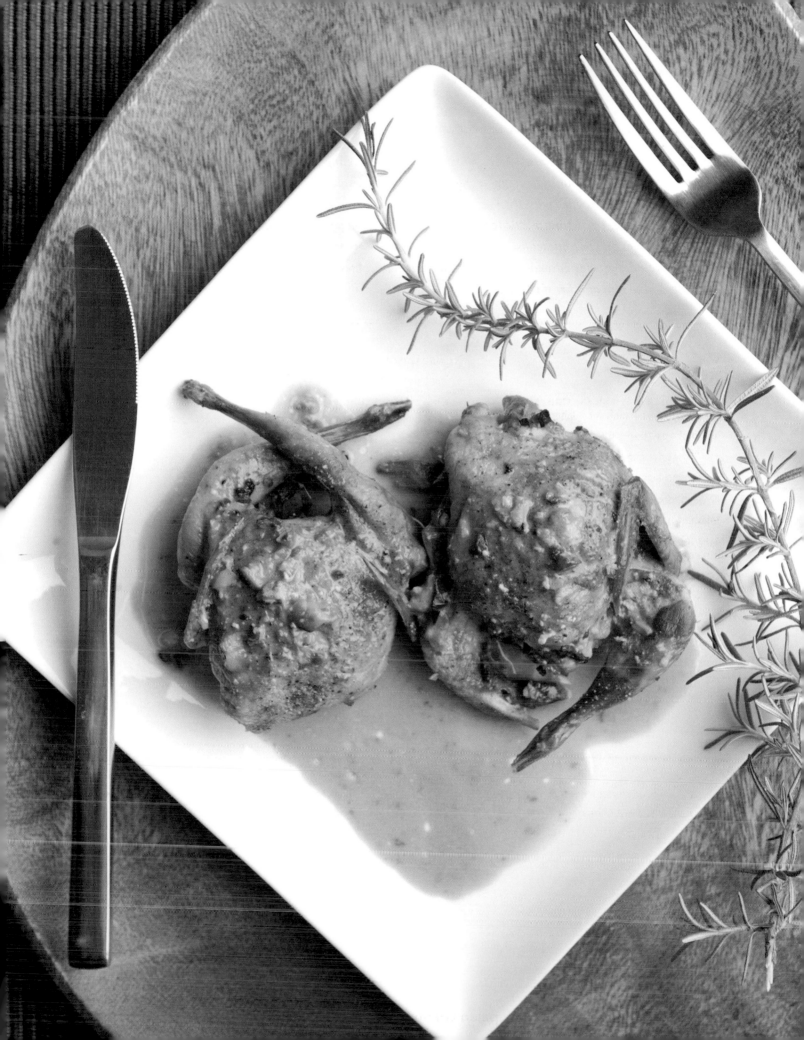

# shrimp and grits

*You might say this is the recipe that broke the caveman's back. Julie had made Paleo Grits only a few days before, and I really wanted to surprise her with a cool meal that incorporated her latest creation. Julie is the real brains behind the apron in our house. So over dinner with Robb Wolf and Nicki Violleti I bragged about my latest creation. Nicki pounded the table and pointed at us. "That's it, you two are writing a cookbook!" Robb and Nicki proceeded to brainstorm how this "Redneck Paleo Cookbook" (as it was once called) could work. We got an e-mail the next morning from Robb's publisher and off we went.*

*History has it that shrimp and grits started as a simple fisherman's breakfast in the Carolina low country, where they would sauté shrimp in bacon grease and serve over grits. Of course, talk to any chef in the South and they'll all have a different interpretation on shrimp and grits. Our interpretation? Try it for yourself and see how you like it. Play around with it and make up one of your own! Who knows? Maybe you'll get the itch to write a cookbook.*

---

| | |
|---|---|
| 4 | slices bacon |
| ½ | cup (125 g) celery, diced |
| ½ | cup (75 g) green onion, chopped |
| ½ | cup (85 g) red pepper, diced |
| ½ | cup (50 g) mushrooms, sliced |
| 2 | teaspoons Cajun seasoning |
| 2 | cloves garlic, minced |
| 1 | pound (450 g) shrimp, peeled and deveined |
| 2 | tablespoons almond flour |
| 2 | tablespoons sherry |
| 1 | cup (250 mL) chicken stock |
| 1 | tablespoon fresh lemon juice |

1. In a large skillet over medium heat, cook the bacon until crispy. Remove bacon to paper towels.
2. Pour off the bacon grease, reserving about 1 tablespoon in the pan.
3. Return pan to heat, and add celery, green onion, red pepper, and mushrooms, cooking until vegetables are softened. Add Cajun seasoning and stir.
4. In a medium bowl, coat the shrimp with the almond flour. Add to pan along with garlic, and sauté until shrimp are just pink.
5. Stir in sherry, chicken stock and lemon juice, being sure to loosen any browned bits on the bottom of the skillet.
6. Simmer for 5–8 minutes to reduce liquid.
7. Serve shrimp over Paleo Grits (recipe page 206).

---

**Plan Ahead**—*Paleo Grits can be made ahead of time and stored in the refrigerator. Simply reheat to serve.*

**Hint**—*This recipe freezes well. Put shrimp and grits in one container.*

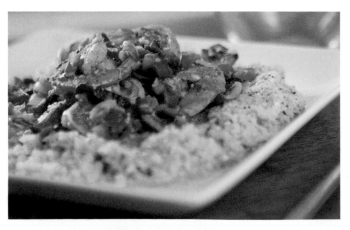

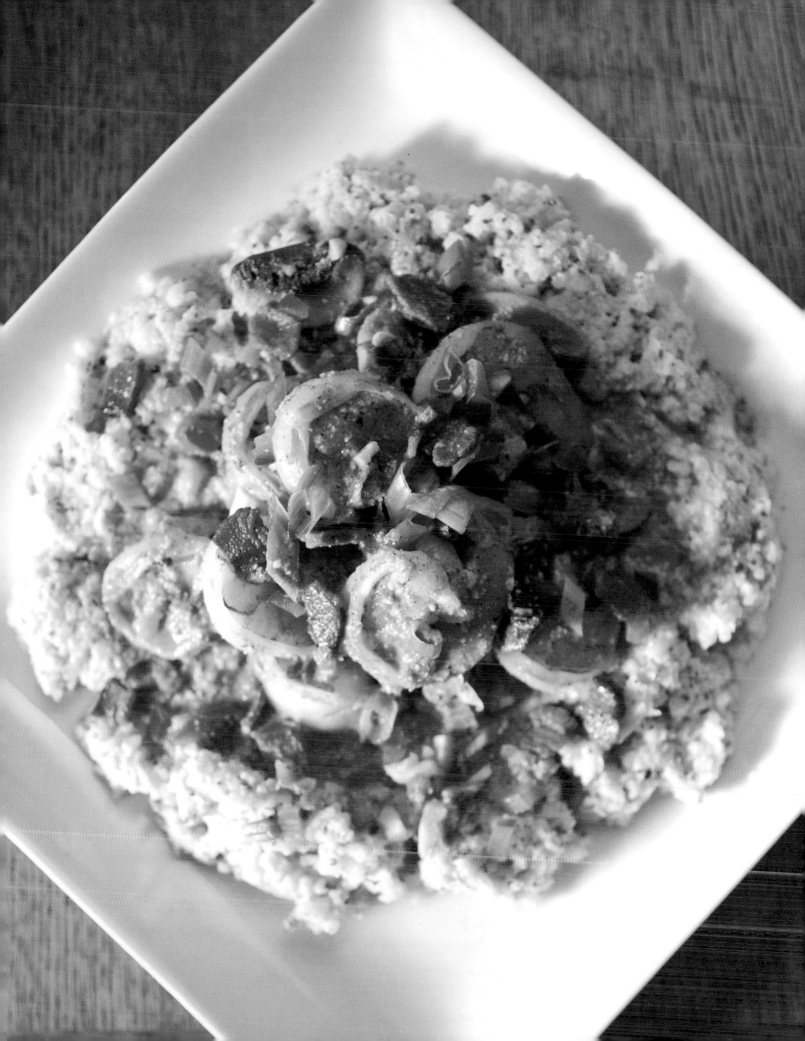

# georgian pecan-crusted trout

*Most restaurants here in Georgia that profess to have a "Southern" flair will have some variation of Georgian trout on the menu. First of all, it's local. Secondly, there's something uber-Georgian about the combination of sweet pecans grown here in the state and trout that makes it twice as Southern—or so it seems.*

*This is a really simple and fast dish, and great for when you want a restaurant-quality dinner, but you don't want to spend hours making it.*

| | |
|---|---|
| ½ | cup (75 g) almond flour |
| ½ | teaspoon salt (optional) |
| ½ | teaspoon pepper |
| 2 | large eggs |
| 1 | cup (50 g) toasted pecans, roughly chopped |
| 4 | 6- to 8-ounce (150–230 g) pieces of trout |
| 2 | tablespoons clarified butter, divided |
| ¼ | cup (60 mL) lemon juice |
| ½ | cup (120 mL) white wine |
| ¼ | cup (45 g) capers, rinsed |
| 2 | tablespoons fresh Italian parsley, chopped |

1. Place the almond flour along with some salt and pepper on a large plate or shallow dish.

2. Whisk the egg whites slightly, and place into a separate dish and put the pecans into a third dish.

3. Working one piece at a time, dredge the trout flesh side down first into the flour mixture, then into the eggs, then into the pecans, pressing down to get nuts to adhere. Set aside and repeat process with other pieces of fish.

4. Heat 1 tablespoon of the butter over medium-high heat. Add the fish (in batches if necessary) skin side up (nuts side down) and cook until golden, about 5 minutes. Carefully flip over and cook another 4–5 minutes until the fish is just cooked through and skin is golden.

5. Remove fish to a platter and cover with foil to keep warm.

6. Add the butter, lemon juice, and wine to the pan, scraping to bring up any of the browned bits from the fish.

7. Add the capers and whisk to combine all, until heated through. Stir in the parsley, and pour sauce over the fish to serve.

**Variations**—*If you can't find trout, some decent substitutions might be bluefish, salmon, or arctic char.*

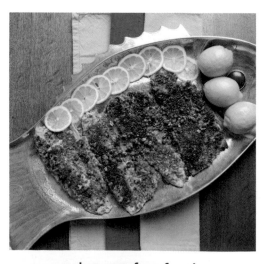

**paleo comfort foods**

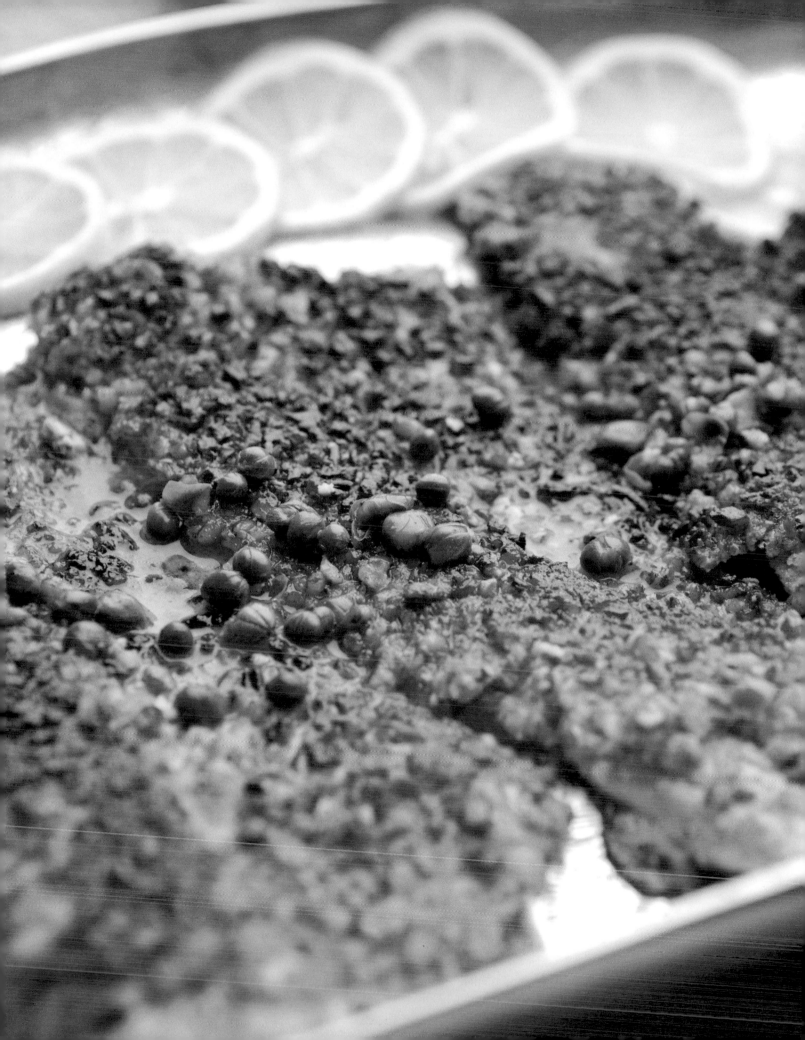

# shrimp skillet

*This is one of those recipes where if you have a bunch of fresh oregano, tomatoes, and peppers in the garden, it's super easy. You can add just about any vegetables in this and it will be so tasty.*

*You'll notice the recipe is written for a full 2 pounds of shrimp. You can absolutely scale this down to 1 pound, but I think you will want lots of leftovers.*

| | |
|---|---|
| 2 | pounds (900 g) medium shrimp, peeled and deveined |
| ~ | zest and juice of 1 lemon |
| 2 | tablespoons fresh oregano, chopped |
| 5 | cloves garlic, minced |
| 3 | tablespoons olive oil + 1 additional tablespoon |
| 1 | medium onion, thinly sliced |
| 1 | red bell pepper, sliced into long strips |
| 4 | tomatoes, seeded and chopped |
| ~ | splash of white wine |

1. Combine the shrimp in a large bowl with the lemon zest and juice, oregano, garlic, and olive oil.
2. Allow to marinate for 15 minutes.
3. Heat a large skillet over medium high heat. Add the additional tablespoon of oil, and add the onion and peppers, cooking until onions are translucent.
4. Increase heat to medium-high and add the shrimp mixture. Stir often and once shrimp have turned pink, add in the tomatoes and splash of white wine.
5. Cook just enough to heat tomatoes through.

**Variations**—*Are you allowing dairy into your life? If so, mix in some feta cheese. It's super tasty with this combination. Don't have oregano? Basil would be great in this recipe too!*

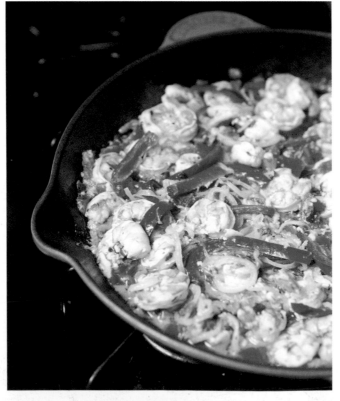

paleo comfort foods

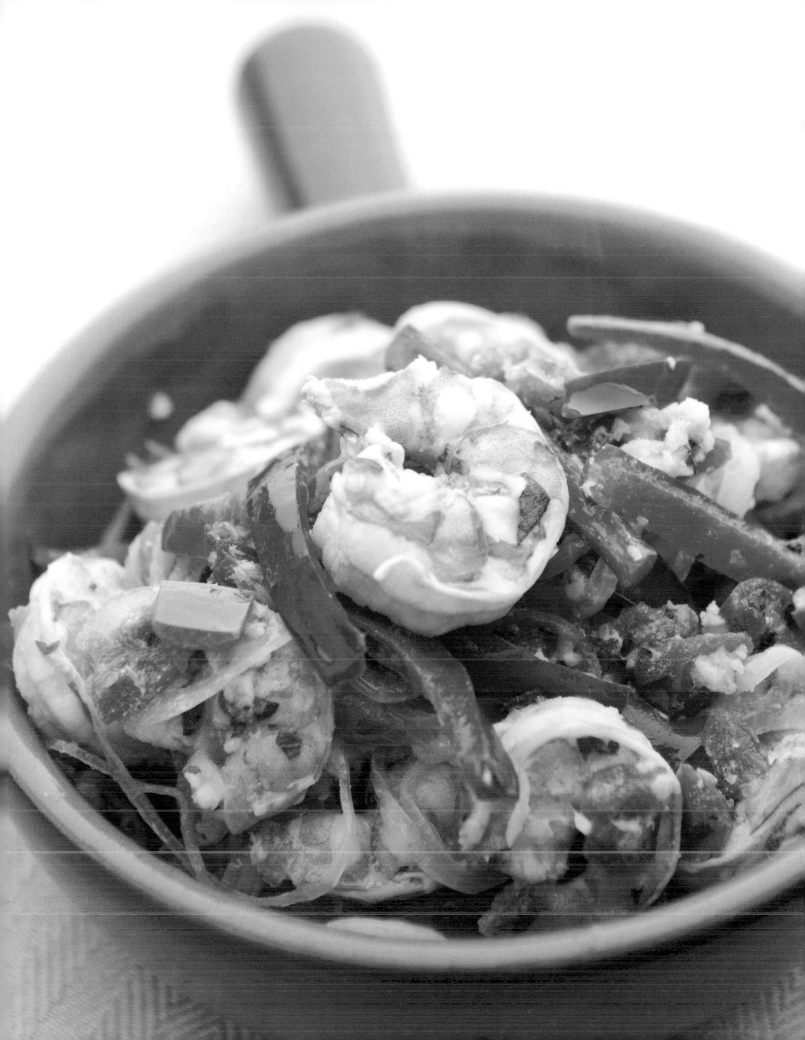

# cedar-plank chipotle salmon

*This is by far one of our favorite salmon recipes. It is relatively easy to make and assuming you have a cedar plank soaked and ready, then you'll be done in less than 45 minutes. This recipe can transform into a dip or appetizer in a snap. Combine fish with Paleo Mayonnaise (page 100) to make a delicious spread to put on sliced veggies.*

| | |
|---|---|
| 1 | cedar plank, soaked in water for at least 30 minutes |
| 1–1½ | pounds (600 g) salmon filet |
| 1 | teaspoon chipotle pepper powder |
| ½ | teaspoon fresh cracked pepper |
| ¼ | teaspoon sea salt |
| 2 | limes, quartered |

1. Grill should be set up for indirect medium-high heat.

2. Remove any bones from salmon. Rinse under cold water and pat dry.

3. Place on cedar plank with skin side down. Mix chipotle, pepper, and salt in small bowl and spread over the fish.

4. Place on grill for 25–30 minutes. Salmon is done when it reaches 135–140°F (58–60°C).

5. Remove from grill and serve immediately from plank, removing skin if desired. Squeeze lime wedge over salmon and garnish with fresh dill or cilantro.

**Tips & Tricks**—*Don't have a grill? Preheat your oven to 325°F (165°C) and stick the plank right in there. Let the salmon cook for 30–40 minutes. Just make sure you place a sheet pan under the plank to catch drippings.*

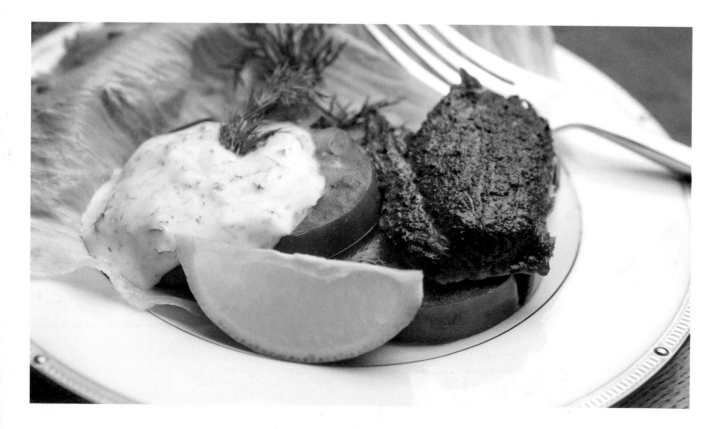

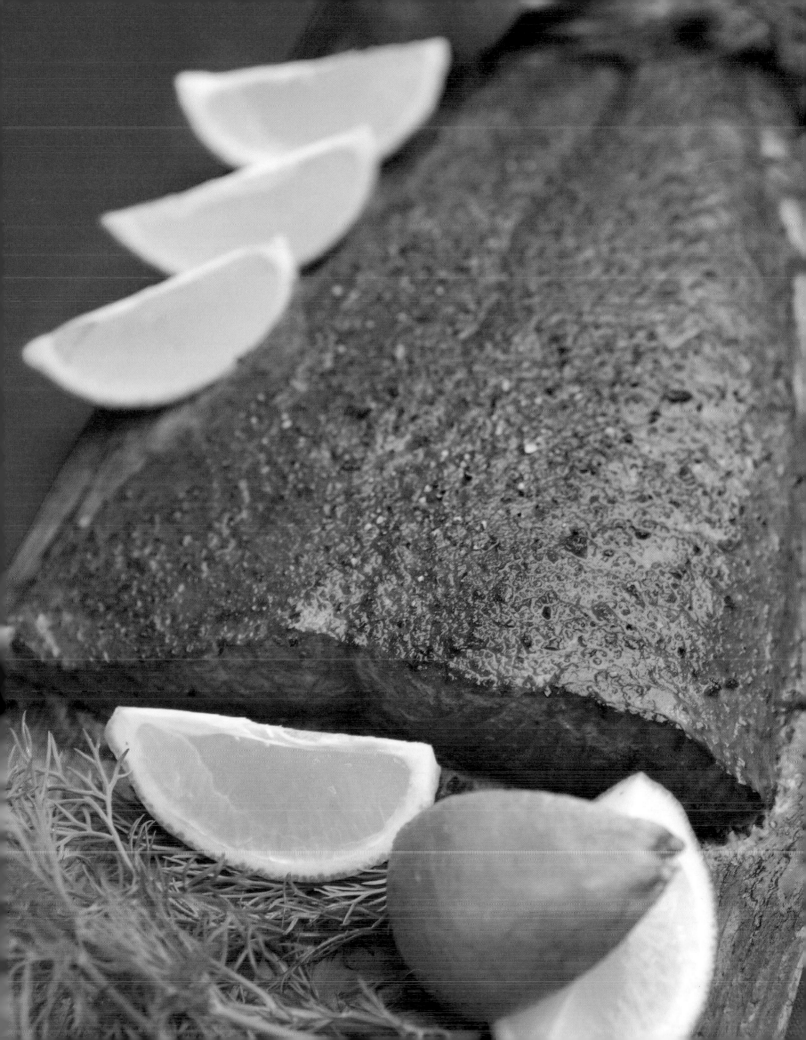

# fish tacos

*One of the advantages of living in Southern California was the access to fish tacos. Let me clarify: access to really good fish tacos. However, the best fish tacos I ever had were on my trip to Mazatlan with friends Heather and Adam, and the fishing trip we went on, where we would drop our fishing line and catch "pez" (fish) just about every single time our line went in the water. We caught a TON of fish. The fishing boat captain instructed us to take the fish back to our hotel, where they would gladly clean and cook up the fish for us. These, in fresh corn tortillas, with the best guacamole you've ever had, made for an amazing meal.*

| | |
|---|---|
| 1 | tablespoon olive oil |
| 1 | teaspoon ancho chili powder |
| ~ | juice of 1 lime |
| 1 | teaspoon cumin |
| 1 | jalapeño pepper, minced (optional) |
| 1–2 | pounds (450–900 g) wild-caught fish of your choice—mahimahi, grouper, red snapper, cod, etc., cut into no bigger than 4-inch (10 cm) pieces |
| 1 | tablespoon avocado or coconut oil |
| 1 | head Bibb, iceberg or romaine lettuce, rinsed with leaves kept whole |

1. Combine the olive oil, ancho chili powder, lime juice, cumin, and jalapeño in a large bowl.
2. Toss the fish into the marinade, and let sit for 15 minutes.
3. Preheat a large skillet over medium high heat, and add avocado or coconut oil.
4. Add the fish, cooking about 5 minutes per side or until fish is flaky.
5. Break the fish into smaller, bite-sized pieces, and serve with Tastiest Slaw Ever (recipe page 190), cilantro, tomatoes, and Chipotle Dipping Sauce (see recipe page 94).

**Variations**—*If you prefer, grill the fish instead of pan frying, or for a crispier fish, dredge fish pieces in egg then almond flour, to get more of a crunch. These tacos are great served in the Coconut Flour Tortillas too (recipe page 118).*

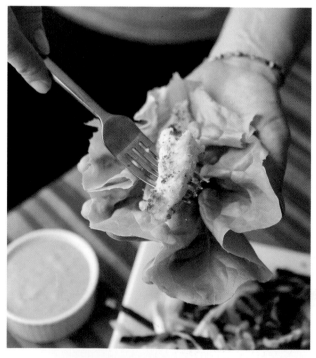

paleo comfort foods

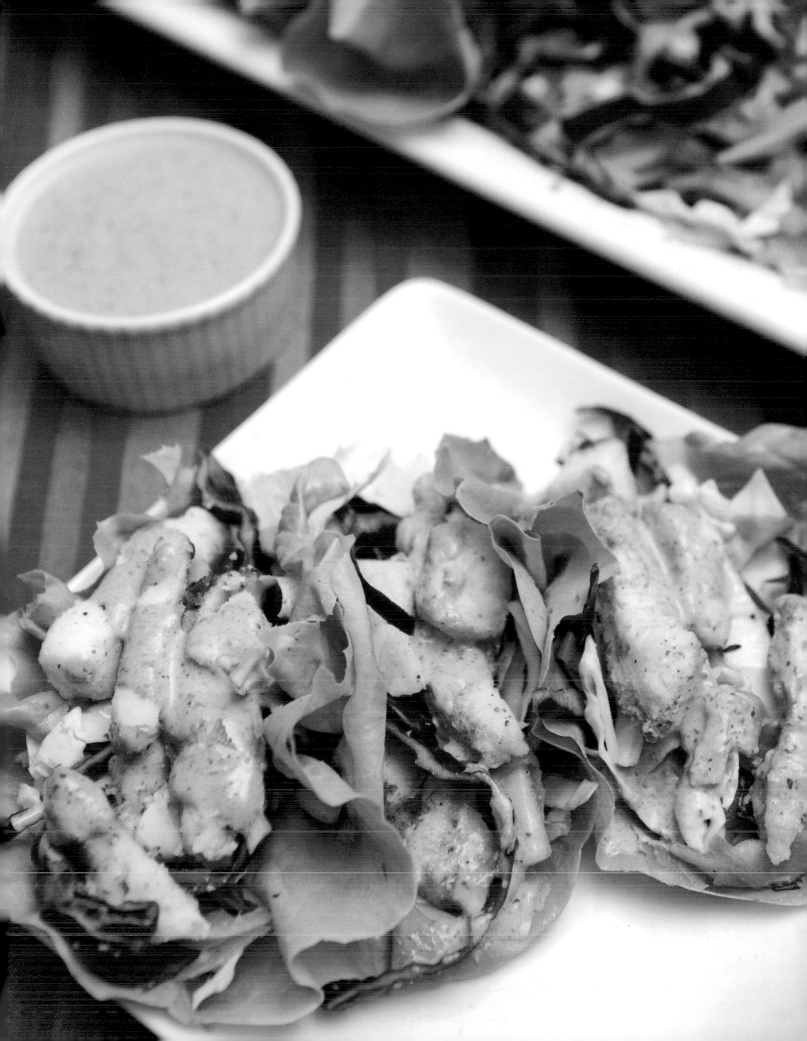

# fish stick-o-licious

*This is the finned version of our chicken fried steak recipe. Fat and protein coming together to conquer taste buds all around the world. Who in the world didn't eat fish sticks as a child? This is a recipe for the entire family to enjoy eating. For more ideas on kid-friendly recipes, you should check in with the talented Sarah Fragoso at everydaypaleo. com. Her Everyday Paleo book and blog have been hugely successful in helping busy families live healthier, paleo lives!*

| | |
|---|---|
| 18 | ounces (500 g) cod or catfish |
| ½ | cup (75 g) coconut flour |
| ½ | teaspoon garlic powder |
| ¼ | teaspoon black pepper |
| ½ | cup (75 g) almonds, finely chopped |
| ½ | cup (50 g) pecans, finely chopped |
| 2 | large eggs |
| 1 | tablespoon olive oil |

**1.** Rinse fish and pat dry with a paper towel. Cut into 3- to 4-inch (7–9 cm) lengths. Try to make them all the same thickness.

**2.** Preheat your oven to 450°F (235°C).

**3.** In a medium bowl, combine coconut flower, garlic powder, and black pepper. Place the finely chopped nuts on a small plate and whisk the eggs in a medium bowl until they begin to froth.

**4.** Coat the fish in the flour mixture and pat to get rid of excess. Dip the floured fish into the egg and then into the chopped almonds. Press the fish into the almonds to they stick well on all sides.

**5.** Place strips on well-oiled baking sheet. Use the olive oil to drizzle on each and bake for about 20 minutes. They'll be golden brown and ready to go.

**Plan Ahead**—*Have Tartar Sauce (recipe page 108) or Cave Ketchup (recipe page 102) ready before you start.*

**Variations**—*Try this with salmon or any flaky fish you can cut into strips.*

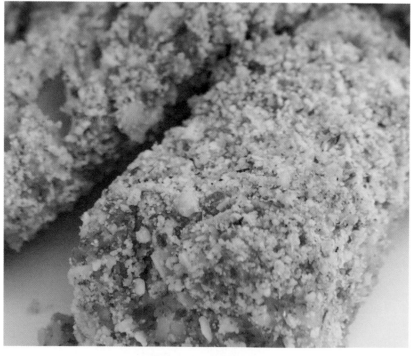

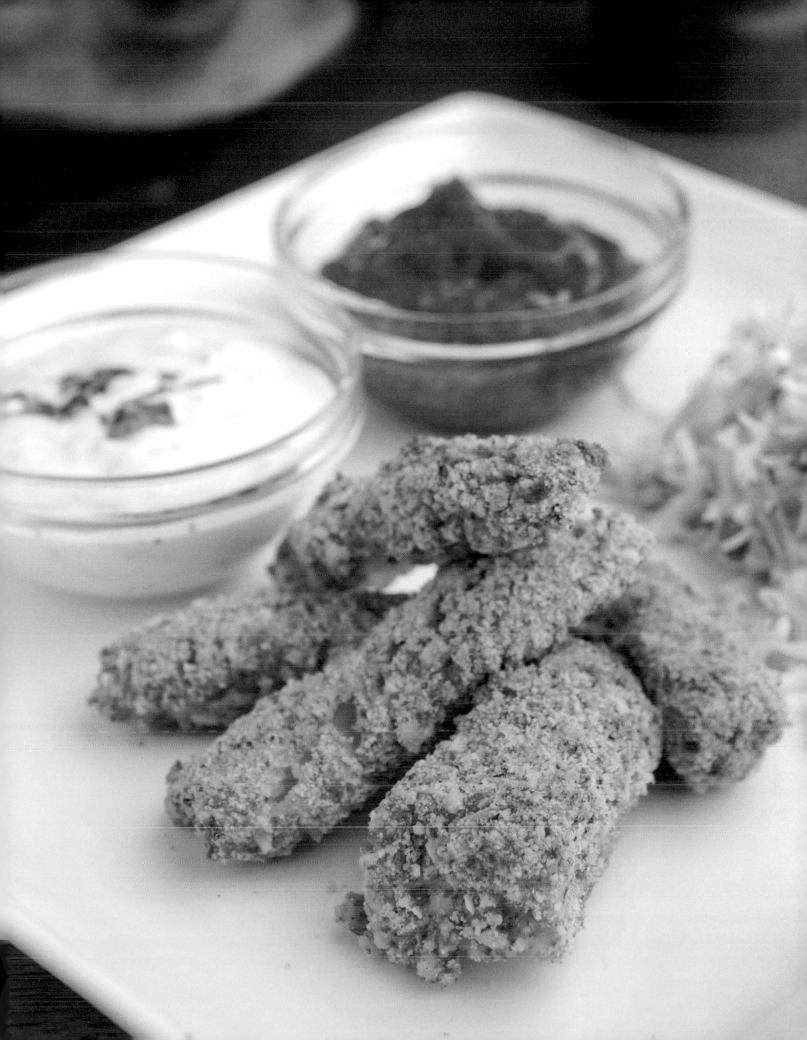

# pork tenderloin—p, b & j

*Taking a classic name and making it even more delicious. The other white meat reigns supreme! If you don't already have a homemade nut butter lying around, this recipe could take an extra few minutes. We almost always have some Pecash butter in our refrigerator. Feel free to use any nut butter combo you want.*

*We prefer a slightly more tart apple when baking most anything. Granny Smiths work really well. If you don't have a food processor, well go get one! If that is not an option, you can get away with chopping the apples up really finely and mixing in a bowl with the other ingredients.*

| | |
|---|---|
| 2 | pounds (900 g) pork tenderloin |
| 2 | apples, peeled and cored, cut into chunks |
| ½ | teaspoon cinnamon |
| 1 | tablespoon honey |
| 1 | teaspoon lemon zest |
| ½ | cup (125 mL) Pecash Butter (see recipe, page 90) |
| 2 | cloves garlic, minced |
| 1 | teaspoon black pepper |
| 1 | pinch salt |
| ½ | cup (125 mL) hot water |

1. Butterfly the pork tenderloin lengthwise and roll out to form a flat, uniform piece of pork . Preheat your oven to 350°F (175°C).

2. Place apples, cinnamon, lemon zest, and honey into food processor and pulse until the mixture looks like a chunky applesauce. Careful not to overdo this. Chunkier is better.

3. Pour the apple mixture onto the flattened tenderloin and spread around evenly. Carefully roll up the pork starting at the long side, then place roll into a baking dish.

4. Bake for 45–60 minutes (about 25 minutes per pound). Remove from oven when internal temperature reaches around 150°F (75°C). Let rest in pan for 10 minutes.

5. Mix Pecash Butter, minced garlic, pepper, and salt in bowl. Slowly add water until you reach the desired consistency (think thick soup).

6. Using a large spatula, place pork on serving dish and pour ½ of your sauce over the top. Serve the remaining sauce in a bowl (or keep it for yourself . . . it's yummy).

**Tips & Tricks**—*Once butterflied, pound the meat into a consistent thickness if needed. You can then more easily fold it like a sandwich or roll it up. You will want to cut the finished product into thick slices before freezing this one.*

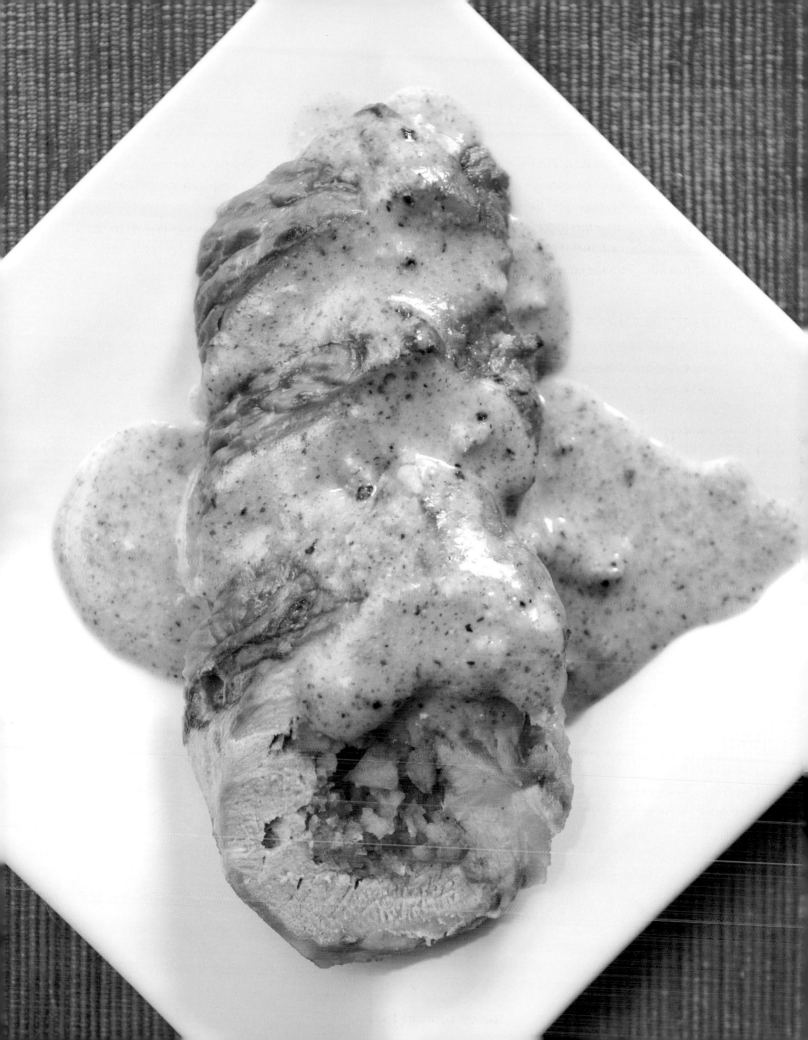

# country curry

*There are four main reasons I asked Julie to marry me: her curry abilities, incredible good looks, extremely caring heart, and her passion for bringing happiness to others (these are in no particular order). Julie's curry recipe was the first time I had ever tried this classic dish. She made it as part of a food swap, which you read about in the introduction of this book. I still have the original recipe she hand wrote for me. Country Curry was my attempt at fusing the flavors and aromas of Thai curry with the smokiness of Southern barbecue.*

| | |
|---|---|
| 2–3 | tablespoons curry paste (red, green, panang, or Massaman are all great in this) |
| 1 | can coconut milk, DON'T SHAKE IT UP |
| 2 | teaspoons garlic, minced (about 2 cloves) |
| 2 | onions, sliced |
| 3 | cups (750 mL) chicken broth |
| 1 | green pepper, chopped |
| 1 | red bell pepper, chopped |
| 1 | yellow squash, cut into chunks |
| 1 | pound (450 g) okra, pieces cut in half crosswise |
| 2–3 | Kaffir lime leaves |
| 1 | pound (450 g) smoked pork butt, shredded or chopped |
| 1 | pound (450 g) andouille sausage, sliced |
| ½ | cup (12 g) Thai basil leaves |
| 10 | Thai peppers (optional) |
| 4 | cups (1 kg) cauliflower rice |

1. Heat curry paste in large Dutch oven until it begins to darken and becomes very fragrant.

2. Add ½ can of coconut milk (should be mostly the thick milk from the top of the can). Incorporate well into the curry paste.

3. When lumps are gone, add garlic and onions and the remaining coconut milk. Stir well and cook until onions soften.

4. Add chicken broth, peppers, squash, okra, and Kaffir leaves to pot and simmer for 10 minutes.

5. Cut/shred your pork into large chunks and add to pot along with your basil and sausage. If you want it "Thai Hot," dice up ½ of your Thai peppers and add them.

6. Simmer for another 20–30 minutes or until okra is tender.

7. Serve over cauliflower rice and garnish with remaining Thai peppers.

**Variations**—*Try with smoked venison or beef, and by all means play around with several curry flavors.*

**Ingredient Notes**—*Sauté your cauliflower rice in 2 teaspoons of fish sauce to serve with this recipe.*

**Hint**—*Freeze this recipe to enjoy days or weeks later.*

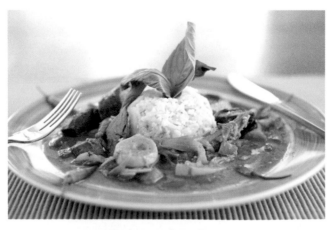

paleo comfort foods

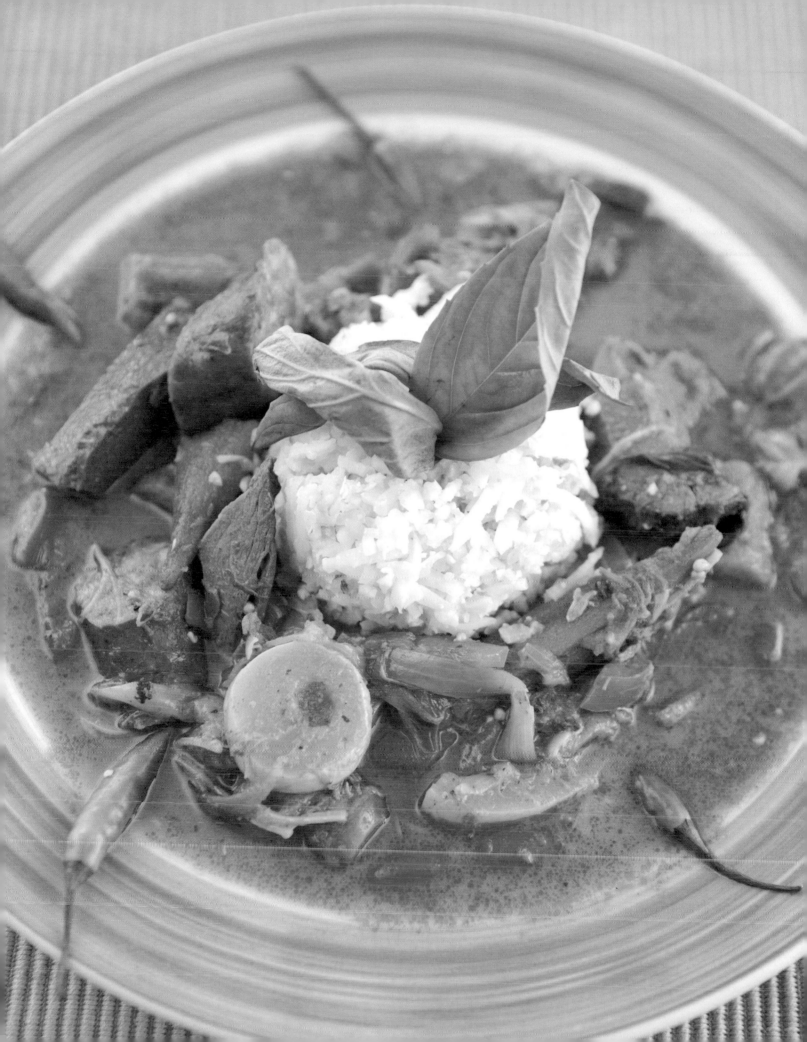

# smokin' good pork spare ribs

*I'm reasonably sure that my dad could make a living cooking things. His tailored smoker has seen its fair share of cooking endeavors. For years the Mayfield-Fisher Fourth of July Hog Cookin' was a must-attend for many of our friends. My earliest accounts of this party (it started when I was not yet 1) were two whole hogs thrown on a pit and cooked to pulled-pork perfection.*

*The interesting thing that Dad discovered around year 23 of this party was this: by cooking the whole hog all at once, you are basically ruining the ribs. Ribs cook much faster, and if they are still attached to said piggy . . . then they'll be mired in drippings and rendered inedible. Needless to say, the Fourth of July party menu got even better when they decided to order the hog already quartered and cooked the ribs separately.*

*Some like 'em dry, some like 'em wet. If you have some wet revelers coming over for dinner, maybe whip up a batch of BBQ Sauce (recipe page 104) for them to pour over their ribs when you serve them.*

---

| | |
|---|---|
| 3–4 | pounds (2 kg) pork spare ribs |
| 1 | cup dry rub (see pages 126–127 for recipes) |

1. Begin by pulling the filmy membrane off the back of the ribs. Spread the dry rub all over.
2. Once covered, place in refrigerator for 2–3 hours (you can leave them overnight if you want). Remove and allow to come to room temperature.
3. Get your grill or smoker running at around 250°F (120°C) with no direct heat to the meat. If you have soaked wood chips, use them. Place a drip pan under your meat underneath your cooking rack filled halfway with water.
4. Place ribs meaty side up onto your rack and over pan. After 1 hour of smoking, flip ribs over.
5. Allow to cook for 1 more hour and then pull ribs from grill. Cover in aluminum foil and put back in the smoker for 1 more hour.
6. Pull from grill and let sit for 10 minutes before cutting into serving sizes.

---

**Variation**—*You can use baby back ribs for this recipe too.*

**Tips & Tricks**—*Don't have a smoker yet? Use your oven with the heat set to the same specifications and follow instructions as if in a smoker.*

**Ingredient Notes**—*Use one of the dry rubs from our book or create your own. We always have some dry rub sitting around waiting for the smoker.*

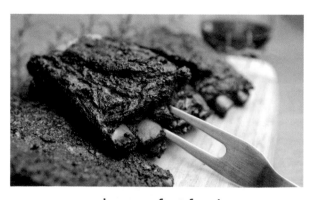

**paleo comfort foods**

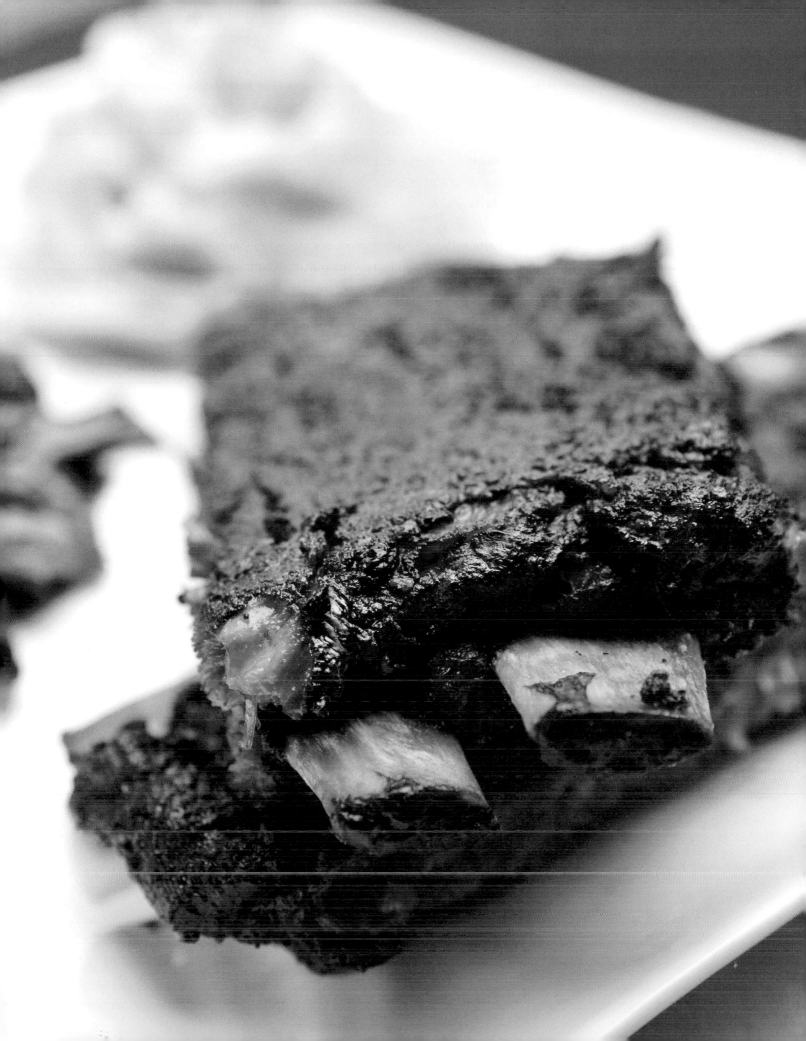

# pulled pork

*This is not a recipe you decide to make for dinner at lunchtime. It takes an investment of time. The good news is that most of the 20–24 hours this takes are not labor intensive.*

*The recipe calls for 5–10 pounds of meat. If you're toward the heavier end of that spectrum, consider doubling the dry ingredients for the rub.*

*It might be time to go back to the chapter on equipment and start thinking about that Big Green Egg!*

---

½     cup (70 g) Dad's Dry Rub (see recipe page 126)

5–10    pounds (2–4 kg) pork butt

### A quick rub in a pinch

1     teaspoon cumin seed, ground

1     teaspoon fennel, ground

2     teaspoons black peppercorns

2     teaspoons garlic powder

1     tablespoon chili powder

1     tablespoon dried rosemary

1. If you don't have a batch of Dad's famous rub laying around, combine you cumin, fennel, and black pepper in a grinder. Once ground, add in garlic powder, chili powder, and rosemary. Cover meat with spices moments before placing on the smoker.

2. Smoker should be ready to rock at 225°F (105°C). Depending on your particular smoker, you may need to add some wood chips every 3–4 hours.

3. Cook meat for 18–24 hours. Remove from heat when internal temp reaches 190°F (88°C), cover and let rest for 45–60 minutes.

---

**Variations**—*You can also use the dry rub recipes from this book (pages 126–127). One book, three dry rub recipes!*

**Tips & Tricks**—*Don't have a smoker or grill? Sprinkle one tablespoon of liquid smoke on your meat before you rub it and place in an oven preheated to 225°F (105°C). Cook for same time as above. Vacuum-seal meat after it has cooled to enjoy later. This is the pulled pork we like to use in our Country Curry (recipe page 270).*

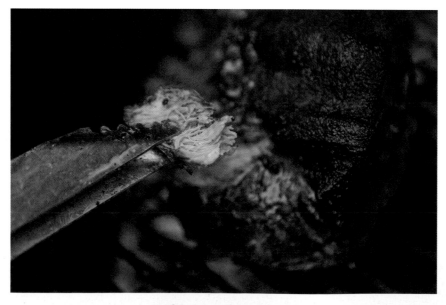

paleo comfort foods

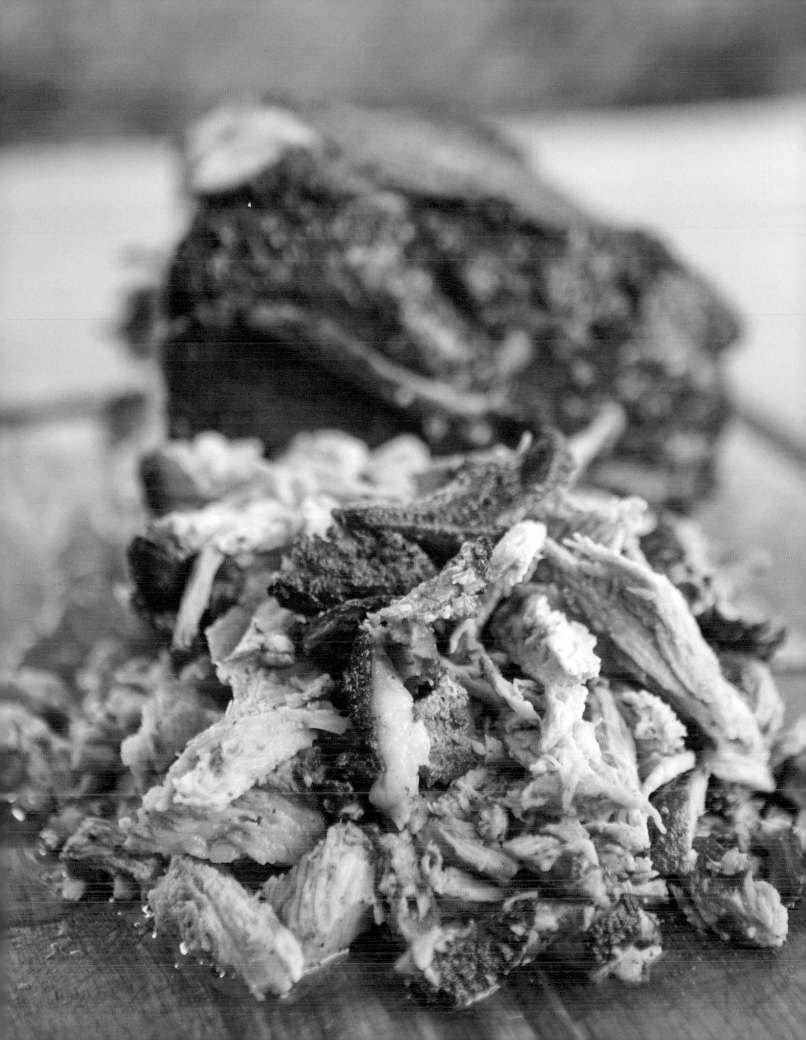

# venison medallions with mustard sauce

*Many years ago, I shot my first deer on some family land of ours in Alabama. My 30/30 lever action Winchester was the weapon of choice, as it was a gift from my dad, who was with me on the hunt. I remember my heart thumping out of my chest, taking a big deep breath in, then squeezing to pull the trigger and landing my first doe.*

*While hunting is definitely a sport, it's also an amazing way to get some of the most natural meat you've ever had. Deer aren't on feedlots, in confined spaces, and there certainly is no guarantee you'll get one (I've had many days where I've come up empty). Deer tenderloin is some of the leanest meat you can find, and there are hundreds of ways you can cook it. While I love smoked deer meat out on the Big Green Egg, and love me some deer jerky, this recipe Julie came up with is also mighty fine.*

| | |
|---|---|
| 1½ | pounds (700 g) venison tenderloin, cut into ¾-inch-thick (1.75 cm) medallions |
| 1 | tablespoon avocado oil |
| 3 | tablespoons Dijon mustard |
| 1 | tablespoon clarified butter |
| 1 | shallot, chopped |
| 1 | cup (250 mL) beef or veal stock |
| ½ | cup (125 mL) dry red wine |
| ~ | salt and pepper to taste |

1. Let meat come to room temperature first.
2. Take 1 tablespoon of the mustard and rub it on the flat sides of the medallions.
3. Heat a large skillet over medium-high heat until very hot. Add in the oil, and when it gives off wisps of white smoke, add the medallions to the pan.
4. Allow the medallions to sear for 4–5 minutes on the first side, then using tongs flip over and cook another 4–5 minutes for medium rare.
5. Remove medallions, place on a plate and let rest.
6. In the skillet you were just using, reduce heat to medium adding the clarified butter and shallots, stirring to release any of the browned bits in the pan.
7. Add the stock, wine, and remaining mustard, and whisk all to create sauce.
8. Pour sauce over the medallions and serve.

**Variation**—*You can easily add mushrooms to your pan sauce to add a little more earthy flavor to things.*

**Ingredient Notes**—*If you don't have venison tenderloin, the backstrap is very similar (but different) and is a fine substitute.*

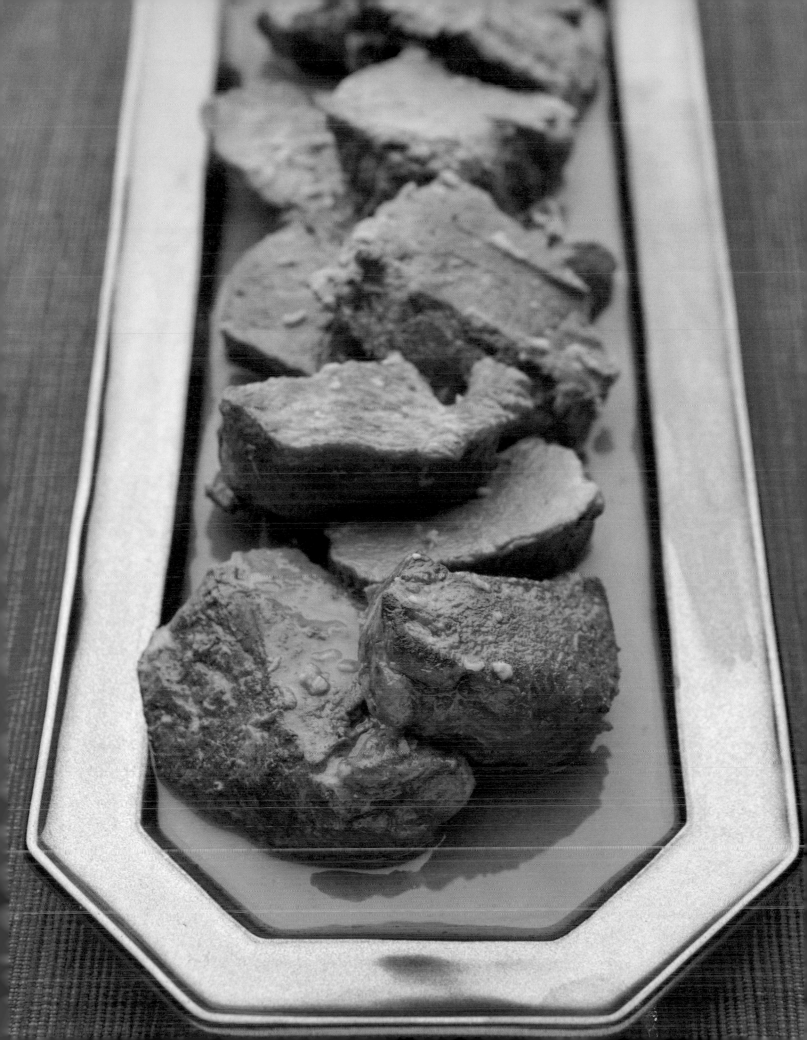

# braised rabbit

*If you should ever have the chance to go on a rabbit hunt, I highly recommend it. The exhilaration of waiting for them to run out in front of you is something you need to witness firsthand. My first rabbit hunt was on Gene Hartman's farm in east Tennessee. It was an especially cold morning and we were blessed with two inches of fresh snow. I had no idea what to expect. Then came the dogs . . . about twelve beagles. They move at a snail's pace, tracking the rabbit and yelping the whole way. When they flush one, you are likely not ready for it, and it's hard to be patient. You're thinking that the rabbit has run off . . . but sure as the sun comes up it will be back.*

*I had never eaten rabbit before that day. We harvested seventeen on the hunt. A man's got to figure out what to do with all that meat. Braising small game like rabbit is a surefire way to get it good and tender. If you're not a rabbit hunter, check the Internet for stores in your area. We have a great spot in Marietta, Georgia, called the Cajun Meat Market. They have wonderful rabbit, quail, and sausage, and they are also the home of the famous Turducken.*

---

| | |
|---|---|
| ¼ | cup (60 mL) coconut oil |
| 1 | 2- to 3-pound (1.25 kg) rabbit, quartered |
| 2 | cups (200 g) onions, thinly sliced |
| 4 | cloves garlic, minced |
| ¼ | teaspoon black pepper |
| 2 | cups (500 mL) chicken stock |
| 2 | teaspoons thyme, chopped |
| 1 | bay leaf |
| 1 | tablespoon coconut flour |
| 1 | tablespoon lemon juice |
| ¼ | cup (60 mL) cold water |

1. Heat oil in large skillet. Place rabbit in skillet and brown on all sides.
2. Remove rabbit and set aside on plate. Sauté onion and add in garlic until tender.
3. Add pepper, stock, thyme, and bay leaf. Place rabbit back in pan and bring liquid to boil.
4. Reduce heat and simmer covered for 35–45 minutes.
5. Remove rabbit, onions, and garlic to serving platter.
6. Mix coconut flour, lemon juice, and cold water until smooth. Stir in to pan sauce.
7. Bring to boil. Simmer for 3–5 minutes stirring frequently.
8. Once thickened, pour over rabbit and serve.

---

**Variation**—*If you haven't been able to book your rabbit hunt yet, chicken works really well in this recipe too.*

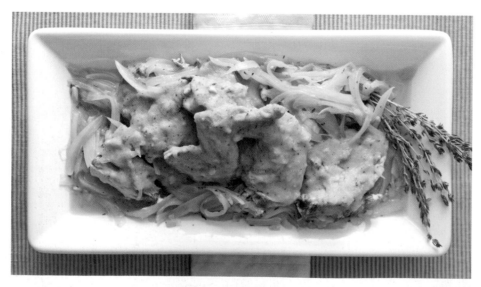

paleo comfort foods

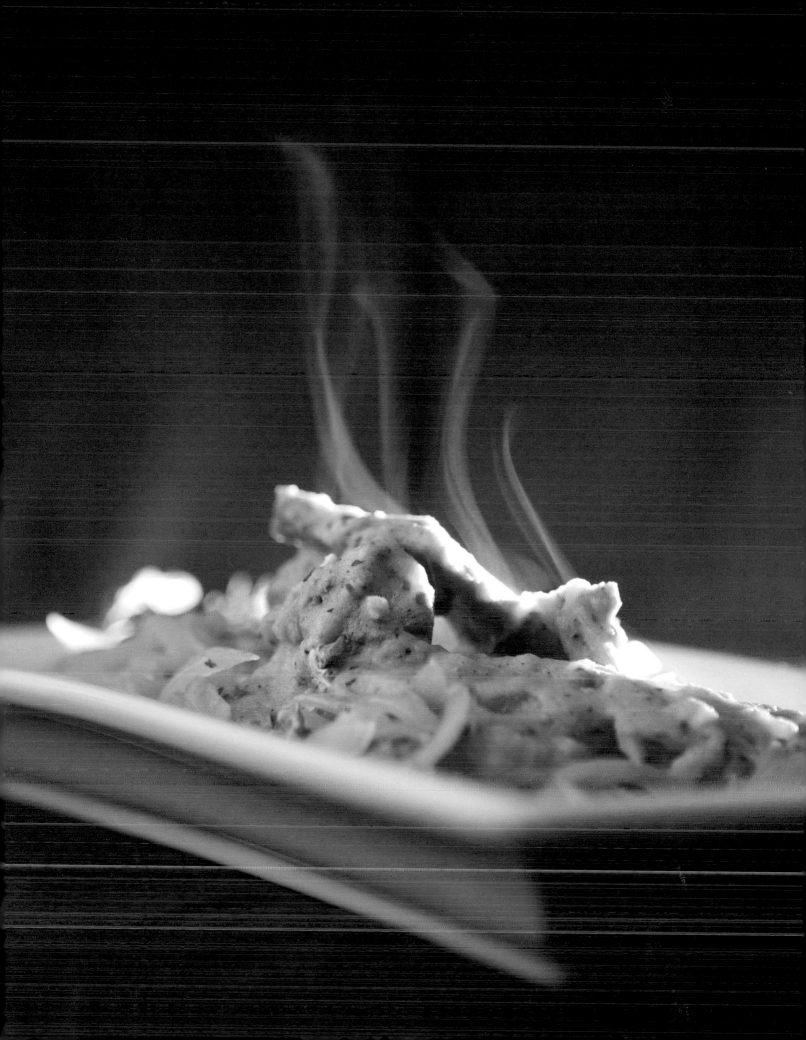

# spaghetti sauce

*Mmmmmm . . . spaghetti. When I was a kid, I called it Ba-scetti. Don't act like you nailed this one right out of the gate. The Italians call this stuff "sauce." We spend at least one weekend a year canning tomatoes and tomato sauce (without the meat added at that point). It is so nice to carry the freshness of vine-ripe tomatoes into the colder months. You'll still get plenty of fantastic flavor by using store-bought tomatoes.*

*Most spaghetti sauces are pretty simple. This one is no exception. The bad guy with most sauces like this isn't the sauce, it's what you pour it over. Serve this little number over spaghetti squash, kelp noodles, or shredded zucchini and squash.*

| | |
|---|---|
| 2 | pounds (900 g) ground beef |
| 2 | teaspoons black pepper |
| 1 | tablespoon olive oil |
| 2 | large sweet onions, chopped |
| 3 | cloves garlic, minced |
| 1 | large green pepper, chopped |
| 1 | quart (1 L) crushed tomatoes |
| 1 | quart (1 L) whole canned tomatoes |
| 1 | 6 ounce (180 mL) can tomato paste |
| 2 | tablespoons fresh basil, chopped |

1. In large pot, brown meat with 1 teaspoon of black pepper. Remove to bowl.
2. Heat olive oil in same pot and add garlic, onions & green pepper. Sauté for 3–5 minutes. Onions and pepper will begin to soften.
3. Add all other ingredients plus the meat and stir well.
4. Bring everything to a slight boil. Cover and reduce to simmer for 30–40 minutes.

**Variations**—*Change out your meat (ground turkey, sausage, deer, etc.).*

**Hint**—*Freeze in small containers. Don't include your noodle replacement, as it won't thaw as well.*

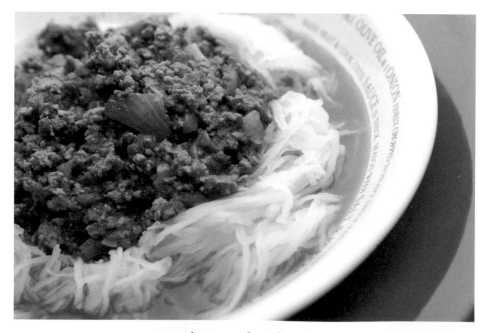

TOMATOES & A PINCH OF RED PEPPER LAKES.

# bangers and mash

*This recipe plays homage to my Irish heritage. At least for me, there's something incredibly comforting about bangers and mash. Maybe it's the thought of ducking into a pub in Ireland on a cold and rainy day and ordering up a plate of these, or just the fact that any pub you go to in Ireland is probably going to have this on the menu.*

*You can get wildly creative with this recipe: note that most typical Irish bangers and mash recipes don't call for mushrooms. I just happen to love mushrooms, so I add them to quite a few recipes! You could substitute leeks for the onions, or add in a bunch of other vegetables to make this your own.*

| | |
|---|---|
| 4 | large sausages (pork, turkey, or chicken) |
| 1 | tablespoon olive or coconut oil |
| 1 | large onion |
| 1 | cup (125 g) mushrooms |
| ½ | tablespoon almond flour |
| ¾ | cup (180 mL) chicken or beef stock |
| ~ | splash of balsamic vinegar |
| ~ | Mashed Cauliflower (recipe page 180) |

1. Heat a large skillet over medium heat. Sear sausages on each side until browned.
2. Add enough water to cover sausage ¾ of the way, and continue cooking until cooked through and water has cooked off.
3. Remove sausages to plate.
4. Add oil, onions, and mushrooms to same pan, scraping up bits from sausages.
5. Cook until onions are translucent and somewhat caramelized.
6. Add in flour and stir, cooking for 3–4 minutes.
7. Add in stock and balsamic vinegar.
8. Add sausages back to onion/mushroom mixture.
9. Serve over Mashed Cauliflower.

**Ingredient Notes**—*Read your labels on the sausages. You never know what ingredients might be in there.*

**Hint**—*You can enjoy this for days or weeks to come by freezing in individual portions.*

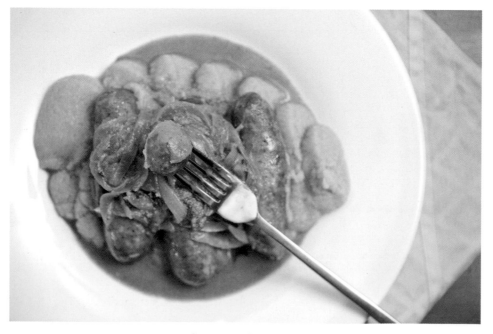

paleo comfort foods

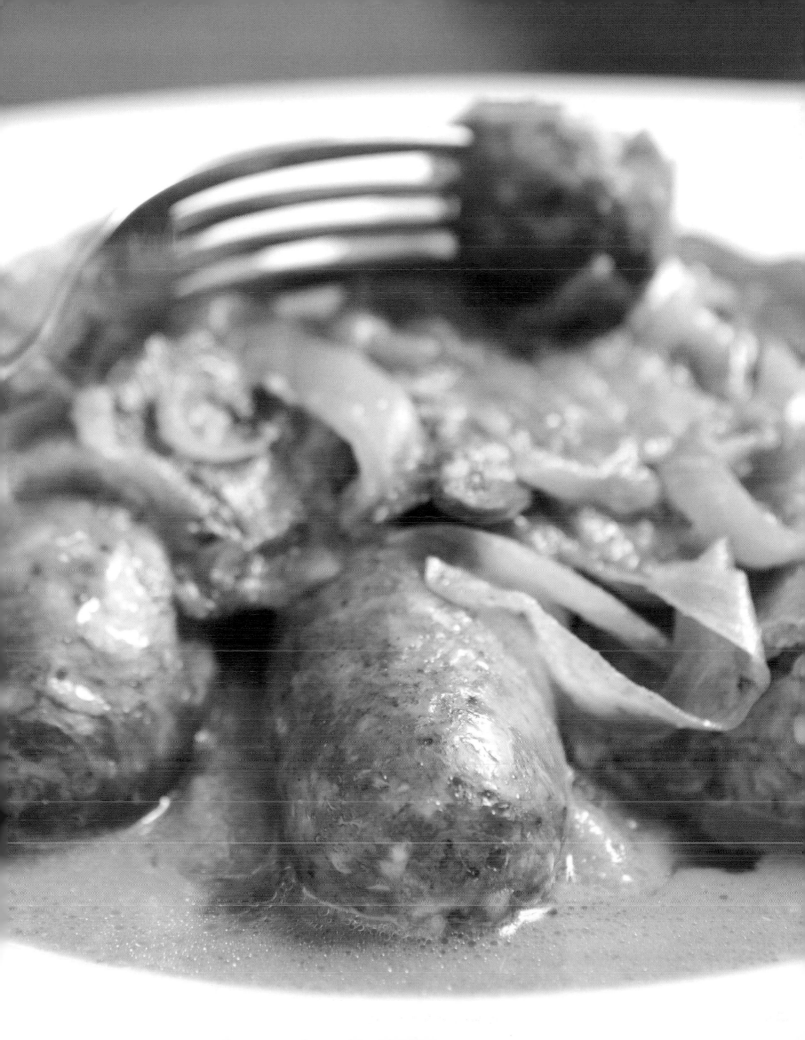

# tacos de lengua

*This authentic Mexican dish is simply amazing. Some cultures consider the tongue a delicacy. One bite into the tasty meat and you'll know why. The meat is fatty and fine textured like pot roast and you can get them at many markets nowadays. Obviously we would prefer that you seek out a grass-fed cow tongue. You'll need to plan ahead for this one. It takes some time to cook the meat.*

| | |
|---|---|
| 1 | beef tongue, 2–3 pounds (1 kg) |
| 3 | cloves garlic |
| 1 | large onion, quartered |
| 2 | bay leaves |
| 2 | teaspoons salt |
| 1 | teaspoon peppercorns |
| 1 | tomato, chopped |
| ½ | red onion, finely chopped |
| ½ | cup (12 g) cilantro, chopped |
| 1 | lime, sliced |

1. Rinse tongue well to prepare. In large pot, cover tongue with water.
2. Add garlic, onion, bay leaves, salt, and peppercorns and bring to a boil.
3. Reduce heat and simmer for about 3 hours. Remove from heat and allow tongue to cool in broth.
4. When the tongue is cool enough, remove it from broth. Peel away the outer skin (it will feel like rubber) to reveal the tender meat inside. Remove any excess fatty tissue and dice up into chunks.
5. Serve in warm Coconut Flour Tortillas (page 118) with tomato, red onion, cilantro, and a fresh squeeze of lime juice. You'll want to have a favorite salsa or two lying around for some extra kick.

**Plan Ahead**—*Have salsas and tortillas already made. Heat tortillas right before you serve.*

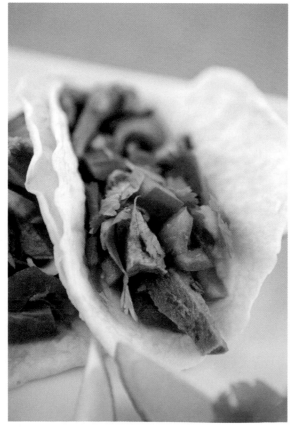

paleo comfort foods

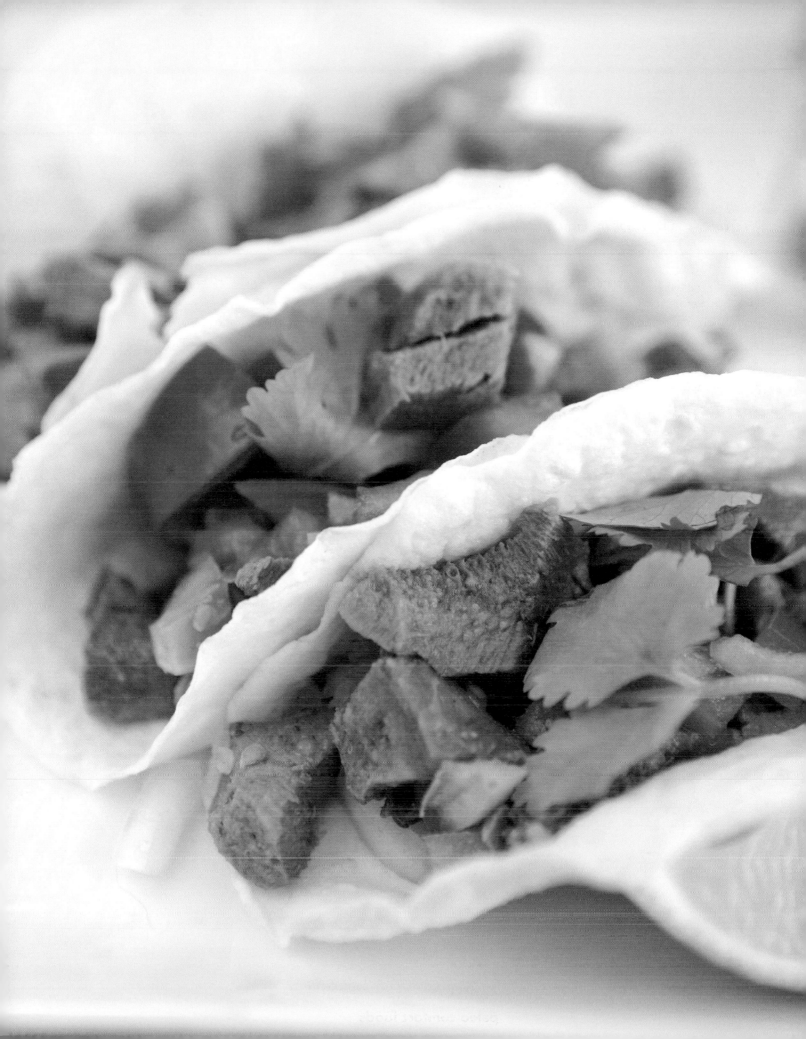

# south of the border stuffed acorn squash

*There are so many great things about this recipe. For one, stuffing with the turkey adds a pack of protein to each of these, so essentially you are creating a full meal with just one stuffed squash. Secondly, taking a Southwestern twist on this is just one way to serve this—you can easily change up the veggies and create a whole new concept. For example, if you have some leftover hamburgers in the fridge, crumble those up along with some mushrooms, tomatoes, maybe some kale, to make it "hamburger-stuffed squash." Thirdly, you can totally make this all ahead of time and just reheat when ready to serve.*

| | |
|---|---|
| 2 | acorn squash |
| 1 | tablespoon olive or coconut oil |
| 1 | onion, minced |
| 3 | cloves garlic, minced |
| 1 | red pepper, chopped |
| 1 | pound (450 g) ground turkey or ground turkey sausage |
| 2 | tablespoons chili powder |
| 1 | tablespoon cumin |
| ½ | cup (100 g) tomatoes, chopped |

1. Preheat oven to 400°F (205°C).
2. Cut the acorn squash in half lengthwise, removing the seeds and pulp. Place facedown in a baking pan, with about ¼ inch (.6 cm) water.
3. Bake for 30–45 minutes or until squash are soft.
4. Heat a large skillet over medium heat, add in oil, and when hot stir in onions and garlic. Cook until onions are translucent, being careful not to burn garlic.
5. Stir in peppers and cook for 3–4 minutes longer.
6. Add in turkey and spices and brown until turkey is cooked through.
7. Strain off any excess liquid from the turkey, and stir in tomatoes, heating through.
8. Pour out any of the water in the pan with the squash, and place faceup. Fill with turkey mixture and serve, topped with your favorite salsa.

**Variations**—*Ground chicken, ground beef, ground bison, or even just some chopped-up chicken breasts would be fantastic alternatives for this recipe.*

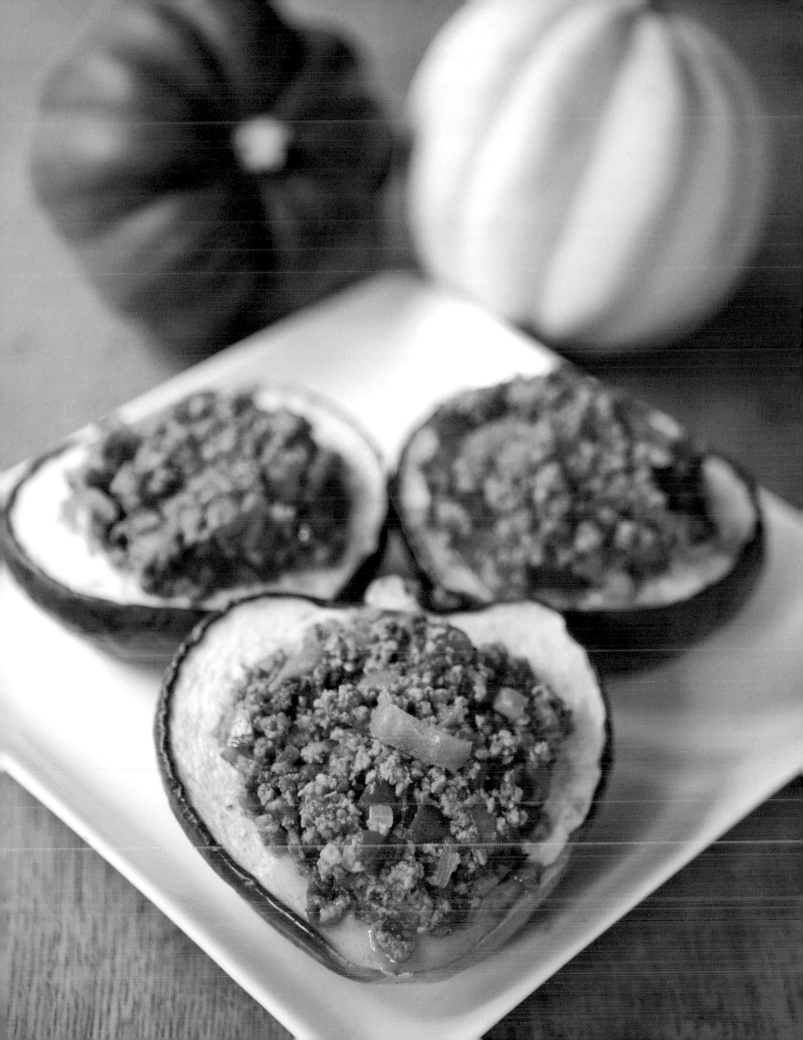

# pot roast

*I can't remember the first time I decided to make a pot roast. I think it had something to do with wanting to use my big old Le Creuset pot. What I do remember is getting this dish tossed into the oven, leaving the house for a few hours, and coming home to this amazing aroma that I could actually smell before I even came through the door.*

*Don't be tempted to shorten the cooking time on this. If the meat does not fall apart, and is not fork tender, let it cook longer.*

*This dish is comfort food at its finest, and freezes exceptionally well.*

---

| | |
|---|---|
| 1 | 3- to 4-pound (2 kg) chuck roast |
| 3 | cloves garlic |
| ~ | salt and pepper to taste (optional) |
| 2–3 | tablespoons bacon grease or olive or coconut oil |
| 2 | cups (300 g) carrots, chopped |
| 1 | medium onion, chopped |
| 3 | cups (300 g) celery, chopped |
| 3 | cups (450 g) mushrooms, sliced |
| 2 | cups (500 mL) dry red wine |
| 1 | 28-ounce (840 mL) can tomatoes |
| 1 | cup (250 mL) water |
| 2 | cups (500 mL) beef stock |
| 1 | tablespoon balsamic vinegar |
| 2 | sprigs fresh thyme |
| 2 | sprigs fresh rosemary |

1. Preheat the oven to 300°F (150°C).
2. Pat the roast dry with paper towels. Cut a few slits in the meat and insert the pieces of garlic into the slits.
3. Season the meat with pepper and salt (if desired). Heat a large Dutch oven over medium-high heat.
4. Add the oil until just smoking, then add roast and sear for approximately 3–5 minutes each side. Remove from heat.
5. Add carrots, onion, mushrooms, and celery and saute until onions are translucent. Add the meat back to the vegetable mixture along with the herbs.
6. Pour in the wine, tomatoes, water, stock and vinegar and bring to a boil.
7. Remove from stove, cover and place in the oven, turning meat over about every hour or so.
8. Cook 3–4 hours, or until meat is fork tender.
9. Serve over Mashed Cauliflower (see recipe page 180).

---

**Variation**—*If you prefer not to cook with wine, you can certainly braise this meat in just beef stock.*

**Hint**—*Freeze pot roast with the cauliflower to enjoy later.*

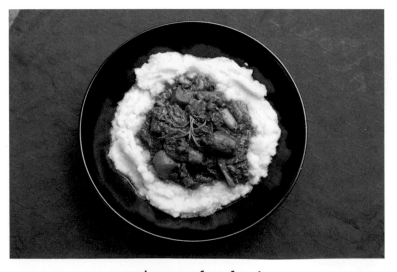

**paleo comfort foods**

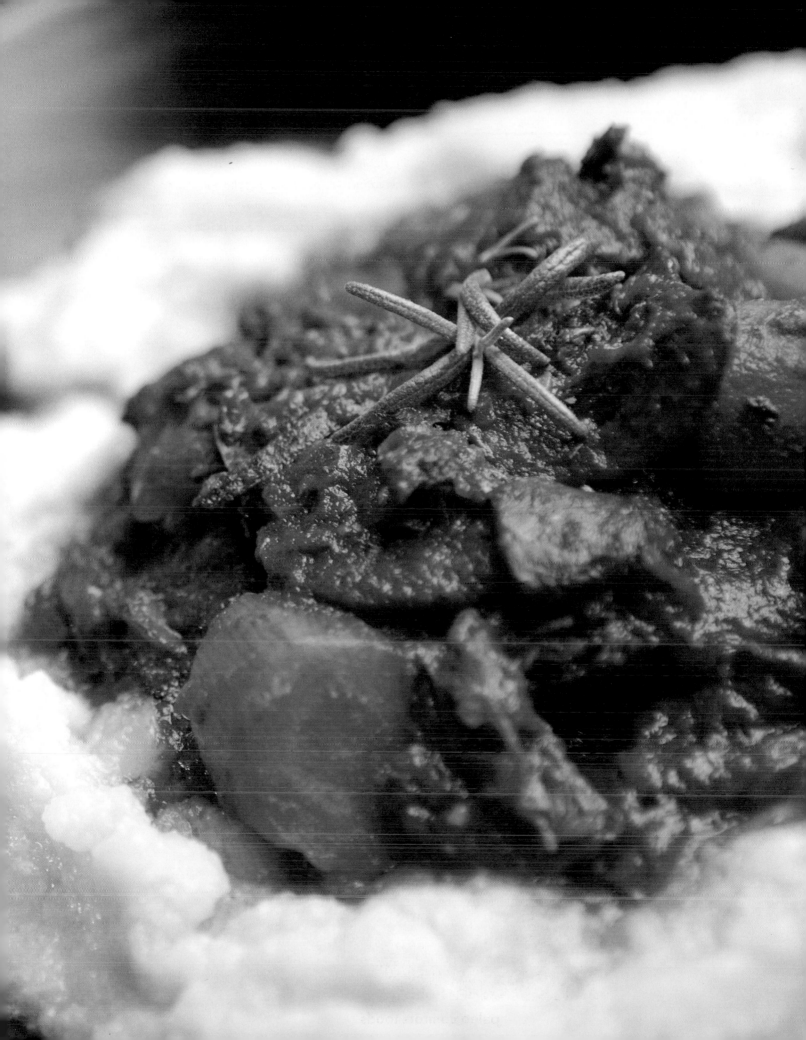

# smoky brisket without the smoker

*Before I met Charles, I did not have an outdoor grill, or a smoker for that matter. Life was very sad in that regard. Which meant getting a bit creative: indoor grill pans that invariably set off my smoke detector, and every now and then using a wee bit of liquid smoke.*

*There seems to be one universal brisket principle that must be adhered to no matter what recipe you're following: low and slow. Some of the outdoor smoker recipes cook for 12–16 hours. Fortunately, this one shortens that a bit, and makes your house smell pretty incredible.*

*Even without the liquid smoke, brisket is some tasty comfort food, and there are literally thousands of recipes out there as to how to prepare.*

---

| | |
|---|---|
| 2 | teaspoons salt (optional) |
| 1 | tablespoon black pepper |
| 2 | teaspoons cayenne |
| 4 | cloves fresh garlic, crushed |
| 1 | 3- to 4-pound (2 kg) brisket, untrimmed |
| 1 | yellow or white onion, sliced |
| ¼ | cup (60 mL) tamari or coconut aminos |
| 1 | tablespoon Worcestershire sauce, optional |
| 2 | tablespoons liquid smoke |
| 2 | tablespoons brewed espresso or dark coffee |
| ¼ | cup (60 mL) apple cider vinegar |
| 1 | cup (250 mL) beef stock |
| 3 | fresh jalapeños, sliced |

**1.** Preheat oven to 250°F (125°C).

**2.** Mix together the salt, black pepper, cayenne, and crushed garlic, and rub all over your brisket. Allow the brisket sit out and come to room temperature.

**3.** In your large roasting pan or a Pyrex 9 inch x 13 inch (23 cm x 33 cm) pan, add in your onions, coconut aminos (or tamari), Worcestershire sauce, the liquid smoke, espresso, apple cider vinegar, beef stock, and some of the jalapeños.

**4.** Set the brisket on top of the onions and jalapeños with the fat side up. Set your remaining jalapeños on top of the brisket.

**5.** Cover the pan tightly with aluminum foil and let bake for at least 4 hours.

**6.** Remove the brisket from the pan, and it should almost fall apart when you touch it. Let it rest outside the pan for at least 20 minutes.

**7.** When ready to serve, trim the fat from the top, and slice very thin against the grain.

---

**Ingredient Notes**—*Liquid smoke comes in all varieties, some with all kinds of additives. You want to find one where its only ingredient is "natural liquid smoke." How is this made in the first place? Manufacturers heat the given wood (typically hickory) over a heat high enough to get it smoldering, and then that smoke is passed through water to create the liquid smoke. It's then refined for impurities and barreled much like whiskey. As with everything in life, there is debate about the safety of liquid smoke. According to the European Commission, "Because smoke flavorings . . . are subject to fractionalization and purification . . . the use of liquid smoke flavorings is generally considered to be less of a health concern than the traditional smoking process." For what it's worth, I surely wouldn't down bottles of this, but a few tablespoons seem pretty reasonable to try and get that smoky flavor.*

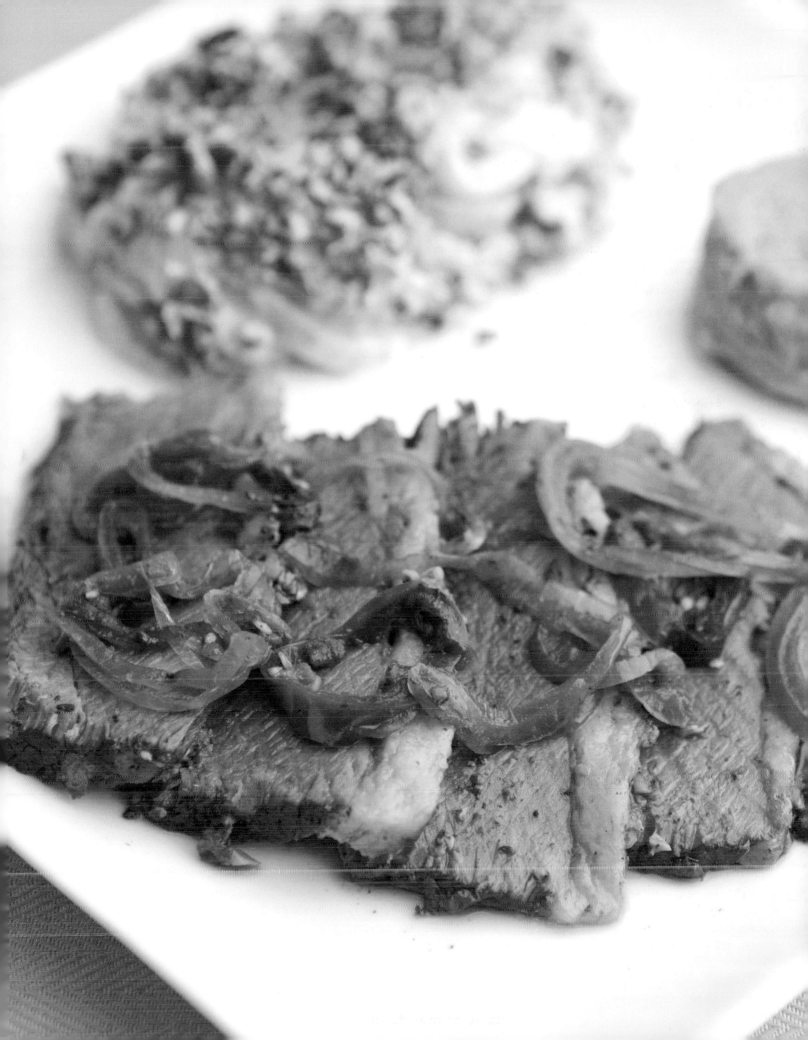

# steak roll

*Long day at the office? Not happy with your neighbors? Don't fret! Pull out your meat mallet and take a few whacks at some meat. This is basically a meat roll-up, so think of some creative things to fill it with and try all sorts of variations.*

| | |
|---|---|
| 2 | beef round steaks, 1 pound (450 g) each |
| 1 | teaspoon black pepper |
| ½ | teaspoon salt (optional) |
| 4–5 | strips bacon |
| 1 | cup (150 g) onion, chopped |
| 1 | teaspoon garlic, minced |
| 1 | cup (100 g) celery, chopped |
| 1 | cup (175 g) mushrooms, chopped |
| ½ | cup (50 g) leeks, chopped |
| 2 | cups (60 g) spinach, chopped |
| ½ | teaspoon thyme |
| ⅛ | teaspoon celery seed |
| 1 | cup (250 mL) beef stock |

1. Pound out steaks into ¼ inch (.6 cm) thickness. Sprinkle with pepper and salt, set aside for use.
2. Preheat oven to 350°F (175°C).
3. Cook bacon in large skillet until crispy. Remove to paper towel and retain grease.
4. In same skillet, sauté onion and garlic in bacon grease for 3–5 minutes. Add celery, mushrooms, leeks, spinach, thyme, and celery seed. Sauté for 5–8 minutes.
5. Chop bacon into small pieces. Combine all filling ingredients in bowl and allow to cool slightly.
6. Lay out each steak and spread mixture across surface to within an inch of the edge. Roll up to most uniform shape. Use a few toothpicks to hold roll in shape.
7. Place rolls in greased baking dish and pour broth over steak. Bake for 1 hour covered.
8. Remove cover and spoon stock over tops of steak. Bake uncovered for another 30 minutes.

**Variations**—*You can use various round cuts or try with tenderloin. Some other favorites we like stuffing these with are kale and chopped apples. You can also cook this on a grill or smoker. You will want to wrap it with kitchen string to keep its shape.*

**Hint**—*Cut the roll into pieces before you freeze it.*

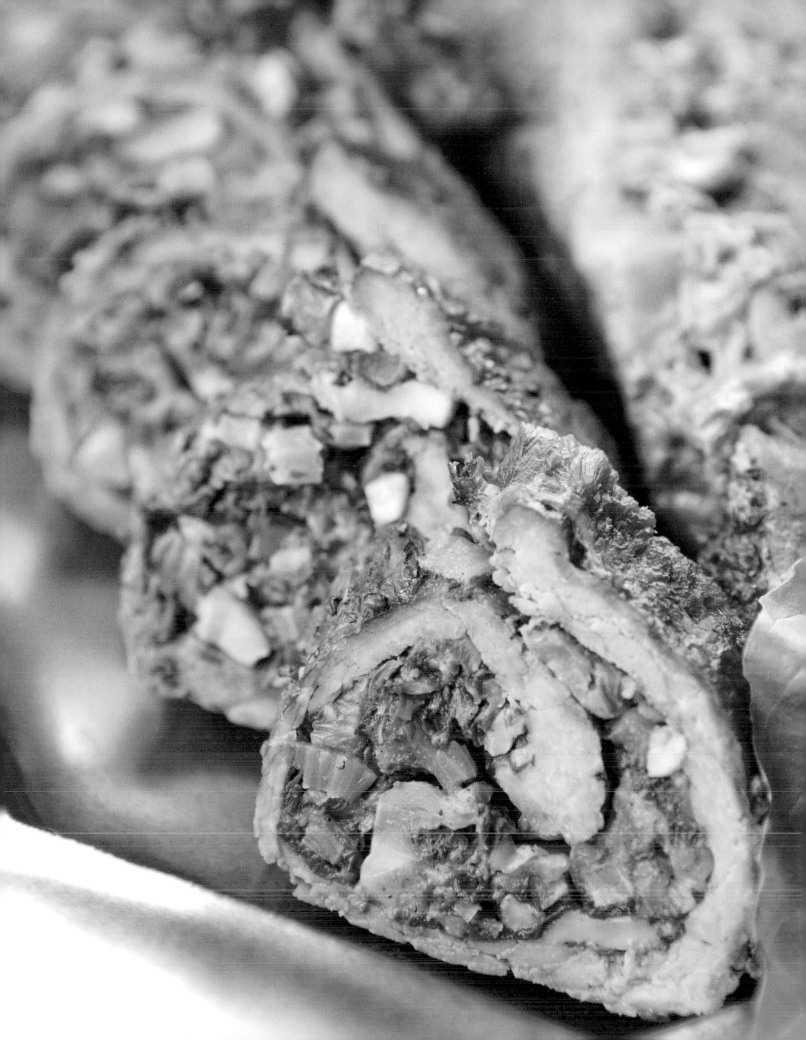

# braised short ribs

*Do not let the directions for this one intimidate you. Yes, there are some steps involved for this, but it is oh-so-worth every bit! Your house will smell amazing for the entire time this is cooking—seriously.*

*The mushrooms are optional, but I love the earthy-meaty veggie addition. Inspired by Suzanne Goin's short rib recipe.*

| | |
|---|---|
| 3–4 | pounds (2 kg) of grass-fed beef short ribs (flanken-style or English cut—both work fine) |
| 2–3 | teaspoons fresh thyme leaves, minced |
| 2 | teaspoons black pepper |
| 2 | teaspoons kosher salt |
| 2 | tablespoons avocado oil |
| 1½ | cups (225 g) onion, chopped |
| ½ | cup (75 g) carrots, chopped |
| ½ | cup (50 g) celery stalks, chopped |
| 4 | sprigs fresh thyme |
| 3 | bay leaves |
| 2 | tablespoons balsamic vinegar |
| 1 | cup (250 mL) marsala wine |
| 3 | cups (750 mL) dry red wine |
| 4 | cups (1 L) beef stock (or veal if you have it) |
| 6 | ounces (150 g) thick-sliced portobello mushrooms (optional) |

1. One hour before you begin cooking, remove the ribs from the refrigerator and their packaging. Season with thyme, salt, and pepper.

2. Preheat oven to 325°F (165°C).

3. In a large Dutch oven, heat the oil over medium high heat. Place the short ribs meaty sides down in the pan, working in batches if needed to avoid overcrowding. Sear until they are nicely browned on each of the meaty sides (no need to brown the rib side). Transfer the browned ribs to a plate and set aside.

4. In the same Dutch oven, reduce your heat to medium, and add in your onion, carrot, celery, thyme, and bay leaves. Stir with a wooden spoon to scrape up all the browned bits in the pot, and continue cooking until vegetables are softened and translucent.

5. Add in the balsamic vinegar, marsala, and wine and stir, bringing heat up to high and letting the mixture come to a boil. Let the liquid boil until it is reduced in half.

6. Pour in the stock and bring liquid back up to a boil.

7. Place the short ribs back in the pan placing the mushrooms on top and cover.

8. Braise in the oven for 3–3½ hours or until the ribs are fork tender and do not resist at all.

9. Remove ribs and mushrooms from the Dutch oven. Increase temperature of oven to 400°F (205°C). Place ribs meat side up on a sheet pan and roast for 10 minutes or until browned.

10. While the ribs are roasting, strain the braising liquid through a fine sieve placed over a bowl to retain all the strained liquid. Press down on the solids in the sieve to squeeze all the liquid out. If you want you can skim off the fat at this point.

11. Return liquid back to the Dutch oven, and bring up to a boil. Simmer until sauce thickens slightly.

12. Return the ribs and mushrooms back to the sauce and serve, spooning sauce over ribs.

**Do Ahead**—*You can do the braising of the short ribs the day before; remove from braising liquid and refrigerate overnight. This will cause the fat to solidify in a layer on the top, which makes it very easy to then skim off.*

**Ingredients**—*There is a big difference between beef short ribs, spare ribs, baby back ribs, etc. When in doubt, ask the nice person selling you your ribs (hoping that's a local farmer!). Tell them what you are making, and say what the recipe is. A local farmer and/or good butcher will be more than happy to help you out.*

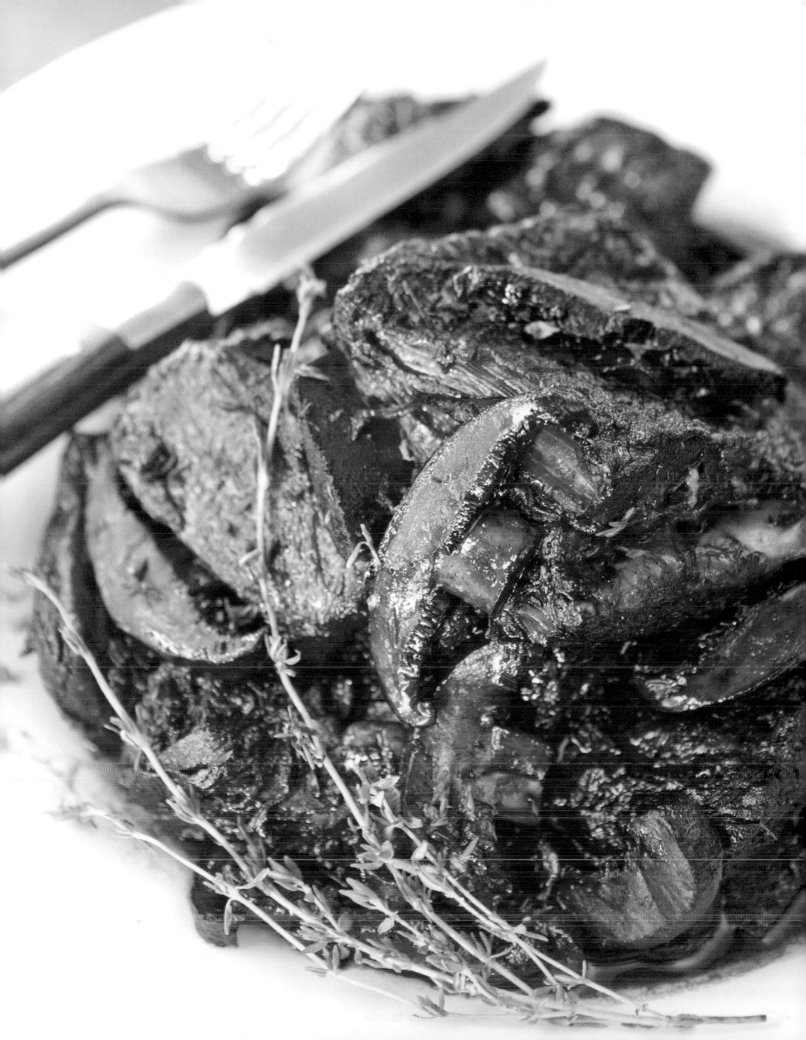

# farmer's pie

*We first made a variation on this shepherd's pie when Charles' mom stocked us full of fresh lamb they had gotten from a friend of theirs in Tennessee. We've since kept this in our recipe rotation. It is a favorite on those cold rainy days. The leftovers reheat exceptionally well too.*

*I credit Lisa—Charles' mom—with always arming us with things like the locally raised lamb and keeping our pantry stocked with her home canned tomatoes.*

| | |
|---|---|
| 1 | tablespoon coconut or avocado oil |
| ¼ | cup (50 g) fresh chopped garlic |
| 2 | pounds (900 g) ground lamb |
| 2 | cups (300 g) onions chopped |
| 2 | cups (250 g) carrots, peeled and sliced |
| 2 | stalk celery, chopped |
| 1 | tablespoon fresh rosemary, chopped fine |
| 2 | teaspoons dried thyme |
| 4 | cups (1 L) canned tomatoes |
| 2 | tablespoons balsamic vinegar |
| 2 | tablespoons Worcestershire sauce |
| 6 | cups (1.5 L) Mashed Cauliflower (recipe page 180) |

1. Preheat oven to 350°F (175°C).

2. Heat a large skillet over medium/medium-high heat. Add the oil and once hot, stir in the garlic, being careful not to burn.

3. Add in the lamb and stir, combining with the garlic. Cook until the meat is browned.

4. Remove the lamb/garlic mixture from the pan, then add in the onions, carrots, celery, rosemary, and thyme.

5. Cook until onions are translucent and carrots and celery softened.

6. Add the meat mixture back into the pan, and stir in the tomatoes, balsamic, and Worcestershire and bring to a simmer.

7. Pour meat/vegetable mixture into a 9 inch x 13 inch (23 cm x 33 cm) baking pan, and with a rubber spatula spread a layer of the Mashed Cauliflower over the top, forming a solid layer of the mash.

8. Bake for 20 minutes or until the mashed cauliflower is slightly browned on top.

**Variations**—*Try this with ground beef, deer, or bison.*

**Plan Ahead**—*Have the Mashed Cauliflower done before you start.*

**Hint**—*This is probably one of our favorite recipes to eat on the go. It freezes really well.*

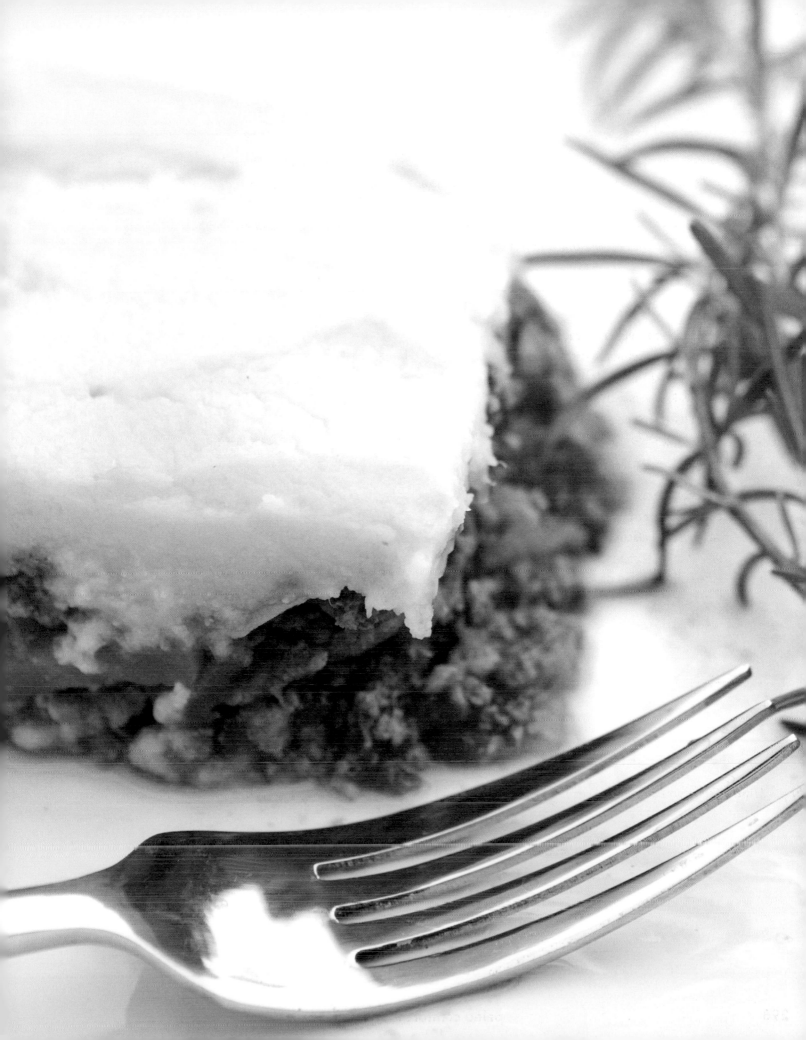

# grilled flank steak

*This is a fantastic recipe for so many reasons. For us, the best part of this tasty marinade is that it gives us the opportunity to mention (again) the Magic Bullet. When it comes to dressings, marinades, and easy cleanup . . . well it is simply the king.*

| | |
|---|---|
| 1 | teaspoon black peppercorns |
| 1 | teaspoon cumin seed |
| 3 | cloves garlic |
| ¼ | cup (60 mL) olive oil |
| 2 | tablespoons lime juice |
| 1 | tablespoon red wine vinegar |
| 1 | tablespoon fresh rosemary |
| 1–2 | pounds (500–900 g) flank steak |

1. Grind peppercorns and cumin seeds (in mortar and pestle, coffee grinder, or Magic Bullet).
2. Combine remaining ingredients (up to steak) in blender (or place in Magic Bullet after grinding). Blend well and pour over flank steak in ziplock bag.
3. Allow to marinate at least 3 hours (preferably overnight).
4. Preheat grill to medium-high heat. Oil the grill grate to prevent sticking.
5. Grill meat for about 5 minutes per side, or you achieve desired doneness.

**Variations**—*If you like your meat a bit on the rare side, try this method. Heat grill to as high as it will go. I can get my Big Green Egg up to up to 850°F (455 °C) pretty quickly. Throw meat on for 90–120 seconds. Flip and cook for another 90–120 seconds. Now turn off all heat and allow to cook for another 4–6 minutes.*

**Tips & Tricks**—*If your flank has a thicker middle, pound out the meat to a consistent thickness so that everything cooks to the same doneness.*

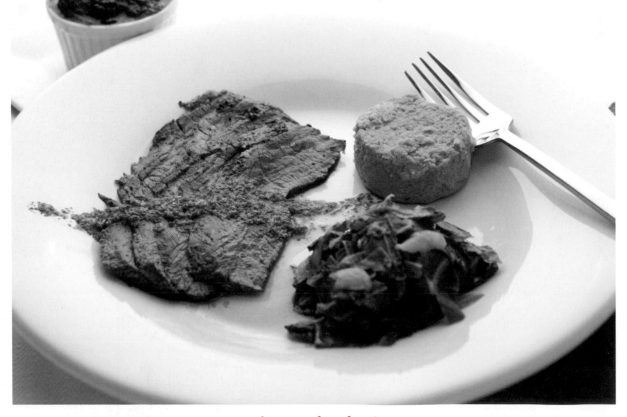

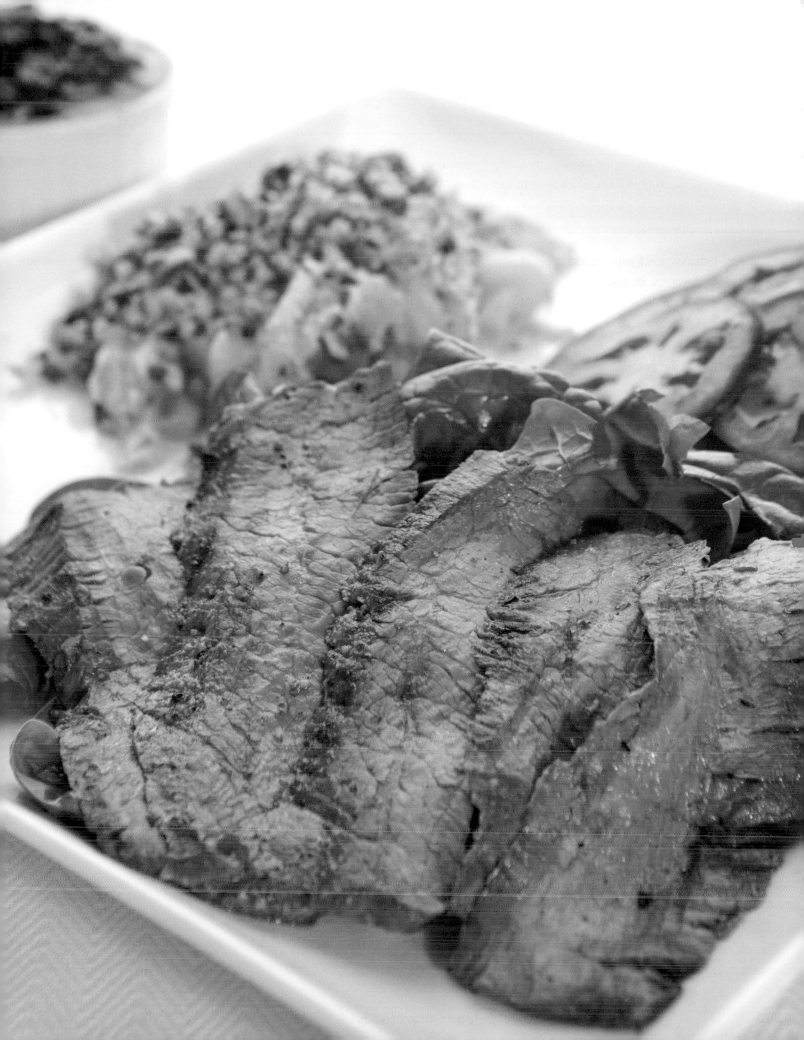

# chicken fried steak

*Throw this one in my top 5 for tasty, comforting, and just plain awesome. This protein and fat amalgamation is sure to make anyone happy. I know what you're saying . . . isn't it going to taste like coconut? If there is a hint of it in there, it's from the coconut milk used in the gravy. For those without a palate for coconut, I recommend substituting ¼ cup heavy whipping cream instead. Yes, it's dairy (though mostly fat), so you're going to have to choose between broadening your palate or taking in a little dairy.*

| | |
|---|---|
| 2 | pounds (900 g) beef round, trimmed of fat |
| 1 | teaspoon salt |
| 1 | teaspoon black pepper |
| 1 | cup (150 g) almond flour |
| ½ | cup (75 g) coconut flour |
| ½ | teaspoon garlic powder |
| 3 | large eggs |
| 3 | tablespoons coconut oil |
| 2 | cups (500 mL) chicken broth |
| ½ | cup (125 mL) coconut milk |
| 1 | teaspoon fresh thyme |
| ½ | teaspoon coarsely ground pepper |

## The steaks

1. Cut meat into ½-inch-thick (1 cm) slices and season both sides with half of your salt and pepper.
2. Mix your flours, garlic powder, and remaining salt/pepper into a pie pan. Set aside 2 tablespoons for gravy. Dredge the meat on both sides in the flour and place on cutting board. Now tenderize each piece with a meat hammer until ¼ inch (.5 cm) thick.
3. Beat eggs in another pie dish or large bowl. Coat each piece of meat in egg, then coat again with flour mixture. Place on plate and allow them to sit for 10 minutes.
4. Preheat your oven to 250°F (120°C).
5. In a large skillet, heat 2 tablespoons of your coconut oil over medium-high heat.
6. When oil is hot, add pieces of meat to pan, being careful not to over-crowd.
7. Cook meat for about 3–4 minutes per side. Remove pieces to a wire drying rack on a cookie sheet. When you have cooked all the meat pieces, place in oven until browned.

## To make the gravy

1. Add the remaining coconut oil to frying pan.
2. Whisk in remaining flour mixture 1 spoonful at a time.
3. Pour in chicken broth and deglaze pan.
4. Continue to whisk pan as you bring mixture to a soft boil and gravy begins to thicken. Add the coconut milk, thyme, and coarsely ground pepper and continue stirring until gravy reaches desired thickness.
5. Serve gravy over the steaks and enjoy.

**Tips & Tricks**—*To save time, purchase cubed steak from your local butcher.*

**Variation**—*This is an excellent recipe for venison and bison.*

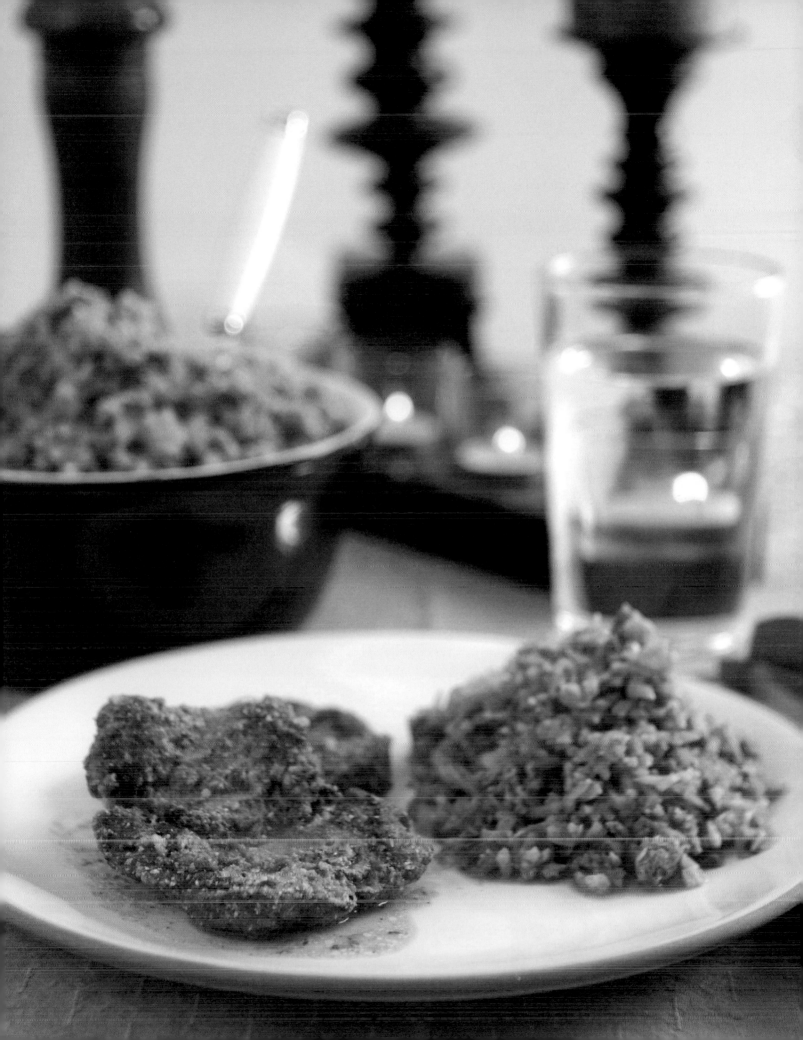

# venison-stuffed peppers

*I look forward to fall for so many reasons. The leaves change color, football is in full swing, and I get to go climb trees in search of venison. Bow season here starts in mid-September. I've owned a bow for years but seemed to always find a reason to keep it in the storage room and just wait for rifle season to open. That is, until two years ago. I'm now officially a bow-hunting fool. I've yet to get one with my trusty Proline, but that won't dampen my spirits. Plus I get to scout out the terrain for rifle season a bit early. Maybe this will be my year for bagging Bambi with a bow. Wish me luck, or compliment my alliteration, your choice.*

| | |
|---|---|
| 6 | bell peppers, assorted colors |
| 4 | strips thick bacon, chopped |
| ½ | pound (225 g) ground pork |
| ½ | pound (225 g) ground venison |
| ¼ | cup (40 g) celery, diced |
| 1 | cup (150 g) onion, diced |
| ¼ | cup (40 g) garlic, minced |
| ½ | cup (75 g) green onion, chopped |
| ¼ | cup (6 g) parsley, chopped |
| 2 | large eggs, beaten |

1. Cut tops out of bell peppers and remove inside seeds. Dice tops and save for later. Soak peppers in boiling water for 5 minutes to soften.

2. Cook bacon in large skillet until crispy to render fat. Once brown, remove from skillet and set aside for later.

3. Add ground deer and pork to skillet. Using a wooden spoon, chop meats well to incorporate.

4. Once meat is thoroughly browned (10–12 minutes), add celery, onion, garlic, and reserved peppers from tops. Sauté for another 10–15 minutes until onions are cooked.

5. Preheat oven to 350°F (175°C).

6. Mix green onion and parsley well with the meat filling. Remove from heat and allow to cool slightly in bowl.

7. Once cooled, fold in the beaten eggs and season to taste with black pepper. Stuff peppers generously with mixture.

8. Place in oven and cook until brown on top (about 30 minutes).

**Tips & Tricks**—*Make sure your peppers can stand up on their own. If not, slice a very thin layer off the bottoms to create a flat surface. You can also put them in a Bundt pan to hold them up—great use for that cake pan that probably is not seeing much action.*

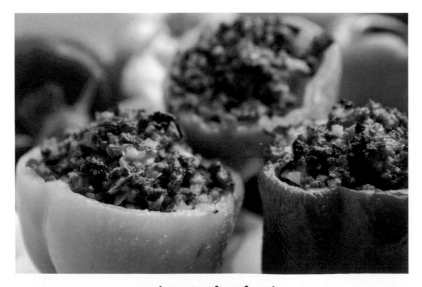

paleo comfort foods

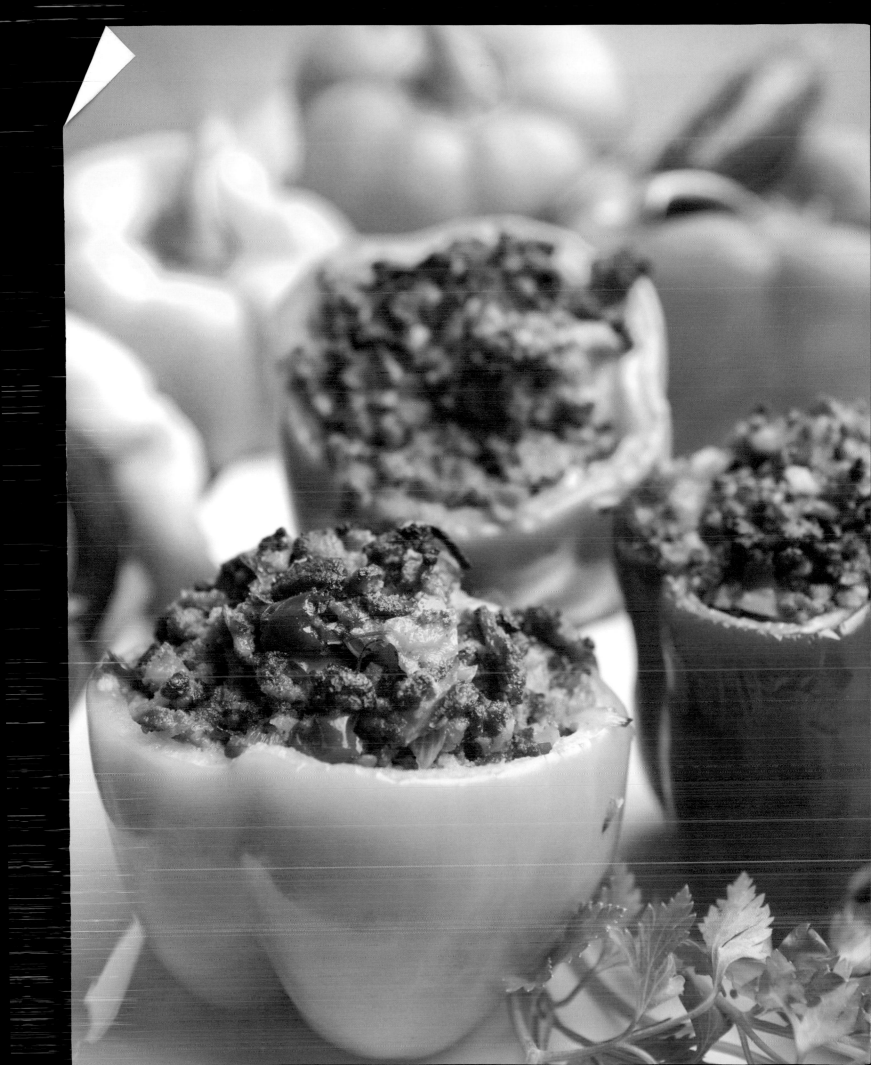

# osso buco

*The name of this classic means "bone with a hole" in Italian. What the name doesn't tell you is that the hole is full of some really tasty bone marrow. The name doesn't say anything about what kind of meat to use. Traditionally, this dish is made with veal. We have thoroughly enjoyed making this with beef shanks. It is a little less expensive, and beef shanks come included with our grass-fed cow order. Braising this tasty cut for a few hours will bring out the triple-threat flavors of marrow, meat, and gelatin. This combination of texture and richness is unforgettable.*

| | |
|---|---|
| 4 | beef shanks |
| ¼ | cup (60 mL) coconut oil |
| 2 | cups (300 g) onion, chopped |
| 1 | large carrot, peeled and chopped |
| 1 | green bell pepper, chopped |
| 1 | red bell pepper, chopped |
| 1 | tablespoon garlic, minced |
| ½ | cup (125 mL) dry white wine |
| 1 | cup (250 mL) chicken broth |
| 1 | tablespoon lemon juice |
| 28 | ounces (794 g) whole canned tomatoes |
| 1 | tablespoon basil, chopped |
| 1 | bay leaf |
| ¼ | teaspoon salt |
| 1 | teaspoon black pepper |
| 2 | sprigs fresh thyme |

## Optional Gremolata

| | |
|---|---|
| ¼ | 1/4 cup (6 g) Italian parsley, finely chopped |
| 2 | cloves garlic minced |
| ~ | zest from 1 lemon |

**Combine ingredients and mix well in sauce. You may also simply garnish individual servings with gremolata.

1. Allow meat to come to room temperature before cooking (about 30 minutes). Dust shanks with a pinch of black pepper and salt.

2. Heat coconut oil over high heat in sauté pan large enough to hold all meat in single layer. Brown both sides of shanks for about 3 minutes each side in pan.

3. Remove shanks and set aside, reducing heat to medium high, and preheat oven to 350°F (170°C).

4. Toss onions, carrots, peppers, and garlic in to sauté until they soften slightly, about 5 minutes.

5. Return temp to high and pour in your wine and broth. Deglaze pan as you add in your lemon juice, tomatoes, basil, bay leaf, salt, and pepper.

6. Reduce liquid by about a third by cooking uncovered. Return the shanks to the pot along with the thyme sprigs.

7. Cover and place in the oven for 90–120 minutes. Remove from oven when meat is extremely tender.

8. Use a slotted spoon or spatula to carefully remove contents to serving platter.

9. Continue to cook/reduce sauce to desired thickness. Pour over shanks when serving.

---

**Variations**—*Use lamb or veal shank instead of beef. You can also replace a pepper with 2 ribs of celery.*

**Tips & Tricks**—*We can't stress enough that you need to be careful removing the meat from the pot. It makes for better presentation and that tasty marrow stays put in the bone. Yes, eat the marrow!*

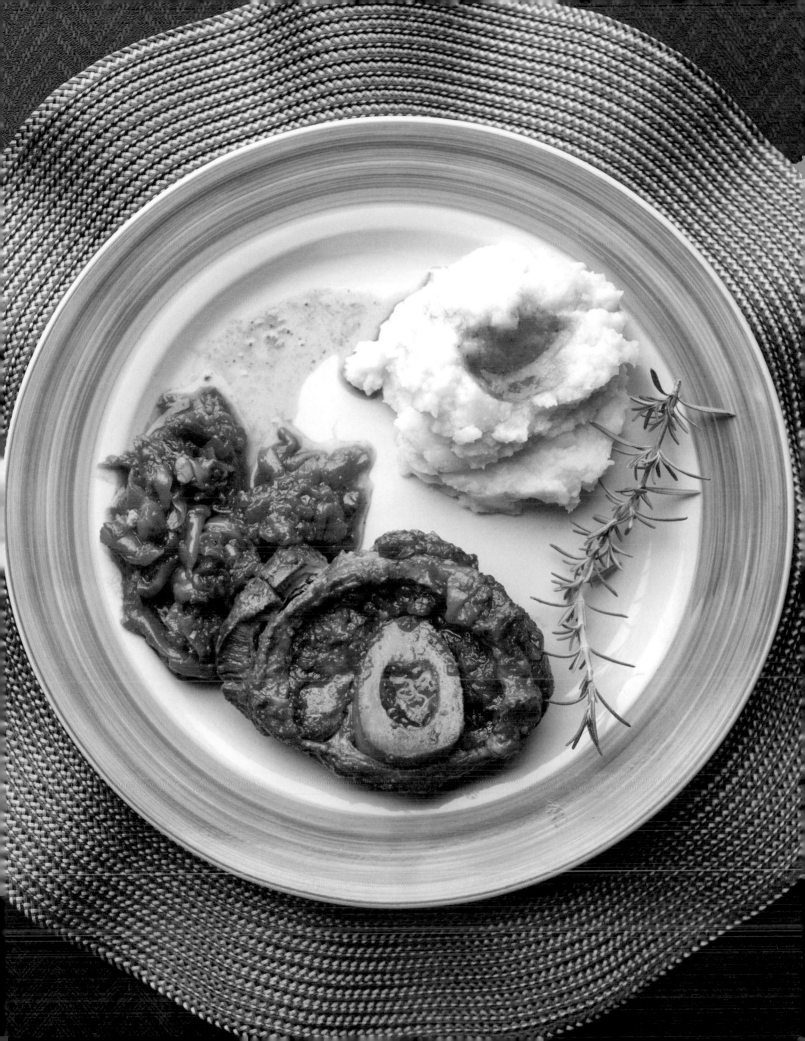

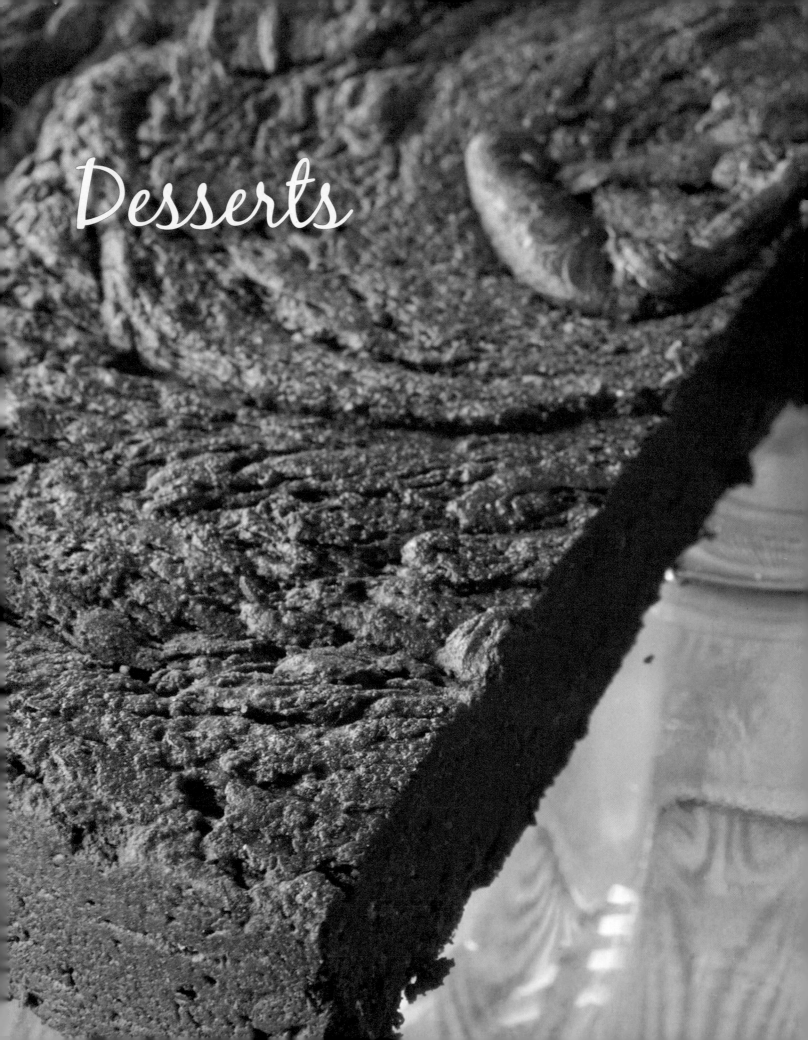

Desserts

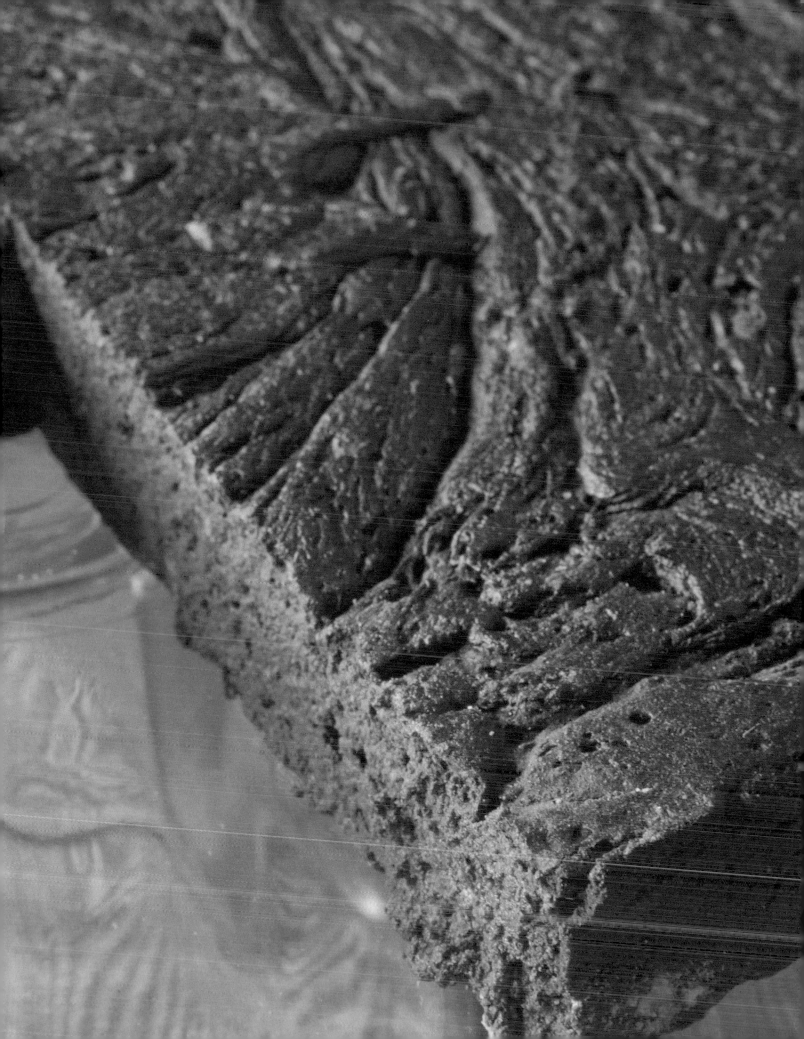

# banana nut bread

*Growing up, I was extremely picky about my bananas. After long swim practices, I would only eat the bananas that had the perfect ripeness (perfect by my standards) which meant just past the green stage, but not one speck of brown. I could not fathom eating browned bananas. Unless, of course, these bananas were used as banana bread. That was the only suitable use for browned bananas and any respectable banana bread will use only the best browned bananas.*

*The only sugar in this bread comes from the bananas. Some of you may wish to add in some honey, but I really don't think it's needed. This is a wonderful loaf to bring as a hostess gift or into one of those pot-luck brunches! Think of this as one of your paleo treats!*

| | |
|---|---|
| 3 | cups (450 g) almond flour |
| 2 | teaspoons baking soda |
| ½ | teaspoon salt |
| ¼ | cup (60 mL) coconut oil, melted |
| 4 | large eggs |
| 2 | very ripe bananas, mashed |
| 3 | teaspoons vanilla |
| 3 | teaspoons cinnamon |
| ½ | cup (50 g) walnuts, chopped |

1. Preheat oven to 350°F (175°C).
2. Combine the almond flour, baking soda and salt in a small bowl.
3. In a separate bowl, mix together the coconut oil and eggs.
4. Mix the flour combination into the oil and eggs, and stir until well blended.
5. Add in the mashed bananas, vanilla and cinnamon. Fold in the walnuts.
6. Pour batter into a greased loaf pan. Bake for 25–30 minutes or until a toothpick comes out clean.

**Variation**—*This recipe also works well as muffins. Just grease 12 medium-sized muffin cups, filling up about ⅔ of the way with the batter.*

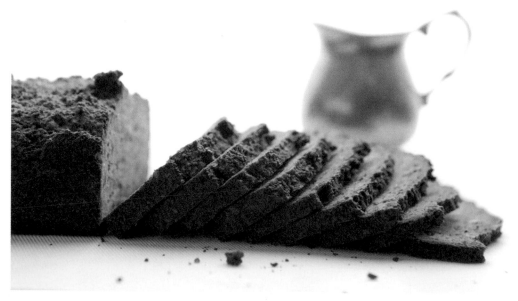

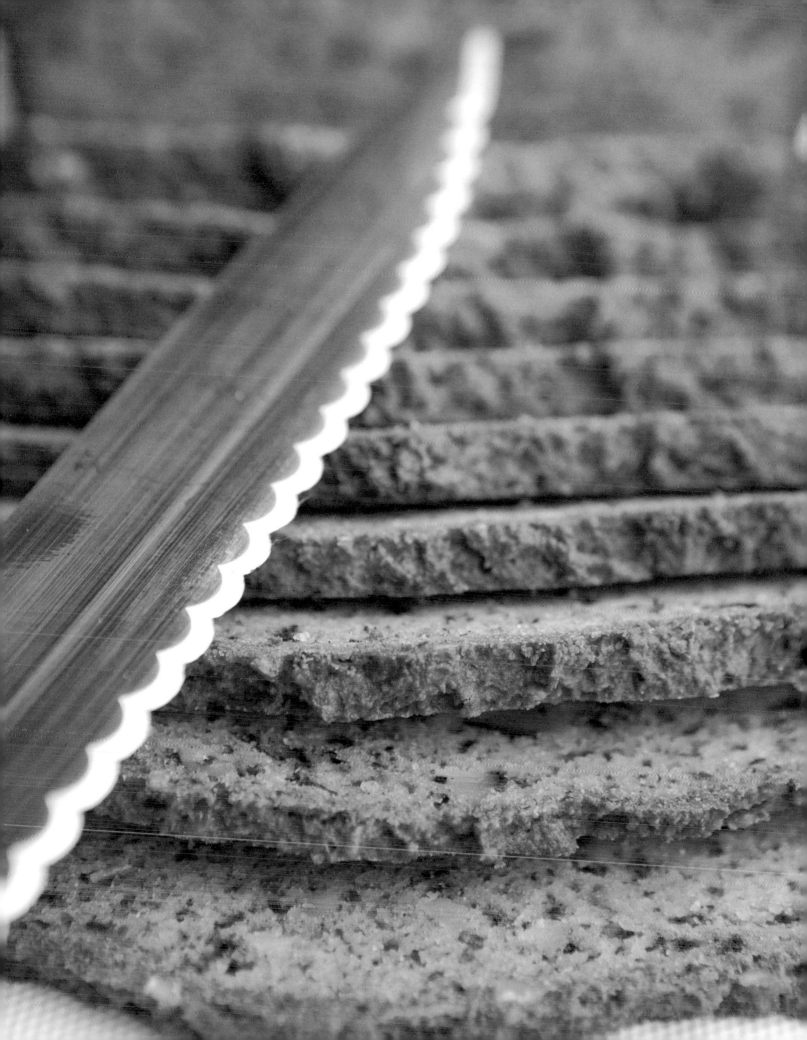

# poached pears

*It's amazing to really utilize fruits with their natural sugars for sweetening things. This recipe is a classic example of just how sweet oranges and pears are on their own—and how much sweeter they get when cooked together. You seriously won't believe that there is no added sugar, honey, etc. in this recipe.*

*To really let the flavors sink in, let the pears sit in the liquid overnight, and serve either reheated or cold.*

| | |
|---|---|
| 3 | cups (750 mL) fresh-squeezed orange juice (no added sugar) |
| 3 | cups (750 mL) water |
| 1 | 2-inch (4 cm) piece ginger, peeled |
| 4 | ripe (but not mushy) Bosc or Anjou pears, peeled and cored |
| 5 | whole cloves |
| 1 | stick cinnamon |
| ~ | zest of 1 orange |

1. Place all ingredients in a small saucepan, ensuring that all the pears are completely covered with liquid.

2. Cut a circular piece of parchment paper that fits inside the saucepan to keep pears from being exposed to air (if the pears are not covered with something—liquid or parchment—they will brown).

3. Bring heat to a simmer, and let poach in liquid for about 30 minutes or until soft—not mushy.

4. Remove pears from liquid, and bring remaining liquid to a boil.

5. Reduce heat to a simmer, and allow to reduce by ½ to ¾, or until liquid is nice and syrupy.

6. Remove cinnamon stick and pour syrup over pears and garnish with a sprinkle of cinnamon and/or some orange zest to serve.

**Tips & Tricks**—*A melon baller works very well at removing the seeds and core from the pears. To do so, just insert the melon baller from the bottom of the pear and work your way up to remove all the seeds.*

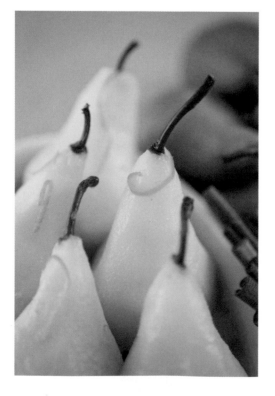

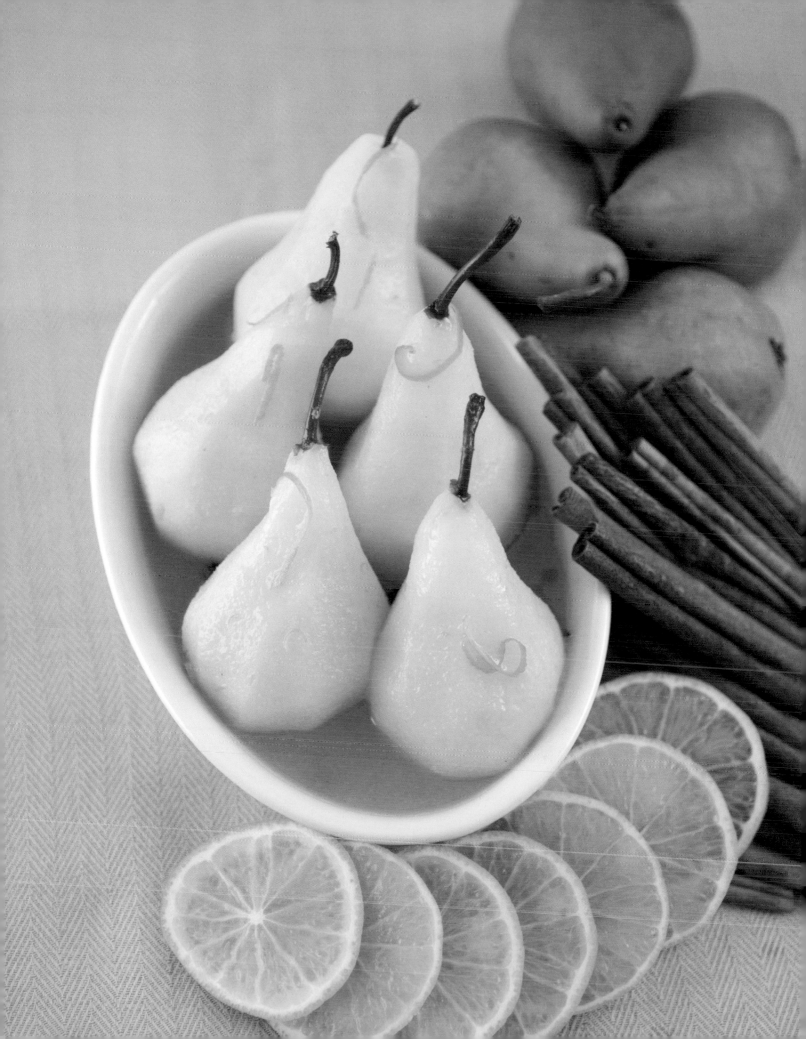

# decadent chocolate cake with a kick

*This is for those times when you are asked to make (specifically) a cake for a work/book club/party event, and you don't want any gluten or massively massive doses of sugar, but you still want to impress the guests. There aren't a lot of ingredients here, it's not too complex, and it is so so so decadent and intense that you really will be happy after even just a small bite.*

*This recipe is loosely based off one in Cook's Illustrated (aka my cooking bible); however, the kinds of chocolate I like to use (a mixture of Trader Joe's 85% and 72% dark chocolate) only come in 3.5-ounce bars. So, a recipe using 14 ounces of chocolate (vs. a full pound) was born. Plus, I suppose I feel a teeny bit less guilty saying that the recipe calls for less than a pound of chocolate. You will be sabotaging your clean eating and nicely regulated insulin levels if you eat this cake every night. Dark chocolate—even the 85% dark stuff—contains some sugar.*

*Good quality, good tasting chocolate makes a difference.*

| | |
|---|---|
| 7 | large eggs, cold |
| 14 | ounces (380 g) bittersweet chocolate, 72%–85% works great |
| 14 | tablespoons butter |
| ¼ | cup (60 mL) brewed espresso or coffee |
| ¼ | cup (40 g) coconut flour |
| 1 | teaspoon pure vanilla extract |
| 2 | teaspoons chipotle powder |
| 1 | teaspoon cayenne pepper |

1. Preheat oven to 325°F (165°C).

2. Line the bottom of an 8- or 9-inch (20- or 23-cm) spring-form pan with parchment. Grease the inside walls and the parchment with butter. Take a very large piece of aluminum foil and tightly wrap the entire outside of the pan (this is to prevent water from seeping into the pan once placed in the water bath).

3. Using either a hand mixer or a KitchenAid stand mixer, beat the eggs until almost doubled in size, about 5–7 minutes.

4. Meanwhile, using either a double boiler or the microwave, melt the chocolate, butter, and espresso together (if using the microwave, use a glass bowl, and heat in 30-second intervals, removing and stirring after each interval).

5. Gently fold in a few spoonfuls of the eggs into the chocolate mixture along with the coconut flour, until few streaks of egg remain. Add about ½ the remaining eggs, folding again, then adding in the rest until combined. Mix in the vanilla, chipotle powder and cayenne until incorporated throughout.

6. Spoon batter into spring-form pan. Place this pan into a large roasting pan or Pyrex baking dish, and fill the dish halfway up the sides of the cake pan with boiling water.

7. Bake for 18–22 minutes, or until an instant read thermometer registers 140°F (60°C). Trust me, you don't want to overcook this cake!

8. Remove pan from water bath, and let sit on a rack to cool. Once it's reached room temperature, remove the sides of the spring form pan, and invert cake onto a plate so as to remove the paper/spring-form bottom.

9. Turn right side up onto a cake stand or platter.

**Variation**—*If you don't want it to have that subtle kick, ditch the cayenne and chipotle powder. Easy enough!*

**Ingredient Notes**—*I attempted this once with clarified butter. While I'd love to say that the results were great, it was kind of an oily result. The milk solids in the butter are important for the mixture, and without it (clarifying the butter removes the milk solids), it just was super oily. I did a version with half butter and half coconut oil, which turned out okay, although a bit on the oily side. If dairy is on your no-no list, you might want to skip over this recipe.*

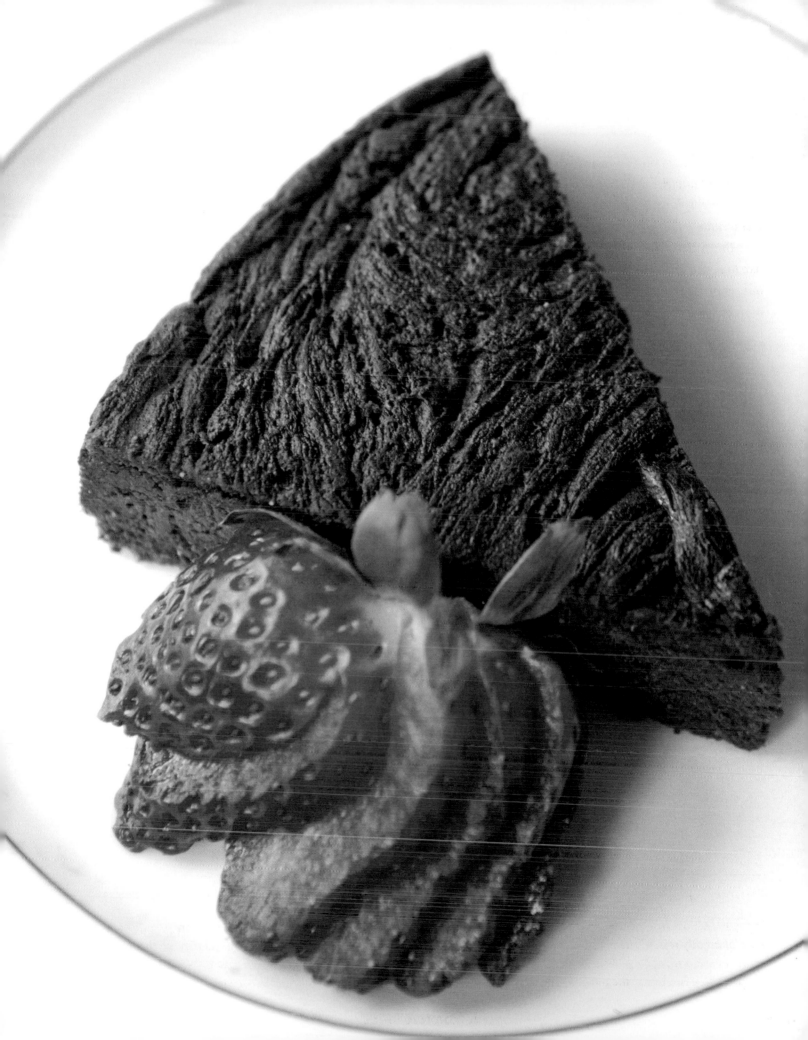

# cool berry tart

*You can serve this tasty treat nearly year round. If berries are out of season, buy the frozen kind and make do. This dessert, like most, packs a pretty potent sugar punch.*

*Let patience rule the day and wait until strawberries and blackberries are in season if you can. Fresh berries are so incredibly sweet you won't need to add the honey to this recipe. Stock up when they are in season and freeze them yourself. My last two batches of tarts have come from berries I froze last season.*

*If you happen to be in East Tennessee in the spring, we highly recommend stopping by Mayfield Farm and Nursery to discover what a real berry is supposed to taste like. My brother's berries are some of the best we have found.*

---

## For the filling

| | |
|---|---|
| 1 | cup (250 mL) water |
| 1 | tablespoon honey |
| 2 | cups (400 g) strawberries |
| 2 | cups (200 g) blackberries |

## For the crust

| | |
|---|---|
| 1½ | cups (225 g) almond flour |
| ¼ | teaspoon salt |
| ¼ | teaspoon baking soda |
| ½ | teaspoon cinnamon |
| ¼ | teaspoon nutmeg |
| ¼ | cup (60 mL) macadamia nut or other neutral tasting oil |
| 1 | tablespoons honey |
| 1 | teaspoon vanilla extract |

**1.** Heat water, honey, strawberries and blackberries in medium sauce pan. Crush berries with potato masher and simmer on medium heat for 15 minutes stirring occasionally. The fruit filling should reduce by a fourth.

**2.** While fruit is simmering preheat oven to 350°F (175°C).

**3.** Combine almond flour, salt, baking soda, cinnamon, and nutmeg in a large bowl.

**4.** Mix oil, honey, and vanilla in a separate bowl and pour the wet ingredients into the dry. Mix until thoroughly combined.

**5.** Press the dough into a pie pan and bake for 10 minutes or until light brown.

**6.** Remove crust from oven and allow to cool for 5 minutes. If you time it right, your fruit filling should be done now and cooling.

**7.** After fruit mixture has cooled a bit, pour in crust and place in refrigerator for 1 hour before serving.

---

**Variations**—*Consider using raspberries in place of either of your other berries. You can also try using small ramekins instead of a big pan. Just press the dough down the sides. Adding dairy in your diet? Consider whipping up a little heavy cream and put a dollop on top when you serve.*

**Tips & Tricks**—*Gently crushing your berries will release the juices and keep the texture intact. If you're looking for a smoother texture, then blend the mixture once reduced.*

paleo comfort foods

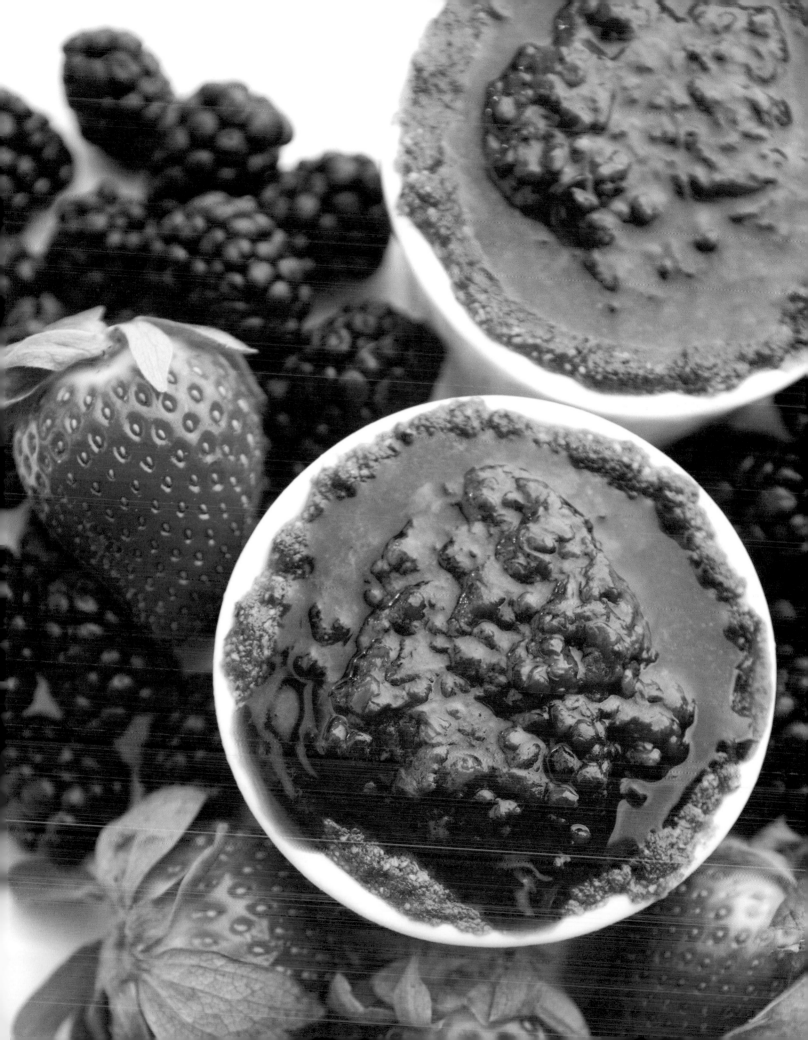

# strawberry shortcakes

*Springtime in the South is a sight to be seen, and I missed it for the eight long years I lived in Los Angeles. Springtime also means super-fresh crops of strawberries—usually starting in late April or early May—and I love strawberries and could eat them by the bowl. The problem is that fresh, local strawberries are typically only available for a few short weeks around April and May. My suggestion is to buy a bunch and freeze them.*

*This recipe is our take on wanting to let the strawberries speak for themselves, while also doing a spin on the classic strawberry shortcake. The "cakes" here are a little bit like scones, little bit like biscuits, and definitely pretty tasty.*

| | |
|---|---|
| 16 | ounces (450 g) fresh strawberries |
| 1–2 | teaspoons honey (optional) |
| 2 | cups (300 g) blanched almond flour |
| ½ | teaspoon baking soda |
| 1 | teaspoon cinnamon |
| 3 | tablespoons cold grass-fed butter or coconut oil |
| 2 | large eggs |
| 2 | tablespoons honey |
| 1 | teaspoon vanilla extract |

1. Wash, hull, and slice the strawberries as small as you desire.

2. Mix in a bowl together with honey, if desired, to somewhat macerate the strawberries.

3. Preheat oven to 350°F (175°C).

4. Line a sheet pan with some parchment paper.

5. In a large bowl, combine the almond flour, baking soda, and cinnamon. Using a fork or knife, cut the butter into the almond flour to form and mix, so that you've formed some small beads of the butter in the dough.

6. In a separate bowl, whisk together the eggs, honey, and vanilla. Stir the wet ingredients into the dry.

7. Using a spoon or measuring cup, drop the dough onto the sheet pan into 8 evenly sized cakes, leaving room in between each cake.

8. Bake for 15–20 minutes until golden brown.

9. Allow cakes to cool, then slice horizontally, and spoon some of the strawberry mixture into the middle, and some extra on the side.

**Variation**—*You know what I'm going to say. If you are allowing dairy into your life, whip up some fresh cream and serve it on these. You won't be disappointed!*

**Tips & Tricks**—*When storing strawberries, moisture is the enemy. Don't wash strawberries until you are ready to eat them.*

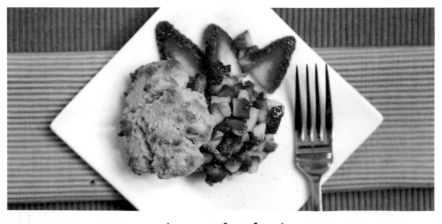

paleo comfort foods

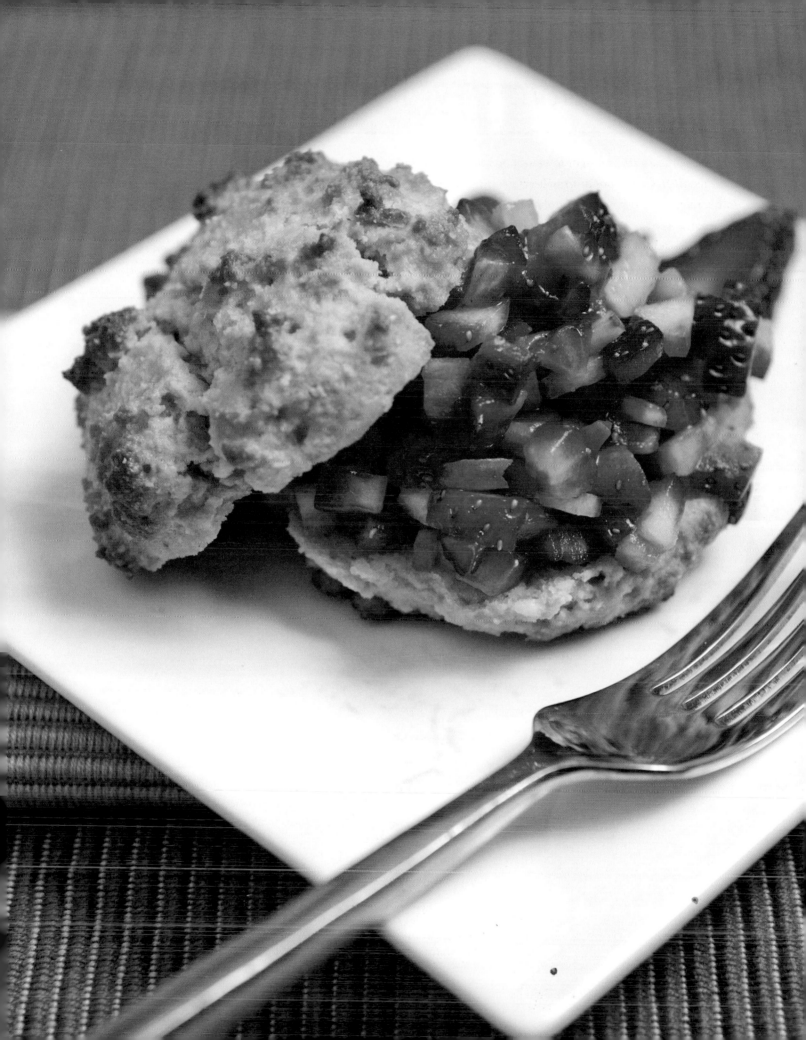

# peachberry cobbler

*Eat your heart out, Martha! We find it amusing how much sugar most recipes call for when making a cobbler. Fresh peaches, blackberries, and blueberries are naturally about the sweetest things in the world. In fact, if they are in season, why not take a trip to a local farm and pick your own? Check the Internet to find out when blackberries and/or blueberries are in season where you live. Both fruits freeze very well, so load up.*

| | |
|---|---|
| ½ | cup (125 mL) butter |
| 1 ½ | cups (180g) finely chopped nuts, such as pecans or almonds |
| ½ | cup (75 g) coconut flour |
| 2 | teaspoons baking powder |
| ½ | cup (125 mL) coconut milk |
| 1 | teaspoon vanilla extract |
| 2 | cups (450 g) fresh peaches, peeled and cut into small pieces |
| 3 | cups (300 g) fresh blueberries or blackberries |

1. Preheat oven to 350°F (175 °C). Meanwhile, allow butter to come to room temperature to soften.

2. In large bowl, mix all dry ingredients. Mix in butter, coconut milk and vanilla and mix very well.

3. Place fruit in deep baking dish and push down until it has a flat surface. Using your fist works really well and you can lick off all the tasty sweetness when you're done. You'll want to release a few of the juices of the berries but still have them maintain their form.

4. Spread the doughy top over the entire surface of the berries and press down to flat.

5. Place in oven and bake for 60–75 minutes. Depending on the size of your dish, your crust may be a little thick and will extra need time to cook all the way through.

6. Serve piping hot.

**Variation**—*Sprinkle a little cinnamon on the berries prior to putting them in the dish.*

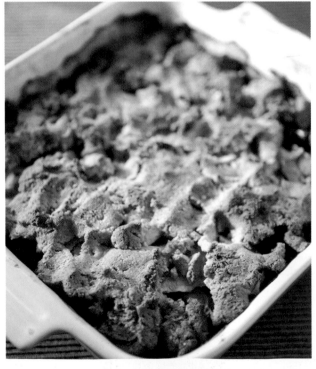

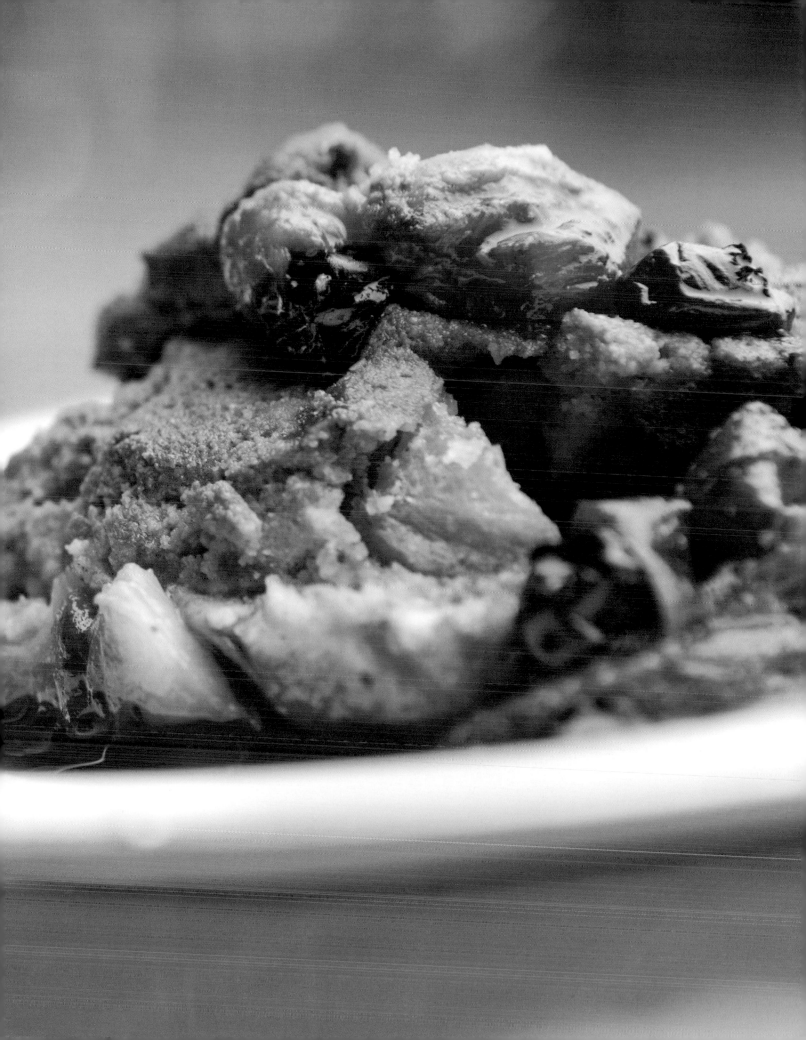

# apple crisp

*"Sullivan's Apple Pie" was a family tradition at Christmas, Thanksgiving, and pretty much any other holiday. People always asked me the secret to the recipe, as it was not an overly sweet pie; rather, it was tart and tangy from the use of the Granny Smith apples (Granny Smiths were the secret). I've been making this pie since high school, and it always reminds me of home (and wondering which family member ate all the crisp topping, leaving the apples behind).*

*I was never really big on pie crust. Just wasn't my thing. For me, it was always about the warm, gooey apples, and the crumb topping. This recipe pays homage to that. Baking this dessert will fill your house with some of the most amazing aromas.*

| | |
|---|---|
| 1 | cup (150 g) almond flour |
| 1 | cup (150 g) Steve's Paleo Krunch, ground into rough meal |
| 3 | teaspoons cinnamon |
| 1 | teaspoon nutmeg |
| 1/3 | cup (80 mL) coconut oil or butter, softened |
| 2 | tablespoons honey (optional) |
| 2 | teaspoons vanilla extract |
| 5–7 | Granny Smith apples, peeled, cored and sliced |
| ~ | juice of 1 lemon |

1. Preheat oven to 350°F (175°C).

2. Combine flour, Paleo Krunch, 2 teaspoons of cinnamon, and nutmeg in a bowl.

3. In a separate bowl, use a fork to combine coconut oil (or butter), honey (if desired) and vanilla. Mix into the flour/Krunch mixture.

4. Scatter apple slices in a 9 inch x 9 inch (23cm x 23cm) baking dish or similar-sized dish, and combine with lemon juice. Stir in remaining cinnamon, and combine well.

5. Sprinkle the almond/Krunch mixture over the apples, cover with foil, and bake for 45 minutes or until apples are soft and bubbly.

6. Remove foil, and bake 10–15 more minutes or until topping is browned.

**Variation**—*If you are allowing dairy into your life, this crisp is absolutely sinful still warm from the oven with some fresh whipped cream on top. Pears combined with apples makes for a tasty crisp too.*

**Ingredient Notes**—*A great substitution for this recipe, if you don't have Steve's Paleo Krunch handy, is 1 cup (120 g) of finely chopped pecans.*

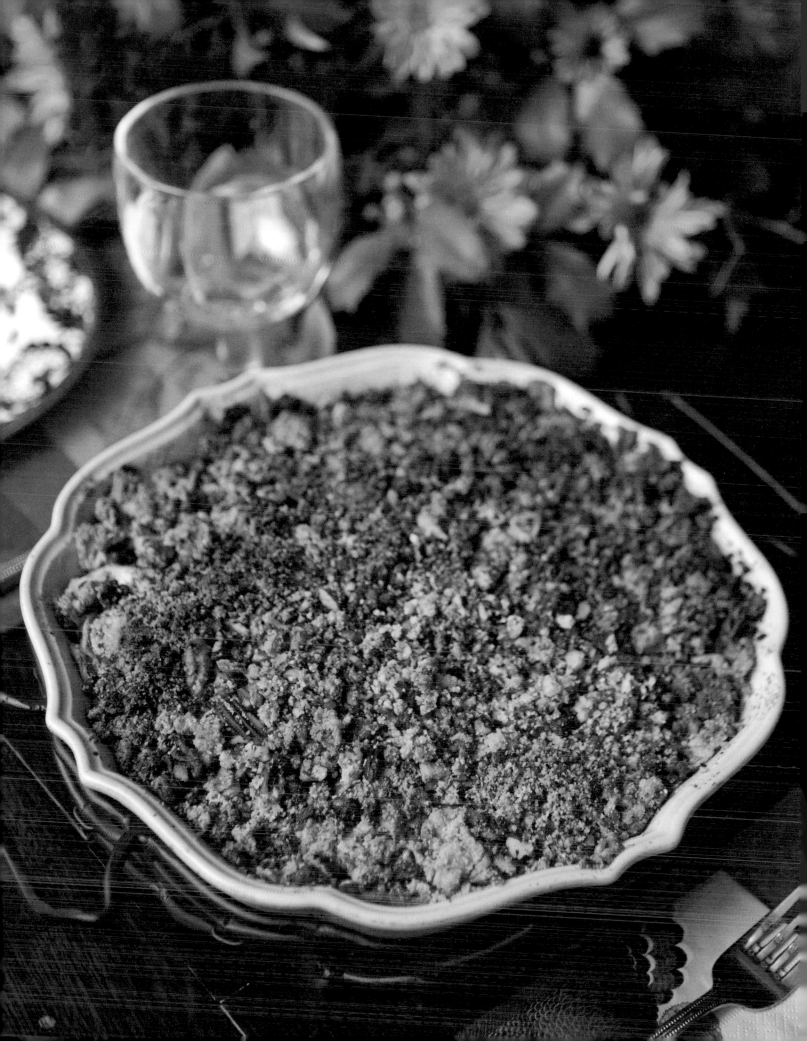

# jules' banana pudding

*Banana pudding is a staple in the South, and typically involves a vanilla cream pudding (sometimes from an instant mix), bananas, and vanilla wafers. While I could have "invented" a vanilla wafer substitute, the point here is to create something that's reminiscent of the old conventional pudding but reframing the flavors and the dish in such a way as to enable folks to enjoy it without the health concerns (sorry all you vanilla wafer lovers out there).*

*While there is no added sugar here, I know you know that bananas are naturally very high in sugar, so again, this is a once-in-a-while treat.*

| | |
|---|---|
| 1 | can coconut milk |
| 2 | large egg yolks |
| 1 | teaspoon vanilla extract |
| 1 | tablespoon coconut oil |
| 1 | tablespoon coconut butter |
| 3 | really ripe bananas (almost black) |
| ½ | teaspoon cinnamon |

1. Whisk coconut milk, egg yolks, and vanilla together over medium heat. Stir constantly with whisk or wooden spoon until mixture starts to thicken.

2. Remove from heat.

3. In a small frying pan, heat the coconut oil and coconut butter over medium heat, and add slightly mashed bananas along with cinnamon. You're just cooking long enough to let bananas start to caramelize somewhat.

4. Pour the coconut milk and egg mixture into a food processor or blender along with the cooked bananas, and process until smooth and creamy.

5. Empty contents into a bowl, and place a layer of plastic wrap directly on the surface. This will prevent a skin from forming.

6. Refrigerate to chill and serve topped with some sliced bananas!

**Variation**—*This is actually really tasty served frozen—almost like a banana ice cream.*

**Ingredient Notes**—*Using bananas that haven't yet ripened all the way will drastically take away from the flavor of this dessert. Be sure to ask the clerk at your grocery store if they have any "extra" ripe ones in back. Most groceries don't keep extra brown bananas on the store shelves.*

**Tips & Tricks**—*To ripen bananas quickly, place them in a paper bag with either a tomato or apple. Seal the bag shut and they should be ripe within 24 hours.*

324            paleo comfort foods

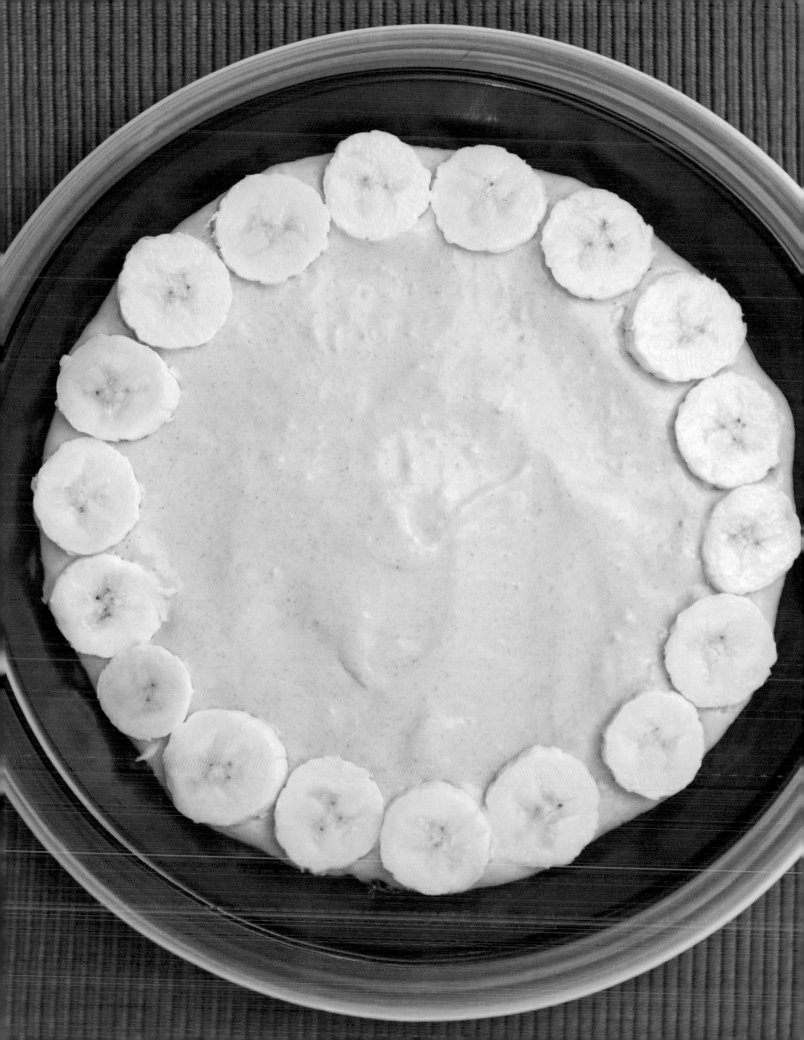

# sweet potato pie

*Why should pumpkin get all the fame and glory when it comes to pie? Sweet potato pie is a Southern comfort staple, whereas pumpkin has much more of a national flair around the holidays. You can easily substitute out the sweet potato for pumpkin, but I for one love the flavor and texture of the sweet potatoes.*

| | |
|---|---|
| 1 | **Nutty Pie Crust recipe** |
| 2 | **cups (400 g) sweet potatoes, peeled, boiled and mashed** |
| 1 | **tablespoon butter or coconut butter, melted** |
| 2 | **large eggs** |
| 1 | **teaspoon cinnamon** |
| ¼ | **teaspoon nutmeg** |
| 1 | **teaspoon baking soda** |
| 1 | **teaspoon baking powder** |
| ¼ | **teaspoon salt** |
| ⅔ | **cup (160 mL) coconut milk** |
| 1 | **teaspoon apple cider vinegar** |
| ¼ | **cup honey (optional)** |

1. Prepare pie crust as stated in Nutty Pie Crust recipe (page 122).

2. Preheat oven to 400°F (205°C).

3. In a large bowl or food processor, mix sweet potatoes and butter. Add in eggs and mix until fluffy.

4. Meanwhile, in a separate bowl, combine cinnamon, nutmeg, baking soda, baking powder and salt.

5. Combine coconut milk, apple cider vinegar and mixture of spices to the bowl containing the sweet potatoes.

6. Mix until fully combined. Add honey if desired.

7. Pour contents into prepared pie crust and bake for 10 minutes at 400°F (205°C), then reduce heat to 325°F (165°C) and bake for 30 minutes or until set.

**Do Ahead**—*Especially if you are making this pie for Thanksgiving or some other holiday, make your crust a day or two ahead of time and keep refrigerated until ready to use. It will make your to-do list that much shorter on your actual holiday! Come to think of it, make the whole thing a day or two before serving. It just lets all those flavors meld together.*

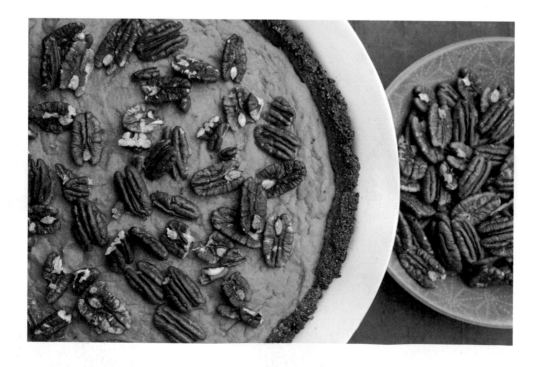

paleo comfort foods

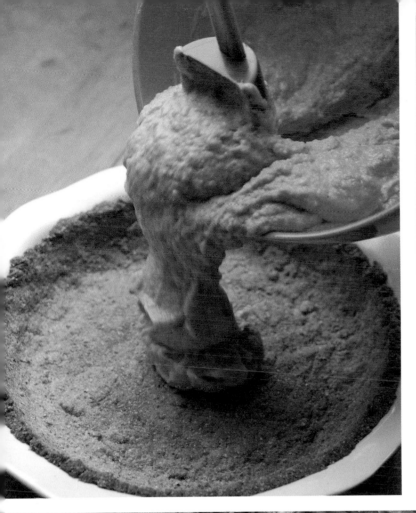

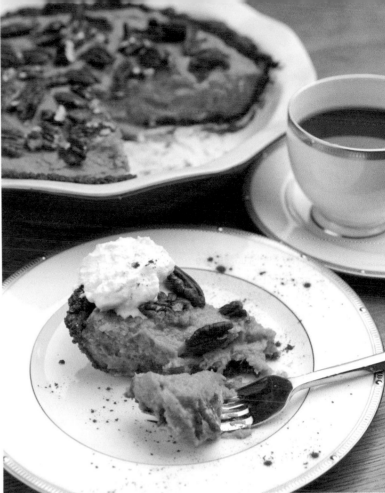

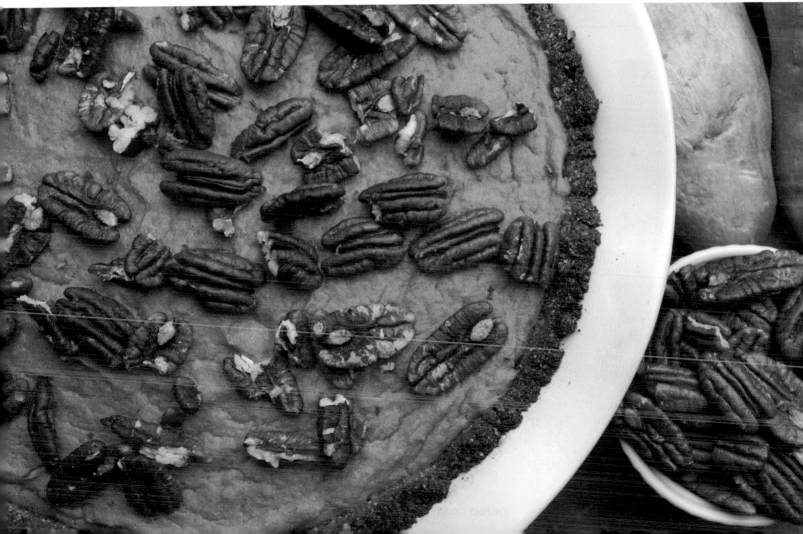

# luscious lemon squares

*Lemon squares are one of those desserts that always made my teeth hurt they were so sweet. Conventional lemon squares recipes typically call for anywhere from 2–3 cups of cane or confectioner's sugar. This variation certainly won't make your teeth hurt, and they don't have nearly as much sugar, but as there is a bit of honey in this (and sugar is sugar after all), it's definitely a treat. Make this once a year for that summertime party you have to go to. It's nice to have a gluten-free dessert to share with all — one that won't mess you up for days like Cousin Betty's peanut butter gluten-bomb brownies.*

| | |
|---|---|
| 1 | cup (150 g) Steve's Original Paleo Krunch |
| ¾ | cup (120 g) raw almonds |
| 1 | tablespoon honey |
| 3 | teaspoons lemon zest |
| 2 | large eggs |
| ¼ | cup (60 mL) coconut oil, melted |
| ¼ | cup (60 mL) butter, melted |
| | |
| 6 | egg yolks |
| ¼ | cup (60 mL) honey |
| ~ | zest of 1 lemon |
| 6 | tablespoons coconut oil or clarified butter |
| ½ | cup (120 mL) lemon juice |

## For the crust

1. Preheat oven to 375°F (190°C) and grease a 9inch x 9 inch ( 23cm x 23 cm) baking pan.
2. Combine the Paleo Krunch and almonds in a food processor and blend until a coarse meal is formed. Add in the honey, lemon zest, eggs, oil, butter and pulse in processor until thoroughly mixed.
3. Empty contents of processor into the baking pan, pressing down to form a crust on the bottom of the pan, and bake for 15 minutes or until golden brown.

## For the lemon custard

1. Combine the egg yolks, honey and lemon zest in a sauce pan. Whisk until combined.
2. Add in coconut oil or butter and turn on stove to medium.
3. Add in lemon juice and continue whisking until mixture starts to thicken.
4. Remove from heat and strain mixture through fine sieve.
5. Refrigerate until cooled completely.

## To make lemon bars

1. Once crust and lemon custard have cooled completely (I suggest waiting until the next day), preheat oven to 350°F (175°C).
2. Spread lemon custard over crust, and place in oven.
3. Bake for 10–15 minutes or until custard looks almost translucent.
4. Allow bars to cool completely, then cut into squares.

**Variation**—*If you don't have Steve's Paleo Krunch, just substitute in almond or any other nut meal.*

**Ingredient Notes**—*Steve's Paleo Krunch is pretty awesome stuff, in that it's like granola/cereal that's paleo friendly, and it supports an awesome organization that provides programs for disadvantaged youth. We highly recommend supporting Steve's Club and getting your hands on some Paleo Kits and Paleo Krunch today. www.stevesclub.org.*

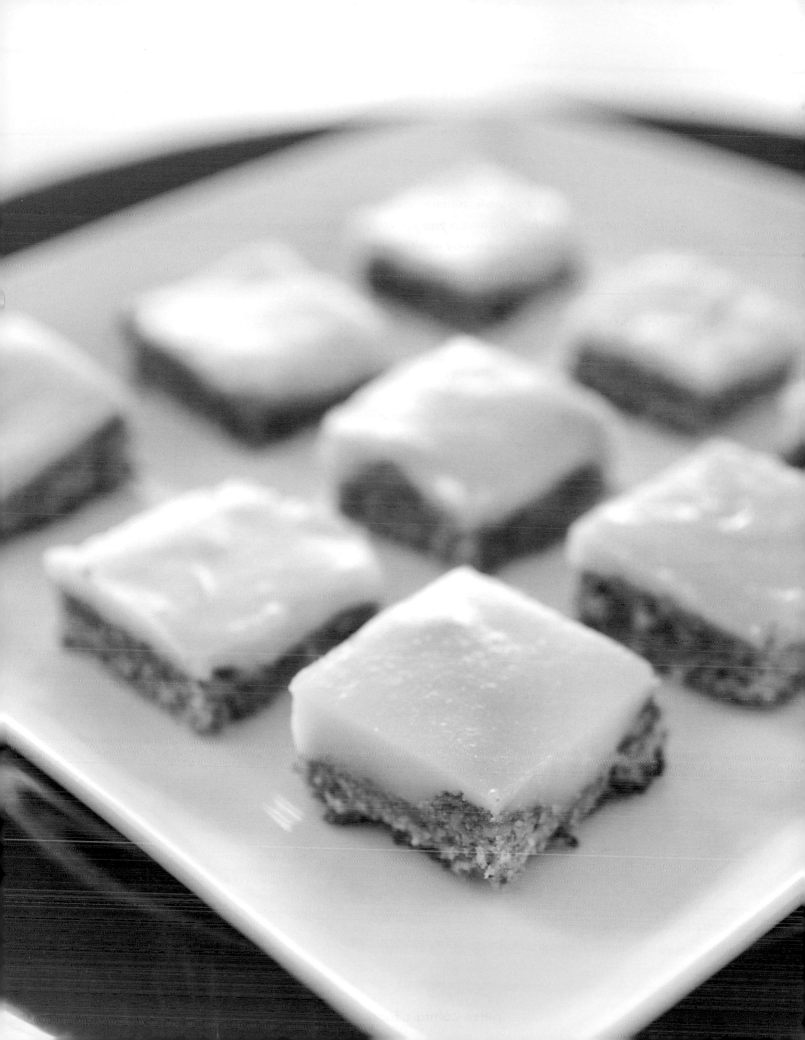

# chocolate coconut pudding

*Mmmmm, chocolate pudding. Great for those days you just aren't feeling so hot and are needing a little something comforting. This isn't your usual "out of the box" pudding, so don't go expecting it. It is, however, decadent, rich, and a sweet treat to have once in a while. We are guessing that even Bill Cosby would approve of this delicious recipe.*

| | |
|---|---|
| 3 | tablespoons high-fat cocoa powder |
| ¼ | cup (40 g) arrowroot powder |
| 1 | teaspoon vanilla extract |
| 1 | can coconut milk |
| 4 | ounces (113 g) good-quality dark chocolate |
| 2 | tablespoons honey |
| 2 | large egg yolks |

1. In a small bowl, combine the cocoa powder, arrowroot powder and vanilla.

2. Add about 2 tablespoons of the coconut milk to combine all and whisk out any lumps.

3. In a medium saucepan over medium heat, bring remaining coconut milk up to a low simmer.

4. Add in the dark chocolate to melt it, stirring often.

5. Mix in the arrowroot/cocoa/vanilla mixture, and whisk continuously.

6. In a small bowl, whisk the egg yolks to break them apart, stir in a little bit of the warm coconut milk mixture, then pour all the contents back into the saucepan, and return to the heat.

7. Whisk all until smooth and the mixture coats the back of a spatula.

8. Pour into small ramekins, place plastic wrap directly on the surface to prevent any skin forming, and put in refrigerator to chill.

9. Serve cold.

**Variation**—*If you prefer not to use honey, puree a really ripe banana in a blender or Magic Bullet to add the desired sweetness to the pudding.*

**Tips & Tricks**—*Cooking the egg yolks in the pudding to a temperature of at least 160°F (72°C) will destroy any bacteria that may reside.*

**Ingredient Notes**—*Penzey's Spices has some amazing high-fat cocoa that really adds the decadent flavor to this. Don't skimp and use poor-quality powdered chocolate.*

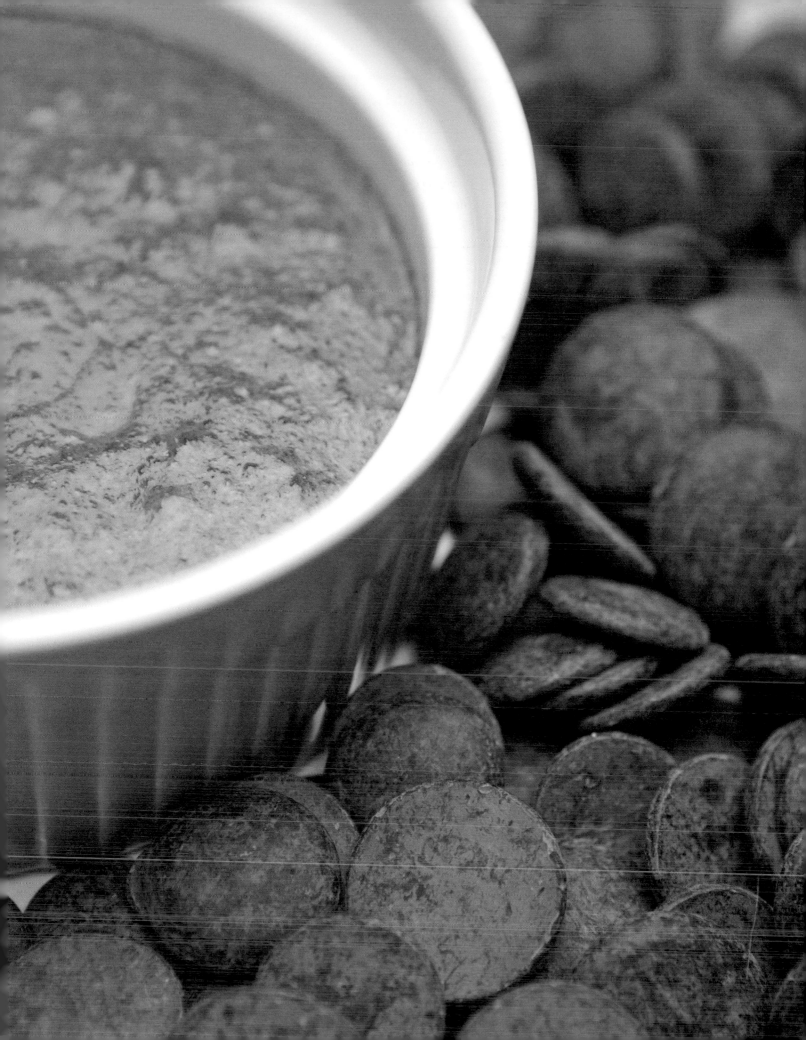

# Index

paleo comfort foods

# Notes